Careers with the Pharmaceutical Industry
Second Edition

Careers with the Pharmaceutical Industry

Second Edition

Edited by
Peter D. Stonier
AXESS Ltd,
Richmond, Surrey, UK

WILEY

Other Wiley Editorial Offices

John Wiley & Sons Inc., 111 River Street, Hoboken, NJ 07030, USA

Jossey-Bass, 989 Market Street, San Francisco, CA 94103-1741, USA

Wiley-VCH Verlag GmbH, Boschstr. 12, D-69469 Weinheim, Germany

John Wiley & Sons Australia Ltd, 33 Park Road, Milton, Queensland 4064, Australia

John Wiley & Sons (Asia) Pte Ltd, 2 Clementi Loop #02-01, Jin Xing Distripark,
Singapore 129809

John Wiley & Sons Canada Ltd, 22 Worcester Road, Etobicoke, Ontario, Canada M9W 1L1

Wiley also publishes its books in a variety of electronic formats. Some content that appears
in print may not be available in electronic books.

Library of Congress Cataloging-in-Publication Data

Careers with the pharmaceutical industry / edited by Peter D. Stonier.– 2nd ed.
    p. cm.
   Previous ed. published with title: Discovering new medicines.
   Includes bibliographical references and index.
   ISBN 0-470-84328-4 (alk. paper)
   1. Pharmacy–Vocational guidance. 2. Pharmacy–Research–Vocational guidance. 3.
Pharmaceutical industry–Vocational guidance. 4. Pharmaceutical chemistry–Vocational
guidance. I. Stonier, P. D. II. Discovering new medicines.

RS122.5.D57 2003
615′.19′0023–dc21   2003041094

British Library Cataloguing in Publication Data

A catalogue record for this book is available from the British Library

ISBN 0 470 84328 4

This book is printed on acid-free paper responsibly manufactured from sustainable forestry
in which at least two trees are planted for each one used for paper production.

Contents

List of Contributors		ix
Preface		xiii
Preface to the First Edition		xv
Acknowledgements		xvii
I	**Background to Medicines Research and Development**	**1**
1	Pharmaceutical Medicine—A Specialist Discipline *Felicity Gabbay*	3
2	The Contribution of Academic Clinical Pharmacology to Medicines Research *Charles F. George*	17
3	A Career in Drug Discovery *David Ellis*	29
II	**Careers in Pre-Clinical and Clinical Research**	**45**
4	A Career in Clinical Pharmacology *Roger Yates*	47
5	Career Opportunities for Physicians in the Pharmaceutical Industry *Bert Spilker*	55
6	The Clinical Research Associate *Gareth Hayes*	67

Careers with the Pharmaceutical Industry, Second edition. Edited by P. D. Stonier.
© 2003 John Wiley & Sons Ltd. ISBN 0 470 84328 4

7   Clinical Trial Administrator and Study Site Co-ordinator—
      Key Roles in Clinical Research   79
      Nicola Murgatroyd, Caroline Crockatt and Gareth Hayes

8   Statisticians in the Pharmaceutical Industry   99
      Christopher Hilton and Trevor Lewis

9   Careers in Data Management   111
      Sheila Varley

10   Working in a Contract Research Organisation   119
      Jane Barrett

III   **Careers in Sales and Marketing**   127

11   A Career in Product Management   129
      Roy Carlisle

12   A Career in Medical Sales and Medical Sales Management   137
      Roy Carlisle

IV   **General Careers with the Pharmaceutical Industry**   149

13   The Role of the Pharmacist in Healthcare   151
      David Jordan

14   Careers for Nurses with the Pharmaceutical Industry   163
      Joyce E. Kenkre

15   The Toxicologist in Pharmaceutical Medicine   177
      Geoffrey Diggle

16   A Career in Clinical Quality Assurance   187
      Rita Hattemer-Apostel

17   A Career in Product Registration and Regulatory Affairs   203
      Pat Turmer

18   Careers in Drug Safety and Pharmacovigilance   213
      Peter Barnes

19   Careers in Medical Information   223
      Janet Taylor

20   Medical Writing as a Career   235
      Brenda M. Mullinger

21   Career Opportunities in Medicines Regulation—The
      Medical Assessor   247
      Nigel Baber

22   Pharmaceutical Law—A Growing Legal Specialty   255
      Ian Dodds-Smith

23   Industry Careers for Pharmacoeconomists   267
     Nick Bosanquet

24   Consultant in Pharmaceutical Medicine   275
     Brian Gennery

V   Career Progression   287

25   Landing that Job—Recruitment, CVs and Interviews   289
     Sue Ransom

26   Career Development in Pharmaceuticals   303
     Roger D. Stephens

27   Opportunities for Education and Training in the
     Pharmaceutical Industry   311
     Peter D. Stonier and Gareth Hayes

     Useful Information   337

Index   341

List of Contributors

Professor Nigel Baber
Medicines Control Agency
Market Towers
1 Nine Elms Lane
London SW8 5NQ
UK

Dr Peter Barnes
Aventis Pharma Pty Ltd
27 Sirius Road
Lane Cove
NSW 2066
Australia

Dr Jane Barrett
The Barrett Consultancy
2 Falcon Way
Wokingham
Berkshire RG41 3HD
UK

Professor Nick Bosanquet
Department of Bioengineering
Imperial College
Bagrit Centre
Exhibition Road
London SW7 2BX
UK

Roy Carlisle
PharmaSolutions Ltd
10 Goddington Road
Bourne End
Buckinghamshire SL8 5TZ
UK

Caroline Crockatt
Intercern Ltd
Linden House
5 High Street
Reigate
Surrey RH2 9AE
UK

Dr Geoffrey Diggle
Formerly Department of Health
Skipton House
89 London Road
London SE1 6LW
UK

Mr Ian Dodds-Smith
Arnold & Porter
Tower 42
25 Old Broad Street
London EC2N 1HQ
UK

Dr David Ellis
Euromedica plc
6a Enterprise House
Vision Park
Histon
Cambridge CB4 9ZR
UK

Careers with the Pharmaceutical Industry, Second edition. Edited by P. D. Stonier.
© 2003 John Wiley & Sons Ltd

Dr Felicity Gabbay
10 Park Lane
Milford on Sea
Hampshire
UK

Dr Brian Gennery
Gennery Associates
Pharmaceutical Consultancy
6 Qualitas
Roman Hill
Bracknell
Berkshire RG12 7QG
UK

Professor Sir Charles F. George
British Heart Foundation
14 Fitzhardinge Street
London W1H 4DH
UK

Rita Hattemer-Apostel
Verdandi AG
Wieslergasse 2
8049 Zurich
Switzerland

Gareth Hayes
nrg pathway
PO Box 9
Appleby-in-Westmorland
Cumbria CA16 6YF
UK

Christopher Hilton
Development Operations
Pfizer Global Research &
  Development
Pfizer Ltd
Sandwich
Kent CT13 9NJ
UK

Dr David Jordan
Pharmaceutical Sciences
Quintiles (Europe) Ltd
Research Avenue South
Heriot-Watt University Research
  Park
Riccarton
Edinburgh EH14 4AP
UK

Professor Joyce E. Kenkre
School of Care Sciences
University of Glamorgan
Research Unit
Pontypridd CF37 1DL
UK

Trevor Lewis
Development Operations
Pfizer Global Research &
  Development
Pfizer Ltd
Sandwich
Kent CT13 9NJ
UK

Brenda M. Mullinger
Wordpower Projects
'Larches'
Shipbourne
Kent TN11 9PL
UK

Nicola Murgatroyd
Phlexglobal Ltd
Dairy House
Churchfield Road
Chalfont St Peter
Bucks SL9 9EW
UK

Sue Ransom
AXESS Ltd
Parkshot House
5 Kew Road
Richmond
Surrey TW9 2PR
UK

Professor Bert Spilker
Bert Spilker & Associates, LLC
8004 Overhill Road
Bethesda, MD 20814-1145
USA

Roger D. Stephens
RSA Consulting Ltd
The Melon Ground
Hatfield Park
Old Hatfield
Herts AL9 5NB
UK

Dr Peter D. Stonier
AXESS Ltd
Parkshot House
5 Kew Road
Richmond
Surrey TW9 2PR
UK

Janet Taylor
Janet Taylor Consultancy Services
19 Nations Hill
Kingsworthy
Winchester
Hants SO23 7QY
UK

Dr Pat Turmer
131 Charlton Road
Kenton
London HA3 9HT
UK

Ms Sheila Varley
Quintiles Ltd
Station House
Market Street
Bracknell
Berkshire RG12 1HX
UK

Dr Roger Yates
Astra Zeneca Ltd
Mereside
Alderley Park
Macclesfield
Cheshire SK10 4TG
UK

Preface

The first edition of this book appeared in 1994 and has been received favourably enough since to warrant a second edition some nine years later. The original title 'Discovering New Medicines' appeared a little opaque for those seeking to learn about careers in medicines research and development. So for this second edition the opportunity has been taken to say it as it is: 'Careers with the Pharmaceutical Industry'. This reflects careers both in the industry, which in the UK employs some 60 000 people, and those supporting, servicing and regulating the industry in its contribution to medicines research, representing up to 250 000 people, in academia, healthcare, government, contract research and consultancy.

As before, it is not possible to cover all the variants of jobs and careers that exist in this complex and evolving industry; notably absent is the manufacturing sector, business management and administration. However, it is hoped there are enough entry points that are recognisable, so that light is thrown on the different career courses in pharmaceuticals, at the core of which are research and development, marketing and sales.

Nine years is not long in the life-cycle of a pharmaceutical product, in that it takes on average 12 years to develop a new medicine from promising new molecules discovered in the laboratory, and those that were in early development when this book first appeared are only now being introduced onto the market for the benefit of patients. The principles of consistent endeavour by professionals achieving incremental progress in knowledge and technical application in new products, which were laid out in the preface to the first edition, are still valid today.

Nevertheless, throughout the 1990s and 2000s there have been many changes in the environment of medicines research; changes in philosophy, direction, organisation, communication, financing and regulation. Much of this perhaps reflects a natural competitive evolution of renewal and re-engineering, responding to the economic business cycle and to the relative merits and successes of individual products, as well as to the potential of future product pipelines. The mapping of the human genome, the growth of information technology through increased computing power and communications via the Internet, and the globalisation of medicines R&D to international standards are just some of the changes which will

Careers with the Pharmaceutical Industry, Second edition. Edited by P. D. Stonier.
© 2003 John Wiley & Sons Ltd

have a major impact on the way we both perceive and conduct discovery research, development and marketing of medicines long into the future.

Change in the business environment and employment, in this as in many industries, means that the concept of jobs for life has been replaced by the need to acquire transferable skills through continuing education and training, and to accept greater flexibility and mobility in career development. Today, temporary project team membership in a matrix organisation can lead to as much goal attainment and job satisfaction as vertical promotion through the organisation did yesterday.

This book sets out to interest those seeking information about a career in medicines R&D, one of our most challenging, stimulating and successful industrial activities. It is hoped it will also be of interest to those already engaged in one area, who seek career development or a move to another sector either within or outside a pharmaceutical company. As before, it might also interest those observers who seek to be informed about how medicines are discovered and developed and the activities of those working in the field.

Peter Stonier
Richmond, Surrey, 2003

Preface to the First Edition

The past 50 years has seen striking success and dramatic growth in the development of new medicines, both from naturally occurring substances in plants and animals, including human, and from purely chemical sources.

These new medicines have allowed doctors to manage a wide range of diseases for which, previously, there was no treatment.

At the same time, scientists have formed a deeper understanding of the normal functioning of the body and how normal processes are changed by illness and disease. Often these two areas of research have interacted so that the use of certain medicines has helped to unravel the workings of the body in health and disease.

Alongside the euphoria of such progress has come the recognition that no medicine is without hazard, at least in some patients. The benefits of successful treatment of an illness must always be balanced against the possible risk of an unwanted side-effect of the medicine. This was tragically illustrated by thalidomide in the early 1960s, when a sedative that appeared to be safer and better tolerated than those already available produced deformities in the babies of some women who had taken the drug for sleep disturbances during pregnancy.

These events more than any others marked a permanent change in the way the world saw medicines research. Government agencies acting in the public interest increased legislation regulating the development, licensing and marketing of medicines, and gradually the public itself was encouraged to take more interest in its health and the medicines used to preserve it. The age of innovation of the 1950s and 1960s gave way to the age of regulation in the 1970s and to the age of communication and accountability in the 1980s.

The coming era of biological innovation and biotechnology, of health care economics and of the application of modern management methods to the research and development process see the 1990s as continuing this evolution, and perhaps also being the start of a new age for medicines.

Whilst today scientific and medical achievements tend to be overshadowed by political and economic considerations affecting medicine and health care services, more patient involvement in treatment and the international rationalisation of research may enable the true benefits of the last 50 years to be integrated with the

Careers with the Pharmaceutical Industry, Second edition. Edited by P. D. Stonier.
© 2003 John Wiley & Sons Ltd

selective demands of informed health care systems to enable progress in treating illness to be continued and to be brought to an even wider population around the world.

The field of pharmaceutical research and development remains one of the hall-marks of the technological age and continues to make innovative progress and to have a profound economic effect on those countries which embrace it. The institutions and companies involved in medicines research have themselves contributed greatly to the increasing standards of research through self-regulation and the imposition of good practices and standard procedures, including audit, to ensure high quality of work. Such actions have not dulled the intellect and skills of a highly trained work-force which forms the focus of so much hope for the future.

For medicines research to evolve and be responsive to the needs of patients and their doctors there must necessarily be an evolution in the breadth and sophistication of the scientific and medical disciplines involved and the teams of scientists, doctors and others contributing to this work. Thus to the research chemists and life scientists conducting basic research and the clinical pharmacologists, pharmacists, physicians and statisticians who traditionally were the conductors of clinical trials, have now been added many long-recognised and some newer specialists—clinical research scientists, data managers, medical writers, research nurses and, increasingly, management specialists, economists, accountants and lawyers.

In parallel with these developments in the scope of medicines research and its management has developed the speciality of pharmaceutical medicine, a discipline concerned with the discovery, development, evaluation and monitoring of medicines and the medical aspects of their marketing. This definition embraces a subject which is both scientific and clinical and includes the many professionals of varied backgrounds mentioned above.

This book contains views from many of the professional disciplines which contribute to pharmaceutical medicine about the jobs involved, and the careers open to those who wish to pursue medicines research in industry and in academia.

Even so, it cannot be all-embracing and, for instance, does not pretend to cover the many contributions made by practising physicians and others whose careful observations at the bedside and in the community have added so much to knowledge of the effects of medicines. Nor does it do justice to the many study volunteers and members of research ethics committees whose unpaid and often unsung work contributes so much to the effort.

Nevertheless it aims to open windows into the world of medicines research, a still widening and growing field, for those without ready information but with career options still unsatisfied and with their futures still to plan.

Peter D. Stonier

Acknowledgements

I would like to thank all those who have contributed to the production of this book, both to the first edition and to this one. I am grateful to the authors, whether they have updated previous chapters or contributed new ones. My assistant, Virginia Moores, has given unstinting and invaluable support, and I thank her. I am appreciative of everyone at John Wiley & Sons who have championed this book and guided it from manuscript to publication.

Careers with the Pharmaceutical Industry, Second edition. Edited by P. D. Stonier.
© 2003 John Wiley & Sons Ltd

PART I

BACKGROUND TO MEDICINES RESEARCH AND DEVELOPMENT

Careers with the Pharmaceutical Industry, Second edition. Edited by P. D. Stonier.
© 2003 John Wiley & Sons Ltd. ISBN 0 470 84328 4

1
Pharmaceutical Medicine— A Specialist Discipline

Felicity Gabbay

Milford on Sea, Hampshire, UK

Introduction

Physicians joined the pharmaceutical industry in significant numbers as early as the 1950s and saw dramatic changes in company and government structures to maintain the introduction of innovative pharmaceutical products whilst ensuring maximum protection to the public. During this period specialist disciplines for physicians and scientists alike have emerged and it can be confusing trying to understand the role of organisations and individuals within pharmaceutical medicine. With respect to pharmaceutical medicine, several chapters in this book endeavour to give an overview of the different opportunities in the discipline, and of the scientific background and specialist training needed to accomplish them.

Pharmaceutical medicine was initially considered to be outside the conventional respected medical and scientific professions. This was despite pharmaceutical physicians' ultimate responsibility for interpreting clinical data to determine whether or not drugs were, or continued to be, marketed. These considerable responsibilities extended nationally and, for some pharmaceutical and regulatory physicians, internationally. The responsibility could be likened to signing prescriptions for whole countries, with some pharmaceutical physicians responsible for the actual signing, many for providing information to ensure the prescription was correct, and others for scrutinising the prescription (through government regulatory departments and committees) once it was written. Pharmaceutical medicine also encompasses scientists qualified in a range of disciplines. People entering the discipline may have degrees or doctorates in pure science subjects such as biology, chemistry or more vocational subjects such as pharmacy or medicine. This chapter summarises the events that led to pharmaceutical medicine becoming the discipline it is and the role played by the professional bodies that support it. Pharmaceutical

Careers with the Pharmaceutical Industry, Second edition. Edited by P. D. Stonier.
© 2003 John Wiley & Sons Ltd. ISBN 0 470 84328 4

medicine has become a respected and exciting discipline and, of those who have joined, few have left.

Pharmaceutical agents have always been at the foundation of medicine and therapeutics. As medicine became professionalised in Europe in the seventeenth, eighteenth and nineteenth centuries, lists of acceptable drugs appeared. The forerunner to the British Pharmacopoeia started life as the London Pharmacopoeia in 1618 (Adam and Passmore, 1980). It included nearly 2000 medicinal agents, few of which had a rationale for their medicinal action that we would recognise today.

The regulation of marketing of recognised medicinal agents was, until the nineteenth century, under the control of the physicians, surgeons and apothecaries. The General Medical Council (GMC), created by the Medical Reform Act (1858), subsequently approved compounds for listing in the British Pharmacopoeia. The amalgamation of physicians, surgeons and apothecaries as a single professional group created the need for skilled specialists to formulate and dispense drugs. Pharmacists filled this role.

During the latter part of the nineteenth century when 'laboratory medicine' made substantial advances, scientists including chemists, pathologists, physiologists and microbiologists identified the causes of a number of diseases. The discoveries coincided with the emergence of large chemical industries utilising the scientific advances in chemistry. Scientists working in the new chemical companies began to turn their attention to applying medical research to develop pharmaceutical agents, and in 1890 general disinfectants, anaesthetics, antipyretics and hypnotics began to emerge. The developments in the pharmaceutical industry around the turn of the century were not limited to national companies and the industry rapidly became an international one. For example, in 1901 Parke Davis, which had a British plant but was an American pharmaceutical company, introduced adrenalin into clinical practice in the UK and in 1914 it was agreed by the GMC to include the word 'adrenalin' in the British Pharmacopoeia (Parke Davis, 1939). Pharmaceutical companies were chemical companies specialising in the production of medicinal agents and were largely run by pharmacists who had established themselves as formulators of medicines—the final stage before dispensing them. Other scientists were, however, also crucial to the work within the companies. These included chemists, toxicologists, pharmacologists and in some companies microbiologists.

Doctors played only a small part in the development of new drugs before the Second World War. Eminent physicians still questioned the value of statistics in the progress of medicine (Armitage and Berry, 1987). Doctors were, however, playing a role in pharmaceutical companies in medical information and clinical interpretation even though they conducted few clinical trials of new medicines. Sir Austin Bradford Hill's book on the principles of medical statistics, published in 1937, was an important milestone (Bradford Hill, 1937) introducing the concept of comparative trials balancing factors that would influence outcome and the main method for performing this in large samples, randomisation.

The emergence of drugs which were clearly efficacious and the ability to demonstrate this in clinical medicine by combining clinical interpretation with medical statistics led to substantial investment, including some government subsidy in the 'pharmaceutical industry' as it was now called (Cromie, 1993). By the 1940s and 1950s there were the first beginnings of clinical trial departments, many staffed by non-medical scientists (who had already been performing animal experiments), as well as physicians. Scientists originally trained in chemistry, biochemistry, pharmacology, pharmacy and many other medically allied sciences have remained to form the largest components of clinical research and medical affairs departments. They fill roles at all staff and managerial levels.

Commercialisation of scientific discoveries led to patents becoming widely applied in many countries, and branding was introduced to protect companies' research and development (R&D) investments (Teeling Smith, 1992). This brought specialised lawyers into the pharmaceutical industry. Companies also now needed to know as soon as possible whether new therapeutic candidates showed clinical effects in patients. Doctors were increasingly recruited to the industry to conduct trials for evaluation of drugs in patients (Cromie, 1993). Branding also brought competition, and companies began to design studies to demonstrate the advantages of the newer therapies against their competitors. This brought physicians and other clinical research personnel into the area of sales and marketing.

An incident in the late 1930s in the USA had a major impact on the development of pharmaceutical medicine. In North America, where there had been relatively less professional control of marketing of pharmaceutical agents, an enterprising but misguided company dissolved sulphanilamide in diethylene glycol, resulting in the deaths of 107 people (Laurence, 1966a). The resulting furore led in 1938 to the setting up of the Food and Drug Administration (FDA), the first of the official full-time bureaucratic agencies dedicated to monitoring the development and marketing of pharmaceutical agents. Within these organisations was born a further specialist breed of physicians and scientists who were devoted to the government assessment of new medicines and the control over the way in which they were marketed. At this stage Europe did not follow suit, thinking the existing controls to be adequate. In the UK these controls included pharmacopoeias, the Therapeutic Substances Act (1925), the Dangerous Drugs Act (1930) and the Cancer Act (1930), all of which were implemented to ensure quality of drugs, control dangerous drugs and protect the public from false claims (Cromie, 1993).

Regulation and patent control brought a national flavour to the companies, dividing up what had been a subject with few geographical boundaries to a subject where most companies now required local affiliates in order to fulfil the requirements for regulation and control in individual countries. Regulation also changed the nature of medical and research departments by demanding levels of evaluation in R&D hitherto not considered.

The impact of patents and branding changed the shape of the pharmaceutical industry (Teeling Smith, 1992). In the 1950s there was a dramatic increase in interest in the commercial behaviour of pharmaceutical companies. In that decade the first broad-spectrum antibiotics appeared in profusion. Many were patented by Lilly and were expensive compared to the unpatented penicillin and spectinomycin.

This generated concern in the USA as to whether patenting and branding were in the public interest or whether they might just lead to companies making huge profits from the sick. This was reported in 1961 by a Senate Committee and resulted in considerable antagonism to the pharmaceutical industry, not just in the USA but also in countries in Europe. Scientists and doctors working in the pharmaceutical industry already suffered a lower professional status than their counterparts in universities or other jobs outside the industry due to general antagonism of the professions to commerce and few would align themselves with the industry in the following decade.

In 1961 thalidomide, marketed in Germany and Great Britain, was shown to be responsible for phocomelia. Not only was the pharmaceutical industry exploiting science by making profit out of the sick, but it was also capable of marketing drugs that had major adverse effects. The physicians working at Distillers (the pharmaceutical company concerned), Drs Denis Burley and Charles Brown, had to evaluate the tragic adverse events (Cromie, 1993). Denis Burley, to whom the first edition of this book was dedicated, remained in the pharmaceutical industry until he retired in 1991. He devoted much of his life to professional organisations linked with pharmaceutical medicine to increase the standards of the subject. He subsequently became President of the Faculty of Pharmaceutical Medicine of the Royal Colleges of Physicians of the United Kingdom but sadly died during his term of office in 1992.

During Denis Burley's lifetime it was to become realised that even if drugs were put through greater toxicological screens than thalidomide, it was impossible to screen out all adverse effects. Furthermore the increased sophistication of data collection and tracking was able to detect effects occurring at very low frequencies (e.g. the effects of practolol in the elderly and the hepatic side-effects of benoxyprofen). A group of pharmaceutical physicians and scientists have devoted their discipline to investigating adverse event frequencies in the population after a drug has been given to tens of thousands of patients. They practise pharmacovigilance and pharmacoepidemiology.

During the 1960s, in response to the thalidomide-related events, regulatory agencies along the lines of the FDA were set up throughout Europe to ensure that rigorous pre-clinical and clinical studies of new chemical entities were conducted before the drugs were marketed. In response, the European drug companies developed groups of clinical scientists who specialised in writing for the regulators (regulatory executives and medical writers), mirroring their American counterparts.

The thalidomide tragedy had damaged the image of the pharmaceutical industry still further and calls in the British parliament for nationalisation of all pharmaceutical companies in Great Britain were part of the Labour government manifesto when it was elected to power in 1964 (Teeling Smith, 1992). The committee set up to look into this in 1967, having examined in detail the economics of R&D and innovation, decided against nationalisation, stating that 'in the absence of the prospect of abnormal profits, private industry would have no special inducement to undertake research to which is attached an abnormal risk of failure'. The committee had discovered that the cost of R&D of a new medicine was extremely high, taking on average 8–10 years to recover from the market. Thousands of drugs may need to be screened to find one suitable candidate. With the introduction of ever more stringent regulations this cost was growing and it has now reached over £350 million for each new drug (www.ABPI.org.uk).

Concerns about the economics of the pharmaceutical industry and its commercial interests have remained and heightened. Ever since the formation of the National Health Service (NHS) in the UK in 1948, the government has been concerned by the cost of drugs, which was, for a long time, estimated to make up about 10% of the cost of health care (Laurence, 1966b). In other countries, governments have introduced systems of reimbursement to help patients pay for drugs, and insurance schemes can also cover the cost of drugs as part of health care. In many countries schemes have been introduced to regulate prices of drugs but at the same time try to ensure continued investment in R&D and innovation by pharmaceutical companies. Initiatives such as the National Institute for Clinical Excellence (NICE) mean that in addition to risk/benefit a government body assesses cost effectiveness and gives guidance on how newly introduced treatments should fit into the clinical armamentarium. These additional assessment bodies now require companies in some countries to demonstrate economic benefit from new pharmacological advances before marketing. The disciplines of health technology assessment and pharmacoeconomics have developed within these fields.

Industry Interfaces

The calls for nationalisation of the industry were accompanied by concerns from academic medicine about the standards of clinical research in industry, questioning the scientific impartiality of pharmaceutical physicians and scientists (Hampton and Julian, 1987). Clinical pharmacology had become a discipline in the 1950s and 1960s and some saw comprehensive drug development as its role. Whilst a symbiosis has developed between universities and industry, it has become clear that the size of the operation involved in the complete development of a new drug is outside the scope of a single university department. Clinical research departments in pharmaceutical companies include specialised clinical research associates, clinical scientists, nurses, data managers, data entry staff, archivists and statisticians, in addition to physicians. The size of one submission to the FDA had grown from about 30 pages in the early 1950s to the volume of paper that would fill a furniture removal van in the late 1970s and is now largely submitted electronically; the number of people working on one clinical research submission had increased to hundreds.

The belief that the industry was likely to suffer from commercial bias did not, however, recede and the FDA increased their demand on the industry to open their doors for inspection. Companies are required to inspect data and data collection procedures using independent auditors who comment on the quality of the data.

Government inspectors also operate in North America and European countries. Harmonised approaches to research and reporting standards between Europe, North America and Japan (International Conference on Harmonisation) have been developed to which many other countries also adhere. These standards require research to be governed by working practices; rules dictated and written by the research group itself but conforming to and called standard operating procedures (SOPs). This sub-discipline, quality assurance and audit in research, has become an important one. Ironically in addition to increasing standards in industry it has unearthed the fact that a small percentage of doctors working in clinical practice under grants are thought to submit fraudulent or severely substandard data (Wells, 1993).

Within the near future all submissions will be made by electronic applications in a harmonised format (the Common Technical Document) and, in addition, Electronic Systems for Transmission of Regulatory Information (ESTRI gateways) will be used for submitting ongoing safety data both in North America and in Europe. Electronic applications involve the deposition with the regulatory agency of all data in electronic form for inspection and sometimes further evaluation. As systems of data capture become more efficient much of the data collected in clinical trials is also recorded from the patient and doctor electronically. Many companies also attach such things as ECGs and X-rays that can be stored digitally. Much of this data capture and transmission is managed through the World Wide Web and has led to incorporation into large trials of web design staff.

One group of pharmaceutical physicians and their teams who deserve special mention are the clinical pharmacologists. Their task is the critical bridge between pre-clinical and clinical studies and the evaluation of what the drug does to the body (pharmacodynamics) and what the body does to the drug (pharmacokinetics) in healthy subjects, in the patient population with the target disease, and also in special populations such as the elderly and children. This is a highly specialised discipline and may be suited to those who already have experience in the subject in clinical medicine.

The co-ordination of the large number of scientists and others involved in a single drug development programme required yet another group of people. Project managers are responsible for ensuring that the many different tasks during clinical development and marketing are achieved. Finance and administration people oversee resourcing of the projects, tracking finance and running the business side of the operation. Finally, and not least, there have to be specialist information technology staff running computer systems that track and integrate the vast amounts of data collected. Numerous other specialists are involved such as designers of case record forms and clinical trials supply pharmacists.

Cost and Complexity in Drug Development

With all the scientific, political and economic evolutions in the pharmaceutical industry the structure of pharmaceutical medicine has become extremely complex and expensive. Small companies have been unable to withstand the expense and the biggest pharmaceutical companies develop many of the compounds brought to the market world-wide. Ninety five percent of drugs marketed in the world are developed by just six countries—the USA, UK, France, Germany, Switzerland and Sweden. Nearly 50% are developed by American companies (Lis and Walker, 1989). Even such companies have found the cost and complexity hard to bear and mergers amongst the top companies have made them even bigger. An alternative solution has been the licensing or co-licensing of drugs between companies, from which a whole specialty of people working in licensing has developed.

Relations between those working in pharmaceutical medicine in the industry and in academia and government have improved beyond recognition in the last two decades. Regulators and academics have realised the immense burden on the industry of demonstrating efficacy and safety. This would clearly be eased if each country did not insist on its own stringent regulations for registering drugs. Pharmaceutical medicine has therefore returned to being a global specialty, most research being part of an overall plan to learn more about an individual drug, with little or no repetition of studies except for confirmatory purposes. The International Conference on Harmonisation (ICH) is among the initiatives to bring all interested parties together to set standards for performing research on new developments. Other initiatives include working parties to produce guidelines for study designs, standard inclusion and exclusion criteria and analytical procedures for individual therapeutic research areas.

Sub-specialisation

In the 1980s, yet another solution to the monolithic pharmaceutical company came into being. This was the formation of smaller service and research companies performing individual activities in pharmaceutical medicine for the pharmaceutical industry as a whole. This has enabled many of the Japanese and smaller biotechnology companies, whose presence in Europe is less dominant than the big companies, to consider developing their own drugs. The service companies are loosely grouped together under the term contract research organisations (CROs), and their functions are as numerous and varied as those within the pharmaceutical industry itself. Some CROs are run by people who have never been in the industry but can offer specialised services needed by the industry such as clinical pharmacology. Although there are estimated to be over a thousand CROs world-wide only a handful offer complete clinical R&D, most specialising in a particular subdiscipline or therapeutic area in pharmaceutical medicine.

The development of pharmaceutical medicine has resulted in a number of subdisciplines referred to elsewhere in this book. R&D of drugs has changed dramatically in the last hundred years and, like other scientifically based commercial developments, the rate of change increased faster as the twentieth century

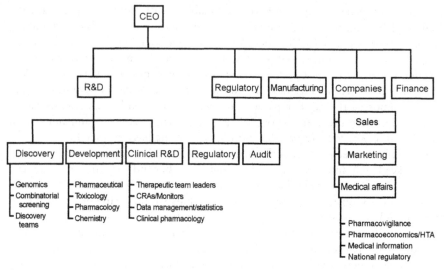

Figure 1.1   Example of the structure of an organisation involved in pharmaceutical R&D and sales

progressed and concluded. In the last two decades there have been dramatic changes in companies, largely driven by developments in information technology, scientific methodology and economics. This has meant an international stream-lining of larger companies and the career progression described, for example, in pamphlets in the late 1980s now bears little resemblance to that within the structure existing in the current pharmaceutical industry and its allied organisations. Figure 1.1 demonstrates, in summary, how pharmaceutical companies may be organised. It demonstrates how physicians and scientists working in different parts of the organ-isation have different highly specialised functions and cannot, as they could in times before, be interchanged. Similarly CROs will offer types of expertise orien-tated towards post-marketing R&D, often in particular therapeutic areas or specialist scientific disciplines, e.g. statistics and data management, but rarely all.

Professional Support

During the nineteenth and early twentieth centuries a number of professional and academic bodies sprang up to support standards in medicine and allied professions. In addition, there was a burgeoning of the number of scientific bodies to encourage innovation in all scientific disciplines. Three types of professional organisation were formed to support the different medical and allied disciplines.

The first two types often coexist in the same organisation. The first provides basic professional support for its members in the jobs that they do. It includes bodies such as the British Association of Pharmaceutical Physicians (BrAPP), one of the first organisations to support pharmaceutical physicians, and there are several others supporting the different disciplines within pharmaceutical medicine. Such organisations bring together professional scientists doing similar jobs, they offer symposia that keep their members up to date with necessary developments and they highlight professional issues that may need to be taken up by other bodies. The second type of organisation is a faculty, college or institute. Examples of these are the Royal Colleges and Faculties of Medicine, and professional institutes such as the Institutes of Chartered Accountants and Surveyors. They are bodies to set standards usually through examination. In pharmaceutical medicine the Faculty of Pharmaceutical Medicine exists to set standards for pharmaceutical physicians through its diploma and its vocational programme for specialist training (Higher Medical Training). In the absence of appropriate standard-setting bodies several of the first type of professional organisations fulfil this role. Examples are many of the physicians' professional organisations in North America and in Europe, the Institute of Clinical Research and the British Institute of Regulatory Affairs (BIRA), which both award diplomas.

Education, Careers and Standards

The standard-setting bodies not only set examinations but also set a list of basic requirements for entry into the career grade. Pharmaceutical physicians need to have at least two years of post-registration general clinical experience before entering pharmaceutical medicine and at least four years of experience in pharmaceutical medicine fulfilling a Diploma of Pharmaceutical Medicine and the requirements of specialist training during that time. Examples of professional organisations and the postgraduate courses offered in pharmaceutical medicine and allied subjects are given in Tables 1.1 and 1.2. Much of the subject matter is similar in pharmaceutical medicine courses. There are many courses available in North America and Europe and they are too numerous to list—these can be found by contacting the professional bodies listed who can put individuals in contact with the appropriate national organisation. Shorter courses are also available and these can be found through the relevant professional bodies or pharmaceutical directories.

Finally, but perhaps most importantly, for it is the way in which any discipline moves forward, there is the academic society. Pharmaceutical medicine is a discipline that is largely concerned with research and development. What then is the role of an academic society doing research into R&D? It is not, as thought by some, to foster research into the therapeutic disciplines themselves as there are ample academic societies for this, but into the methods used to perform research and development. As has been explained in the early part of this chapter, the complex task of bringing together all the scientists and other professional staff involved in bringing a drug to the market place requires sophisticated methodology and

Table 1.1 Professional support groups in pharmaceutical medicine

Disciplinary group	Professional support organisation	Professional educational standard-setting body	Websites
Clinical research staff	Institute of Clinical Research	Institute of Clinical Research (UK) Association of Clinical Research Professionals (USA)	www.instituteof clinicalresearch.com
Medical information	Association of Information Officers in the Pharmaceutical Industry; Information Managers in the Pharmaceutical Industry	AIOPI	www.aiopi.org.uk www.impi.org.uk
Medical writers	American Medical Writers Association; European Medical Writers Association		www.emwa.org
Pharmaceutical physicians	International Federation of Associations of Pharmaceutical Physicians*	Faculty of Pharmaceutical Medicine of the Royal Colleges of Physicians of the UK	www.brapp.org.uk www.ifapp.org www.fpm.org.uk
Statisticians	PSI, Statisticians in the Pharmaceutical Industry		www.psiweb.org
Auditors	British Association Research Quality Assurance; European Federation Good Clinical Practice	BARQA	www.barqa.com www.efgcp.org
Data managers	Association of Clinical Data Managers	ACDM	www.acdm.org.uk
Regulatory	British Institute Regulatory Affairs; European Society Regulatory Affairs	BIRA	www.bira.org www.esra.org www.raps.org
Pharmacoeconomics	International Society of Pharmacoeconomic and Outcomes Research		www.ispor.org
Pharmacovigilance	International Society for Pharmacoepidemiology		www.pharmacoepi.org

*A complete list of international associations for pharmaceutical physicians can be found on their website.

Table 1.2 Available postgraduate courses in pharmaceutical medicine

Professional body	Courses	University
Pharmaceutical medicine	Postgraduate Course in Pharmaceutical Medicine	University Wales Institute of Science and Technology
	MSc Pharmaceutical Medicine	University of Surrey
	Postgraduate Diploma in Pharmaceutical Medicine	Autonomous University of Barcelona, Spain
	Academic Specialty in Pharmaceutical Medicine	Complutense University of Madrid, Spain
	European Course in Pharmaceutical Medicine (ECPM)	University of Basel, Switzerland
	Postgraduate Programme in Pharmacology and Pharmaceutical Medicine	Free University of Brussels (ULB)
	Postgraduate Study Course in Pharmaceutical Medicine	University of Witten/ Herdecke, Germany
	European Diploma in Pharmaceutical Medicine (EUDIPHARM)	University of Lyon, France
	Course in Pharmaceutical Medicine	New University of Lisbon Portugal
	Pharmaceutical Medicine Course	Karolinksa Institut, Sweden
Information management	Diploma in Information Management	City University, London
Clinical research	Certificate of Professional Development Postgraduate Certificate Postgraduate Diploma MSc	John Moore's University, Liverpool
Data management	Postgraduate Certificate Postgraduate Diploma MSc	Kingston University, Surrey
Regulatory affairs	Diploma MSc	University of Wales
Quality assurance	Diploma MSc	East Anglia Polytechnic University
Pharmacovigilance	MSc	University of Hertfordshire

teamwork. Whilst the current emphasis on evidence-based medicine has increased the understanding of clinical research study designs, many tasks must be performed by people who are not necessarily versed in the art of performing the trials to the standards demanded by national and international standard-setting bodies. The importance of minor changes in study design and the detail in Good Clinical Practice (GCP) set by the ICH are often rigorously demanding. For standards to be set, studies must be conducted to validate the methods we use. This is the 'R&D' of R&D. Academic societies provide a forum for the presentation of research into new and as yet unvalidated methods that challenge the way in which we currently work. It is quite difficult for each professional group to find the resource to support all the kinds of professional organisations described and therefore in pharmaceutical medicine these working groups are often set up through a variety of other academic societies and there are some specialising entirely in pharmaceutical and regulatory medicine such as the Drug Information Association (www.diahome.org) and the Society of Pharmaceutical Medicine (www.socpharmed.org).

Conclusion

In the last 50 years radical changes have occurred in pharmaceutical medicine. When one considers that there have been dramatic changes in therapeutics over this period this is not surprising: the introduction of broad-spectrum antibiotics in the 1940s and 1950s, the introduction of drugs based on receptor theory in the 1970s, in the 1980s the first biotechnology products, in the 1990s radical new approaches to drug design and targeting and now the first gene therapy products emerging. In the last few years these developments have been spurred by cracking of the human genome and will make even greater advances with the development of proteomics. The constant search for new therapeutics, their development and the evaluation of their performance throughout the product lifetime have generated a group of highly skilled people whose sole task is to bring effective treatments to the market and to monitor their use.

References

Adam, H.M. and Passmore, R. (1980) Introduction, in *A Companion to Medical Studies: Vol. 2. Pharmacology, Microbiology, General Pathology and Related Subjects* (eds R. Passmore and J.S. Robson), Blackwell Scientific Publications, London.

Armitage, P. and Berry, G. (1987) The scope of statistics, Ch. 1 in *Statistical Methods in Medical Research*, Blackwell Scientific Publications, London.

Bradford Hill, Sir A. (1937) *Principles of Medical Statistics*, Edward Arnold, London.

Cromie, B. (1993) The evolution of pharmaceutical medicine since the 1950s. *Pharmacol. Med.*, 7, 127–137.

Hampton, S.R. and Julian, D.G. (1987) Role of the pharmaceutical industry in major clinical trials. *Lancet*, **Nov. 28**, 1258–1259.

Laurence, D.R. (1966a) Drug control, drug names, in *Clinical Pharmacology*, Churchill, London.

Laurence, D.R. (1966b) Drug therapy: the thalidomide disaster, in *Clinical Pharmacology*, Churchill, London.

Lis, Y. and Walker, S.R. (1989) Novel medicines marketed in the UK (1960–1980). *Br. J. Clin. Pharmacol.*, **28**, 333–343.

Parke Davis (1939) *Analecta Therapeutica*, Parke Davis & Co., London.

Teeling Smith, G. (1992) The British pharmaceutical industry: 1961–1991, in *Innovative Competition in Medicine* (ed. G. Teeling Smith), Office of Health Economics, London.

Wells, F.O. (1993) Fraud and misconduct in clinical research, in *The Textbook of Pharmaceutical Medicine* (eds J.P. Griffin, J. O'Grady and F.O. Wells), Queen's University, Belfast.

2

The Contribution of Academic Clinical Pharmacology to Medicines Research

Charles F. George

British Heart Foundation, London, UK

Introduction

Clinical pharmacologists have a major role to play in the pre-marketing phase of drug development. Specifically, their knowledge and skills equip them for:

1. Studies on dose–response relationships;
2. Studies in special groups, e.g. the elderly, those with liver or renal disease, and of pharmacogenetics;
3. Studies of drug interactions;
4. The estimation of compliance;
5. Other activities.

Studies on Dose–Response Relationships

Although policies within individual companies differ one from another, there can be no doubt that the industry and the recipients of their products have suffered when new chemical entities have been used in too high a dose. There are many examples, which could be cited, but I shall confine myself to two. The first is the treatment of hypertension with benzothiadiazine (thiazide) diuretics. Despite careful studies by Cranston *et al.* (1963) showing that low, intermediate and high doses of bendrofluazide, cyclopenthiazide and chlorthalidone were equieffective in lowering blood pressure, most doctors prescribed intermediate or high doses for their

Careers with the Pharmaceutical Industry, Second edition. Edited by P. D. Stonier.
© 2003 John Wiley & Sons Ltd. ISBN 0 470 84328 4

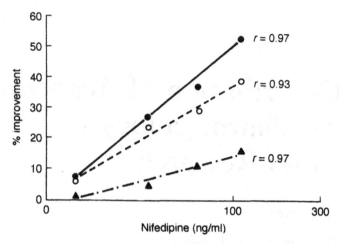

Figure 2.1 Relationship between plasma nifedipine concentration and antianginal effects in patients already receiving atenolol. ●———●, time to pain; O– – –O, time to 1mm ST depression; ▲–·–▲, maximal exercise tolerance. Reproduced from the *British Journal of Clinical Pharmacology*, with kind permission of the editor (Challenor *et al.*, 1989)

patients. Diuretics of this type produce hypokalaemia but the significance of the latter and the risks of long-term glucose intolerance were not appreciated until much later (Murphy *et al.*, 1982; Lant, 1987). Nevertheless, when used in low dose, diuretics remain an effective, economic and simple treatment for hypertension, while their risks are minimised.

Similarly, the first angiotensin-converting enzyme inhibitor to be marketed, captopril, was initially given in large doses (Lant, 1987), often to people in whom we would now prefer to avoid its use, e.g. those with renal artery stenosis and collagen vascular disease. Problems such as rashes and agranulocytosis arose as a consequence of the high doses used compared with those recommended (Romankiewicj *et al.*, 1983). Better methodology (Wellstein *et al.*, 1987) should allow a more detailed study of the extent of inhibition of the angiotensin-converting enzyme in vivo. Such information is of use in exploring the dose–effect relationship and deciding upon an appropriate one (as well as the dosing interval for a new compound).

By contrast, in the sphere of angina pectoris (and hypertension) Pritchard and Gillam (1971) carried out pioneering studies to show the importance of dosage titration. Thus, in angina pectoris studies comparing the efficacy of full dose (average 417 mg/day; range 80–1280 mg) a half, one-quarter and one-eighth of that amount showed a clear-cut dose–response relationship. Originally, it was thought that this might be a reflection of poor absorption in some patients. However, studies by Paterson *et al.* (1970) using radiolabelled propranolol showed that the absorption was almost complete.

Subsequently, Shand *et al.* (1970) demonstrated identical plasma concentration–time curves after intravenous administration to five healthy volunteers but seven-fold difference in the plasma concentrations obtained after oral dosing. This provided evidence for extensive pre-systemic drug metabolism and marked inter-individual differences in its extent. This knowledge was used subsequently to demonstrate the importance of dosage titration in the control of cardiac arrhythmias (Woosley *et al.*, 1979).

The identification of pre-systemic drug metabolism and the likelihood of a short duration of action (as well as individual variability) led to subsequent more rational investigation of other cardiovascular acting drugs. In my laboratories we worked extensively on the dihydropyridine calcium channel-blocking drug, nifedipine.

We demonstrated a close relationship between the response in angina pectoris (time to onset of pain, time to 1 mm ST segment depression and the maximum duration of exercise) and the logarithm of the plasma nifedipine concentration (Challenor *et al.*, 1989) (Figure 2.1). However, even with modified release preparations, twice-daily dosing was insufficient to produce an adequate response throughout a 24-hour day, the benefits wearing off by 12 hours after dosing.

Studies in Special Groups

The elderly

The elderly consume a disproportionate number of medicines (Ridout *et al.*, 1986; Cartwright and Smith, 1988). This is particularly true of drugs intended for use in cardiovascular medicine, others with an action on the central nervous system (e.g. anti-parkinsonian remedies) and for agents with an action on the musculoskeletal system.

Historically, the elderly have run into problems with agents with an action on each of these three systems. Examples include various antihypertensives (Jackson *et al.*, 1976), anti-parkinsonian therapy (Williamson and Chopin, 1980), benzodiazepines (Castleden *et al.*, 1977; Greenblatt *et al.*, 1991) and benoxaprofen (Hamdy *et al.*, 1982). If it is likely that a new medicine will be used by old people then it is essential to perform adequate studies of its pharmacology in that population.

Within my group we (Robertson *et al.*, 1988) performed studies of nifedipine's pharmacology in this age group. After an intravenous dose the initial concentrations achieved were similar to those in healthy young individuals but the clearance was diminished from 519 ml/min to 348 ml/min ($P < 0.05$). After oral administration, plasma concentrations were higher in the elderly than in young people due, in part, to an increased bioavailability from 46% to 61% consequent upon diminished pre-systemic metabolism. But the area under the concentration–time curve was increased also by delayed systemic clearance.

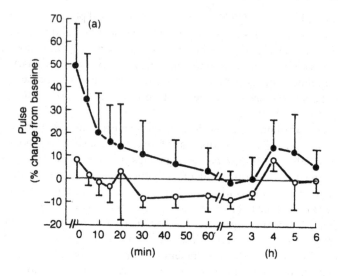

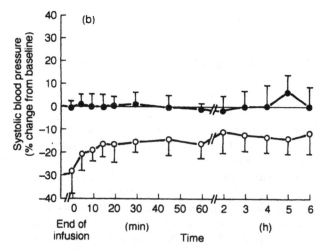

Figure 2.2   Effects of nifedipine on (a) heart rate and (b) systolic blood pressure in young (●) and elderly (○) subjects. Reproduced from the *British Journal of Clinical Pharmacology*, with kind permission of the editor (Robertson *et al.*, 1989)

In addition to these age-related variations in pharmacokinetics, the drug had different effects after intravenous administration. In young people it produced a brisk tachycardia with no drop in blood pressure (Figure 2.2). By contrast, in the elderly there was no increase in heart rate but a pronounced reduction in blood pressure. Such differences reflect not only a decline in baroreceptor function with age (Reid *et al.*, 1971) but also altered adrenoceptor sensitivity (Buckley *et al.*, 1986; Scarpace, 1986; Montamat and Davies, 1989).

Given the increased prevalence of Parkinson's disease in the elderly (Robertson and George, 1990), it is perhaps surprising how little was done to examine the pharmacology of L-dopa in this age group. There are, however, major differences in the pharmacokinetics of L-dopa (Robertson *et al.*, 1989) which, in part, explain the increased incidence of adverse effects encountered.

The elderly tend to complain more about problems with sleeping than do younger people. This is partly because their pattern of sleep is different and because they take 'cat naps' during the day, use less energy than their younger counterparts and require less sleep. Many studies have shown that the elderly are at greater risk from hypnotic drugs than are younger persons, and Greenblatt *et al.* (1991) have made elegant studies of the effects of benzodiazepines in this age group. They demonstrated that the plasma concentration of triazolam needed to produce a particular effect is roughly one-half of that which would produce the same action in younger persons. In addition, hangover effects of benzodiazepines are more common in this age group (Castleden *et al.*, 1977).

The prevalence of arthritis, particularly osteoarthritis of the knee, increases markedly with age (Blackburn *et al.*, 1994). As a consequence elderly people suffer considerable pain and limitation of their mobility. They therefore seek refuge in analgesic compounds.

Although there is relatively little evidence that the non-steroid anti-inflammatory drugs are required they are nonetheless frequently prescribed for patients in this age group. It is therefore vitally important that such agents are properly studied in healthy old people, those who have disease and others who are taking additional drug therapy. In collaboration with three other centres we (George *et al.*, 1986) studied the compound isoxicam in 108 people, of whom half were elderly. Half of the old people were healthy volunteers, while the remainder were patients taking other treatments. Despite differences in age and concurrent disease, there were no significant differences in the pharmacokinetics of this compound between young and old people. By contrast, benoxaprofen was particularly hazardous for old people, especially those with renal dysfunction (Hamdy *et al.*, 1982).

Renal failure

Studies could be undertaken either by nephrologists or clinical pharmacologists. The important point is to define the proportion of drug (or active metabolite) excreted in the urine, and to document any changes in systemic clearance with renal dysfunction so as to make appropriate dosage modification in patients with renal failure. Amiloride is a good example of an initial failure to act upon these principles. The drug is cleared unchanged via the kidneys (George, 1980) and will accumulate in patients with renal disease. Such patients are at risk of hyperkalaemia, and death occurred in a few during the early stages of drug development. Similarly, the acetyl metabolite of acebutolol is active and its clearance is diminished in patients with significant renal disease (Smith *et al.*, 1983), thereby contributing to its overall effects and long duration of action. Other water-soluble, 8-adrenoceptor antagonists have produced problems in patients with renal dysfunction. Although attempts were made to identify the most appropriate dose and dose frequency for atenolol in hypertension, when it was first marketed it was available only in 100-mg doses. The prescription of these to old patients sometimes produced profound bradycardia and syncope. Only subsequently have 50-mg and 25-mg tablets become available.

Liver disease

The majority of drugs which are subject to metabolism within the human organism meet their fate in the liver. Disease of the latter organ can lead to:

1. Diminished albumin synthesis and hence protein binding;
2. Reduced metabolising capabilities due, in part, to shunting of blood through portosystemic anastomoses;
3. Increased end-organ effects.

It is necessary to address most, if not all, of these parameters if a new chemical entity is likely to be used in people with hepatic disease. Clinical pharmacologists may have access to such patients and can help with the design and interpretation of such studies. However, in general it is patients who show diminished synthetic ability for albumin, who are jaundiced or show evidence of liver failure with ascites and encephalopathy who are particularly at risk (George et al., 1992).

Genetic polymorphism

Until comparatively recently there were few examples of how genetic mutations could result in subpopulations with quite widely differing abilities to carry out certain metabolic reactions. Among these, variations in the activity of N-acetyl-transferase were the best documented.

Genetic polymorphism in this case affects the metabolism of substrates, which include hydralazine, isoniazid, procainamide and sulphonamides (George and Waller, 1993).

More recently, genetic polymorphisms have been demonstrated for drug oxidation reactions. Thus, in 1977 'abnormalities' of 4-hydroxylation of debrisoquine were described (Mahgoub et al., 1977; Tucker et al., 1977). Since then, studies have identified numerous drugs which are subject to metabolism by the cytochrome P450 isoenzyme known as CYP2D6. Phenotypically poor metabolisers are subject to a variety of adverse effects, such as orthostatic hypotension from debrisoquine, nausea and vomiting from bufuralol, excessive duration of action of metoprolol and propranolol and possible central nervous system toxicity from a variety of tricyclic antidepressants (George *et al.*, 1992). Most of these discoveries have stemmed from work in academic departments of clinical/biochemical pharmacology. Several departments have established banks of human liver tissue, cell lines, purified enzymes and specific antibodies which allow the detection of potential metabolic pathways. Moreover, selective inhibitors of CYP2D6, including quinidine and propafenone, have been identified which allow the significance of this enzyme to be studied in vivo.

Twenty human isozymes have been cloned and characterised/sequenced in full. Among the most important ones to exhibit genetic polymorphisms are CYP1A2, CYP2B6, CYP2C, CYP2D6 (see above), CYP2E1 and CYP3A4, all of which have been shown to metabolise clinically important drugs (Cholerton *et al.*, 1992). Substrates for these enzymes include caffeine, theophylline; testosterone, tolbutamide and phenytoin; debrisoquine, metoprolol; chlorzoxazone; and nifedipine, erythromycin and ciclosporin.

An alternative technique for defining genetic polymorphism is based upon statistical/modelling approaches for data obtained in vivo on large populations (Jackson *et al.*, 1989). Clinical pharmacologists (mostly based in academia) have contributed much to our understanding of the appropriate use of these techniques (Grevel *et al.*, 1989).

The significance of genetic polymorphism is further developed in the next section.

Studies of Drug Interactions

Traditionally, interactions were studied in 'blunderbuss' fashion. As a consequence, pharmaceutical companies undertook expensive, sometimes meaningless, studies of around 50 compounds with which their product might, in theory, interact. It is my belief, and that of colleagues both in academic clinical pharmacology and in the pharmaceutical industry, that we need to target our studies more meaningfully. In so doing, we should not only satisfy regulatory authorities but also undertake a more informed, ethical and appropriate series of studies. Hopefully, these should be cheaper and take less time than the more traditional approach.

When studying the fate of a new chemical entity in man it should be possible (by a combination of studies performed in vivo and in vitro) to establish the major pathways of metabolism/elimination. Thus, the demonstration that a new benzodiazepine is, like triazolam, metabolised by CYP3A (Kronbach *et al.*, 1989; Gascon and Dayer, 1991) should lead to the initiation of specific interaction studies. Firstly, enzyme inducers such as carbamazepine will need to be studied—perhaps in epileptics, since we know that this same enzyme is responsible for the metabolic degradation of felodipine (Capewell *et al.*, 1988). Interactions with citrus juices may need to be undertaken (Bailey *et al.*, 1991) and a variety of other inhibitors studied, e.g. cimetidine, calcium channel-blocking drugs, ketoconazole and the macrolides, e.g. erythromycin. Interactions may need to be undertaken also with non-sedative antihistamines, with the selective serotonin reuptake inhibitors and ciclosporin. Had it been recognised that astemizole and terfenadine were metabolised by this same cytochrome P450 system, studies might have been undertaken with specific inhibitors, e.g. erythromycin, and the *torsade de pointes* form of ventricular tachycardia recognised earlier than 1992 (Honing *et al.*, 1992).

Estimation of Compliance

There are four main variables, which influence the effects of medicines:

1. Pharmaceutical, e.g. the formulation;
2. Pharmacokinetic factors;
3. Pharmacodynamic factors;
4. Patient's medicine-taking behaviour (compliance).

Non-compliance can take several forms, including not taking enough medicine, not observing the correct intervals between doses, not observing the correct duration of treatment, and taking additional medication (either prescribed or non-prescribed). Each of these forms of non-compliance can affect the outcome of drug treatment and is particularly important when assessing the effects of new treatments. Traditionally physicians have relied on their patients giving honest answers to questions such as 'Do you ever forget to take your medicine?' Answers to these and other questions have been supplemented by pill counts which estimate the amount removed from the container. However, this technique assumes that whatever has left the bottle goes through the patient and this may not always be the case.

In recent years blood and urine tests have been used to identify the likely causes of failure to respond to drug treatment. Low blood concentrations mean either a failure to comply with treatment or poor absorption due to pharmaceutical factors and/or extensive pre-systemic drug metabolism. Repetition of the measurement under a period of supervised medication intake can lead to a more accurate assessment of the contribution of non-compliance to the low blood concentrations found.

Compliance with other drug therapy has been assessed by the incorporation of a substance such as riboflavin, which is excreted in urine. Subsequent screening of urine for the presence of riboflavin (by fluorescence under ultraviolet light) was used in the USA to select patients for inclusion in trials of antihypertensive medication (Veterans Administration Cooperative Study Group on Antihypertensive Agents, 1967). Unfortunately there is no foolproof method for assessing compliance but containers with microprocessors built into their lids can identify the precise time of container opening, the demonstration of 'drug holidays' and early cessation of therapy.

Other Activities

In this chapter I have attempted to show some of the ways in which clinical pharmacologists can help the development of new chemical entities. There are, however, other ways in which they contribute to the development of new medicines. First, many act as consultants to the pharmaceutical industry. Second, they contribute also to drug development through their activities as members of ethics committees and drug regulatory bodies such as the Committee on Safety of Medicines and the Medicines Commission. Third, they have devised new techniques for the study of medicines in man.

References

Bailey, D.G., Spence, J.D., Munro, C. and Arnold, J.M.O. (1991) Interactions of citrus juices with felodipine and nifedipine. *Lancet*, **337**, 268–269.

Blackburn, S.C.F., Ellis, R., George, C.F. and Kirwan, J.R. (1994) The impact and treatment of arthritis in general practice. *Pharmacoepidemiol. Drug Safety*, **3**(3), 123–128.

Buckley, C., Curtin, D., Walsh, T. and O'Malley, K. (1986) Ageing and platelet Ct2 adrenoceptors. *Br. J. Clin. Pharmacol.*, **21**, 721–722.

Capewell, S., Freestone, S., Critchley, J.A.J.H., Pottage, A. and Prescott, L.F. (1988) Reduced felodipine bioavailability in patients taking anticonvulsants. *Lancet*, **ii**, 480–482.

Cartwright, A. and Smith, C. (1988) *Elderly People, their Medicines and their Doctors*, Routledge, London.

Castleden, C.M., George, C.F., Marcer, D. and Hallett, C. (1977) Increased sensitivity to nitrazepam in old age. *Br. Med. J.*, **i**, 10–12.

Challenor, V.F., Waller, D.G., Renwick, A.G. and George, C.F. (1989) Slow release nifedipine plus atenolol in chronic stable angina pectoris. *Br. J. Clin. Pharmacol.*, **28**, 509–516.

Cholerton, S., Daly, A.K. and Idle, J.R. (1992) The role of individual human cytochromes P-450 in drug metabolism and clinical response. *Trends Pharmacol. Sci.*, **13**, 434–439.

Cranston, W.I., Juel-Jensen, B.E., Semmence, A.M., Handfield Jones, R.P.C., Forbes, J.A. and Mutch, L.M.M. (1963) Effects of oral diuretics on raised arterial pressure. *Lancet*, **ii**, 966–970.

Gascon, M.-P. and Dayer, P. (1991) In vitro forecasting of drugs which may interfere with the biotransformation of midazolam. *Eur. J. Clin. Pharmacol.*, **41**, 573–578.

George, C.F. (1980) Amiloride handling in renal failure. *Br. J. Clin. Pharmacol.*, **9**, 94–95.

George, C.F. and Waller, D.G. (1993) Drug treatment, in *Clinical Heart Disease in Old Age* (eds A. Martin and J. Camm), Wiley, Chichester.

George, C.F., Renwick, A.G., Darragh, A.S., Hosie, J., Black, D., van Marle, W. and Frank, G.J. (1986) A comparison of isoxicam pharmacokinetics in young and elderly subjects. *Br. J. Clin. Pharmacol.*, **22**, 129S–134S.

George, C.F., George, R.H. and Howden, C.W. (1992) The liver and response to drugs, in *Wright's Liver and Biliary Disease*, 3rd edn (eds G.H. Millward-Sadler, R. Wright and M. Arthur), Saunders, London.

Greenblatt, D.J., Harmatz, J.S., Shapiro, L., Engelhardt, N., Gouthro, T.A. and Shader, R.I. (1991) Sensitivity to triazolam in the elderly. *N. Engl. J. Med.*, **324**, 1691–1698.

Grevel, J., Thomas, P. and Whiting, B. (1989) Population pharmacokinetic analysis of bisoprolol. *Clin. Pharmacokinet.*, **17**, 53–63.

Hamdy, R.C., Mumane, B., Perera, N., Woodcock, K. and Koch, I.M. (1982) The pharmacokinetics of benoxaprofen in elderly subjects. *Eur. J. Rheumatol. Inflamm.*, **5**, 69–75.

Honing, P.K., Woosley, R.L., Zamoni, K., Conner, D.P. and Cantilena, L.R. (1992) Changes in the pharmacokinetics and electrocardiographic pharmacodynamics of terfenadine with concomitant administration of erythromycin. *Clin. Pharmacol. Ther.*, **52**, 231–238.

Jackson, G., Pierscianowski, T.A., Mahon, W. and Condon, J. (1976). Inappropriate hypertensive therapy in the elderly. *Lancet*, **ii**, 1317–1318.

Jackson, P.R., Tucker, G.T. and Woods, H.F. (1989) Testing for bimodality in frequency distributions of data suggesting polymorphisms of drug metabolism: histograms and probit plots. *Br. J. Clin. Pharmacol.*, **28**, 647–653.

Kronbach, T., Mathys, D., Umeno, M., Gonzales, F.J. and Meyer, U.A. (1989) Oxidation of midazolam and triazolam by human liver cytochrome P450IIIA4. *Mol. Pharmacol.*, **36**, 89–96.

Lant, A.F. (1987) Evolution of diuretics and ACE inhibitors, their renal and anti-hypertensive actions: parallels and contrasts. *Br. J. Clin. Pharmacol.*, **23**, 27S–41S.

Mahgoub, A., Idle, J.R., Dring, L.G., Lancaster, R. and Smith, R.L. (1977) Polymorphic hydroxylation of debrisoquine in man. *Lancet*, **ii**, 584–586.

Montamat, S.C. and Davies, A.O. (1989) Physiological response to isoproterenol and coupling of beta-adrenergic receptors in young and elderly human subjects. *J. Gerontol.*, **44**, M100–105.

Murphy, M.B., Lewis, P.J., Kohner, E., Schumer, B. and Dollery, C.T. (1982) Glucose intolerance in hypertensive patients treated with diuretics: a fourteen year follow-up. *Lancet*, **ii**, 1293–1295.

Paterson, J.W., Conolly, M.E., Dollery, C.T. and Hayes, A. (1970) The pharmacodynamics and metabolism of propranolol in man. *Pharmacol. Clin.*, **2**, 127–133.

Pritchard, B.N.C. and Gillam, P.M.S. (1971) Assessment of propranolol in angina pectoris: clinical dose–response curve and effect on electrocardiogram at rest and on exercise. *Br. Heart J.*, **33**, 473–480.

Reid, J.L., Calne, D.B., George, C.F., Pallis, C. and Vakil, S.D. (1971) Cardiovascular reflexes in parkinsonism. *Clin. Sci.*, **41**, 63–67.

Ridout, S., Waters, W.E. and George, C.F. (1986) Knowledge of and attitudes to medicines in the Southampton community. *Br. J. Clin. Pharmacol.*, **21**, 701–712.

Robertson, D.R.C. and George, C.F. (1990) Drug therapy for Parkinson's disease. *Br. Med. Bull.*, **46**, 124–146.

Robertson, D.R.C., Waller, D.G., Renwick, A.G. and George, C.F. (1988) Age related changes in the pharmacokinetics and pharmacodynamics of nifedipine. *Br. J. Clin. Pharmacol.*, **25**, 297–305.

Robertson, D.R.C., Wood, N.D., Everest, H., Monks, K., Waller, D.G., Renwick, A.G. and George, C.F. (1989) The effect of age on the pharmacokinetics of levodopa administered alone and in the presence of carbidopa. *Br. J. Clin. Pharmacol.*, **28**, 61–69.

Romankiewicj, J.A., Brogden, R.N., Heel, R.C., Speight, J.M. and Avery, G.S. (1983) Captopril: an update review of its pharmacological properties and therapeutic efficacy in congestive heart failure. *Drugs*, **25**, 6–40.

Scarpace, P.J. (1986) Decreased β-adrenoceptor responsiveness during senescence. *Fed. Proc.*, **45**, 51–54.

Shand, D.G., Nuckolls, E.M. and Oates, J.A. (1970) Plasma propranolol levels in adults, with observations in four children. *Clin. Pharmacol. Ther.*, **11**, 112–120.

Smith, R.S., Warren, D.J., Renwick, A.G. and George, C.F. (1983) Acebutolol pharmacokinetics in renal failure. *Br. J. Clin. Pharmacol.*, **16**, 253–258.

Tucker, G.T., Silas, J.H., Iyun, A.O., Lennard, M.S. and Smith, A.J. (1977) Polymorphic hydroxylation of debrisoquine. *Lancet*, **ii**, 718.

Veterans Administration Cooperative Study Group on Antihypertensive Agents (1967) Effects of treatment on morbidity in hypertension. *JAMA*, **202**, 1028–1034.

Wellstein, A., Essig, J. and Belz, G.G. (1987) A method for estimating the potency of angiotensin converting enzyme inhibitors in man. *Br. J. Clin. Pharmacol.*, **24**, 397–399.

Williamson, J. and Chopin, J.M. (1980) Adverse reactions to prescribed drugs in the elderly: a multicentre investigation. *Age Ageing*, **9**, 73–80.

Woosley, R.L., Kornhauser, D., Smith, R., Reele, S., Higgins, S.B., Nies, A.S., Shand, D.G. and Oates, J.A. (1979) Suppression of chronic ventricular arrhythmias with propranolol. *Circulation*, **60**, 819–827.

3
A Career in Drug Discovery

David Ellis

Euromedica plc, Cambridge, UK

Introduction

The modern life-saving pill, which is the product of the therapeutic revolution of the second half of the last century, is a symbol of the innovative success of research conducted mainly in the pharmaceutical industry. Despite this inventive track record, however, the challenge for drug researchers to find new and improved therapies has never been greater, due to the combination of rapidly changing economic and social pressures and an ever-increasing complexity of science and technology.

Thus, on the one hand, the cost constraints imposed by finite national healthcare budgets will tend to favour the prescribing of cheaper, generic or over-the-counter (OTC) products rather than the usually higher priced new drugs, unless the latter have a demonstrated therapeutic advantage. On the other hand, to achieve the scientific breakthroughs required for the discovery of genuinely more effective new drugs, pharmaceutical companies must continue to increase their research and development budgets dramatically, in order to meet the challenges presented by more complex biological and chemical problems. This requirement comes at a time when patent expiry will shortly expose some $30 billion of sales to generic competition in the USA alone. *A priori*, it follows that in the future only those pharmaceutical companies that are able to address major medical needs, through harnessing the results of innovative, cost-effective research and development, will survive.

The emergence of the biotechnology industry with its new technologies and research philosophy has had dramatic effects on pharmaceutical research. The traditional pharmaceutical industry was quick to adopt all of the molecular biology, genetics, proteomics and other biotechnology company technologies. Indeed, the use of these approaches by traditional pharmaceutical companies has long since blurred the distinction between them and biotechnology companies to such an extent that we could now, arguably, refer to all of them more properly as

Careers with the Pharmaceutical Industry, Second edition. Edited by P. D. Stonier.
© 2003 John Wiley & Sons Ltd. ISBN 0 470 84328 4

healthcare companies. Genomics and high-throughput screening are often projected as the answer to the healthcare industry's problems but, in reality, they represent the industrialisation of target and lead identification alone. The subsequent stages of biological testing and lead optimisation in drug discovery plus all of the required safety assessment, clinical testing, formulation and process development remain to be done as before. Indeed, the importance of target validation by biologists and rational drug design by medicinal chemists is greatly enhanced by the need to reduce the huge number of potential targets and chemical hits to manageable programmes. These must be properly resourced if significant numbers of new therapies are to emerge from this largely unproven approach.

Pharmaceutical company innovativeness, in the context of addressing major medical needs, is essentially linked to the discovery of:

- Safer and more effective variants of known therapies;
- Alternative drugs acting by novel biochemical or pharmacological mechanisms;
- Novel therapies for major diseases such as cancer, AIDS, neurodegenerative diseases, osteoporosis and immune-inflammatory diseases.

Consequently, the survival and growth of pharmaceutical companies will depend on their ability to discover, develop and market products which fall into one or more of these three categories.

This presents an exhilarating challenge for scientists interested in embarking on a career in drug discovery. In fact, the major costs of research and development (R&D) are biased towards development rather than research, and these are increasing dramatically due to a more demanding regulatory environment. Nevertheless, the fact remains that it will be the improved effectiveness of research in discovering new chemical entities (NCEs) with different and/or more selective biological properties that will focus these development resources on those new agents most likely to lead to quantifiable therapeutic benefits. In addition to this, researchers in the pharmaceutical industry are also working at the leading edge of current international biological and high-throughput chemistry/screening developments, which are surely undergoing the most explosive growth in its history.

Key Elements in Pharmaceutical R&D Strategy

First of all, it is instructive to provide some definitions for the broad activities encompassed by drug discovery and drug development.

The discovery phase of R&D is normally considered to involve all of the research activities which culminate in the identification of a lead compound with a sufficient combination of potency and selectivity, as defined by specific biological tests in animals, for it to have the potential to become a new medicine.

The development phase of R&D (both non-clinical and clinical) includes the complex interwoven sequence of activities required to convert a chemical lead into a marketable medicine, which is both safe and effective in man.

The precise demarcation between discovery and development activities will vary in different companies. Thus, in some companies development encompasses all activities, including safety studies and clinical pharmacology, after the primary biological activity has been established in in vitro and in vivo tests in animals. In other R&D groups it will commence after clinical pharmacology has established safety and pharmacokinetics in man. Perhaps the most important consideration, however, is not the definition of the precise demarcation but the need to ensure that scientists in discovery research collaborate very closely with clinical pharmacologists, toxicologists and process research chemists in defining the critical path for the rapid evaluation of new compounds in exploratory development.

The most important hurdle for a new compound to overcome before it is a serious development candidate is its assessment up to the end of phase I studies and, therefore, it is vital to obtain this assessment as quickly as possible. The close involvement of discovery scientists is likely to aid this fast-track development phase, since the chemical and biological knowledge gained in discovery will be critical in establishing the parameters and checkpoints in the early development plan.

Drug discovery

The most important ingredient for successful drug discovery is probably the most difficult and intangible to define, namely the presence of an innovative working climate within the research group. Experience to date has indicated the superiority of small, flexible research groups with a high degree of autonomy. This philosophy is still most appropriate in small and niche companies. In large corporations the huge investment in core technologies militates against this and the greatest management challenge is to facilitate flexibility and innovation in the current climate.

In some ways we can regard the genomics, high-throughput chemistry and high-throughput screening-related technologies as part of a discovery process which should accelerate the generation of validated targets, chemical hits and leads. Against this background, therapeutic area biologists continue their basic physiological and disease state research while medicinal chemists drive the lead optimisation and drug candidate selection process once the necessary biological hypothesis has been confirmed. However, it is essential that these groups function as an effective team, that they are all very innovative and work to the highest standards of academic excellence and with cutting edge technologies in their respective disciplines.

Some or all of the following elements are necessary to produce this environment and it will be the recognised responsibility of senior management to encourage its creation and survival:

- Freedom for senior scientists to choose projects or areas of research;
- Effective collaboration between scientists in different disciplines, particularly between chemists and biologists;
- Concentration and focus of research resources to acquire knowledge and critical mass;
- Creation of small, highly interactive teams within the overall resource, i.e. to reproduce the biotechnology company culture;
- Informal communication and decision-making to minimise organisational and bureaucratic impact;
- Encouragement of professional recognition;
- Collaboration with external groups to broaden the scientific base of experimental activities;
- Encouragement of peer group evaluation and criticism;
- Condoning of 'risky research' and receptivity to new ideas;
- Toleration of non-conformity;
- Company recognition for project success;
- Interactive, challenging and interested research management;
- Motivation driven by both individual and team goals.

Many of these are recognisable ingredients in successful academic research groups. However, the fact that the pharmaceutical industry research group has a primary objective, namely the discovery of a new drug, differentiates it from the normally less goal-orientated endeavour of academic research.

In essence, drug research is an interactive team game, but with a large amount of freedom for each discipline group, and each scientist within each group, to develop new ideas and approaches. Once the leads are identified, the excitement in the research team is derived from the discovery of more selective and more active compounds. As these emerge, the biologists are presented then with the new challenge of characterising their biological properties more exactly and deciding whether the central biological hypothesis needs to be modified. Assuming that these later compounds possess the required activity profile, further structural modification will then be undertaken to provide a drug candidate with the right profile for exploratory development.

Development

The development process is inherently different in its aims and *modus operandi* from that of discovery research. The main objective of drug development is to assess the therapeutic potential and obtain marketing approval for new chemical entities with maximum speed, optimum cost and high quality of the package submitted to regulatory authorities. Key ingredients include:

- Detailed planning with fast track to phase I studies in man;
- Product profiles clearly defined and agreed with marketing;
- Strong input from regulatory affairs and medical marketing;
- Project managers with good organisational, communication and analytical skills;
- Project team members with good technical, problem-solving and communication skills, coupled with follow-through ability;
- Checkpoints, milestones and management systems to assess project progress;
- Effective use of information technology;
- Flexible use of resources to create and disband teams when required;
- Effective links between process research and production to aid the early involvement of production.

In addition to the need to plan and organise the development process there is also a clear need for innovation and creativity in the solving of defined, but often technically difficult, problems associated with developing a new drug. Thus, although the need for an innovative climate is not as critical as in discovery, it is recognised that development scientists must be given the opportunity to stay at the forefront of their disciplines through the practice of state-of-the-art science and publication of research findings as well as via collaborative interaction with other scientists in R&D.

Management of Discovery and Development

Numerous senior scientists and pharmaceutical industry analysts have noted that small, flexible, highly interactive discovery research groups were the most successful in finding many of the major top-selling drugs, such as penicillins, cephalosporins, beta-blockers, anti-asthma drugs and H2-receptor antagonists, discovered and developed by the UK-based pharmaceutical industry. In addition, the inventive success of the US biotechnology sector, as evidenced by the large number of clinical candidates submitted for regulatory approval, is probably linked to the fact that research in these companies is conducted by small, entrepreneurial and highly interactive teams, which have close links with academic centres of excellence.

This recognition that an innovative climate is often produced in smaller, less tightly managed research groups led some of the larger pharmaceutical companies to separate discovery activities from the rest of the company organisation, including development. At the same time, they gave some autonomy to relatively small research programme teams, therapeutic area teams or satellite research groups, with encouragement to establish close working interactions with academic groups.

However, there are inherent dangers in separating discovery from other company activities and in particular the development process. Thus:

1. The critical collaborative interaction between scientists in discovery and development could be diminished or lost;
2. There is a potential to create an 'ivory tower' mentality in discovery, if links with the 'real world' are made more tenuous; and
3. Development will be less accessible as a future career opportunity to scientists than discovery.

In fact, the success of biotechnology companies in exploiting basic science is almost certainly partly dependent on the close link between the research and business objectives of these companies. The challenge, therefore, for the large R&D groups is to create the required interactive, innovative teams within all parts of R&D, while retaining the ability to organise critical mass resources, particularly in development, to bring products to the market place.

In some companies this has been achieved with greater in-house flexibility by contracting out large parts of the more routine development work under the tight control of experienced company project managers, while solving critical development problems in-house through the creation of specific 'ad hoc' project teams comprised of scientists selected from both discovery and development on the basis of their relevant skills. As with the biotechnology sector, this can then lead to much more overlap between scientists from all areas of R&D with a possible benefit to overall R&D effectiveness. One corollary, and possible additional benefit, of this approach is the resulting reduction in the total numbers of permanently employed staff in R&D and increased flexibility in the spending choices for sizeable development budgets.

Core technologies

The complexity of modern-day science demands that discovery and development programmes will only be successful if 'state-of-the-art' scientific knowledge is brought to bear effectively on the problems to be addressed. This requires a realisation that all R&D groups require to build, develop and exploit a range of core technologies relevant to their scientific focus. These technologies may form an integral part of each department or project team involved in R&D or, alternatively, may exist separately as a broad-ranging support function which provides a collaborative resource to project teams as and when required. Examples of such core technologies might include genomics/gene chip technology, DNA sequencing, bioinformatics, DNA cloning, 'in situ' hybridisation, immunohistochemistry, proteomics, computational chemistry or macromolecular science. Whatever the method of involvement of technologies of this type that a successful R&D strategy must address, the need is to utilise them and ensure that the scientists involved are sufficiently well resourced to remain at the forefront of the development of their respective technology.

Research alliances and product licensing

Most R&D groups in the pharmaceutical industry recognise that, however large their resources, there is a need to network efficiently with other research groups in order to increase the options for the selection of development candidates. This interaction with outside groups may take the form of a collaborative strategic research alliance with another company, close involvement with an academic research group or simply the in-licensing of intellectual property or candidate compounds for development. These activities are now accepted as an essential part of R&D strategy for most pharmaceutical companies and represent the method by which the R&D resource can be broadened without necessarily increasing in-house R&D facilities.

For scientists in discovery research these activities present exciting opportunities to establish links with other research groups and expand their expertise and knowledge into new areas of research.

The Discovery Process

Organisation and management of research

In practice the two main ways of organising and managing drug discovery research within a pharmaceutical R&D group have been: (1) via project or programme teams consisting of scientists drawn from different discipline departments such as medicinal chemistry, pharmacology and biochemistry; and (2) via project or programme teams created from larger multidisciplinary therapeutic area teams which assume most of the additional functions normally associated with separate departments. To these we should now add: (3) via a genetics research department which is charged with providing validated drug targets to project and programme teams. Such departments must contain, or have access to, all of the multidisciplinary expertise required for the validation process.

In one approach a matrix project management system runs across a primary department structure within research. Recruitment, training, staff development, technical performance and resource allocation are the prime remit of departments, while the remit of the research project teams is to conduct the collaborative research aimed at discovering a specific type of new drug. Project teams are managed by project leaders who are accountable, in turn, to the research director, usually via a research committee. In some organisations department heads also act as project leaders for specific research projects.

Both systems of managing discovery research have potential advantages and disadvantages. Thus, powerful departments can subvert and frustrate the work of project teams through the emphasis of overriding and often conflicting loyalties. On the other hand, the absence of a department structure can lead to a drop in scientific standards since peer group interaction and criticism are diminished. In addition, departments provide a natural focus for creative interaction between members of different project teams.

The non-departmental approach to managing research is, to some extent, a contrived one since most project teams will include certain key members who will also work in discipline-based departments. For instance, in particular, support scientists such as physical organic chemists, molecular modellers and molecular biologists may provide critical input, as a more central resource, to more than one project in discovery research. Consequently, provided that the matrix project system is given strong support from the research directorate, there appears to be no reason to dispense with a primary department system since this provides an important additional input in the organisation and management of research, the maintenance of professional standards and productive interaction between scientists working in different project areas.

The birth of research projects

Target identification

Most previous research in the pharmaceutical industry started from an idea based on published or patented results or on in-house or academic research findings. The idea could come from any member of a research group or team and in most progressive organisations encouragement is given to younger scientists to suggest new ideas or approaches which may lead to new research proposals. For instance, based on the selective effects of known or newly synthesised molecules acting on pharmacological receptors or cellular enzymes, the relevance of a particular biological mechanism to an important physiological process in man may be suggested. Often the idea will relate to a way of improving the properties of a known drug or a compound being developed by a competitor company. Alternatively, a company may decide that some commitment to basic research in a particular biological field or therapeutic area is required. This may generate the essential new research results that will lead, in turn, to the testable hypothesis and identified target needed to justify a new project. Such strategies do, of course, remain valid and will continue—especially in smaller companies and those operating in niche areas which rely on specialist in-house knowledge/expertise in a specific therapeutic area or when an obvious target emerges from published research.

In the earlier programmes compounds structurally related to known drugs or biological agonists were screened in biological assays in which these agents were known to be active. Other programmes randomly screened compound libraries in a variety of bioassays looking for a hit to exploit. Structures which were found to be active, together with analogues from the company's own library, others purchased from chemical suppliers and those designed and synthesised in-house were then subjected to a Hansch analysis, in an effort to relate molecular form and functionality to biological activity, by medicinal chemists. The identification and acceptance of structurally definable receptor/ligand or enzyme/inhibitor interactions believed to be of importance in a particular disease, together with major advances in molecular graphics and computational chemistry, facilitated the development of rational drug design and medicinal chemistry as we know it today.

Concomitant with this approach automation technology was also developed, which allowed the screening of whole company compound libraries in such binding site/in vitro enzyme/cell-based assays. This high-throughput screening had the potential to provide hits on which rational drug design could be based when there were no obvious chemical or biochemical starting points.

Pharmaceutical industry research teams embraced, and in many cases pioneered, the use of emerging biotechnology, combinatorial chemistry, high-speed analytical and high-throughput screening technologies. Recently the developments in molecular biology, protein biochemistry and genomics have allowed genetics research to become another driver of research. In part because of the resulting plethora of potential drug development targets the parallel developments in high-throughput (combinatorial) chemistry and high-throughput screening have been essential enabling technologies.

Although it is inappropriate to go into detail here, we can outline a general scenario to indicate the role and influence of genomics and related technologies in drug discovery. In essence the in-house genetics department can sequence genes from patient material and bioinformaticians can compare these with those in public or commercially available databases. Abnormal genes, or genes which are over/under-expressed can be identified, cloned by molecular biologists, expressed by biotechnologists and their expression profiles derived. Discussions with cell biologists, biochemists, pharmacologists and others with specialist therapeutic area knowledge then lead to selection of those gene products that represent potential targets of importance in the disease state. The choice of these targets may well involve the development of animal models (such as a knockout mouse) and clinical genetics amongst other areas.

It is essential that chemistry strategy be decided as early as possible with involvement of both high-throughput and medicinal chemists. High-throughput screeners must also agree what assays they can and must develop if chemical libraries are to be screened. The best target ever identified would be totally useless without a chemistry strategy or a relevant biological assay.

Initial research on targets

Biology

Invariably, the first phase of any research project will involve a feasibility study which may entail further basic research. Biologists must also establish sufficiently sensitive and effective assays for measuring biological activity. Ideally, one or more of these should be adaptable as a high-throughput screen. The basic hypothesis, which may require receptor subtypes or specific isozymes to be identified, will need to be verified first of all. At this early stage one or two biologists (usually pharmacologists, biochemists or cell biologists) will be involved and contributions from a collaborative academic research group may be important. Traditionally this work would be based in discipline departments but could now also take place within a genetics research or equivalent group according to the particular company organisation.

Within discovery research a whole new area of biology has been developed without which the link from genetics research to project status would be impossible. This is based on expression of the full-length DNA clone in *E. coli*, insect, yeast or mammalian cells. Each has its own merits but mammalian cell expression is essential when the protein is the proposed therapeutic agent. The same group will be responsible for protein production, protein purification, protein biochemistry and the production of reagents (such as proteins and monoclonal antibodies) for use in high-throughput screens. When the therapeutic agent is a human protein, or other biological, the iterative medicinal chemistry approach is clearly not applicable although chemical modification may still be required. The project team will, however, still be needed to guide the development phase in order to ensure that efficacy, safety and all other regulatory requirements are met.

Medicinal chemistry

Medicinal chemistry will synthesise any key compounds such as active prototypes, natural transmitters, hormones or substrates needed for target validation work. Once the biological basis for the proposal has been proved (by establishing the importance of a particular mechanism) and a possible method of testing the hypothesis in man identified, significant chemistry resources must be committed. Medicinal chemists will now be in a position to propose a chemical strategy aimed at designing novel compounds which will act selectively on a specific biological target (e.g. as a receptor antagonist or enzyme inhibitor). At this point a new research project is born and the project team formed with a nominated project leader.

There are two main objectives which drive the creative dialogue between chemists and biologists. The first involves the attempt to relate affinity for the target receptor or enzyme (derived from primary ligand binding, enzyme, isolated cell or organ bath assays) to chemical structure, with the aim of designing new compounds with increased affinity and activity. Molecular modelling techniques and the measurement or calculation of physicochemical properties (e.g. lipophilicity, pK_a, electrostatic potential) are routinely used to develop and exploit this link between structure and ligand affinity. The second involves optimising in vivo activity (usually after oral administration) by utilising an understanding of those chemical

properties which influence drug absorption, distribution, metabolism and elimination. Again, this is likely to utilise selected physicochemical parameters,
together with some additional biological in vivo measurements such as blood
levels.

High-throughput chemistry

Prior to the advent of combinatorial chemistry, the average successful drug project
resulted in the synthesis of 1000–10 000 compounds by medicinal chemists. As
individual medicinal chemists are expected to complete 20–25 complex syntheses
per year this implies investing 40–400 man-years per drug. Clearly this is not
sustainable given the large numbers of targets and projects to be supported.

One solution to this has been provided by the high-throughput chemistry
approach. The early solid phase methods used to such great effect for peptide
library production are still preferred for longer syntheses. Liquid phase techniques
were first applied to the production of large maximum diversity libraries of
mixtures. These were screened as mixtures and deconvoluted later if hits were
found. Automation has now been developed that allows the production of more
relevant, smaller libraries of single compounds (say 100–1000 structures) by a core
group of users. High-throughput chemists may also train medicinal chemists in
high-throughput techniques which the latter now use routinely for the production
of small numbers of closely related analogues. Data management, automated mass
spectrometry or NMR analysis and library storage have been recent enabling
developments.

The aim of high-throughput chemistry is to plan a campaign which maximises
the variety of small arrays of chemotypes in manageable libraries. Families of
libraries related to, for example, receptor class rather than subtypes are particularly
valuable. Focus libraries can then be developed based on hits to provide leads for
medicinal chemistry. It is, however, important to recognise the necessity for using
medicinal chemistry insight in guiding the high-throughput chemistry campaign.

High-throughput screening

Integral to this process has been the parallel evolution of high-throughput
screening. Once reliable assays are established, the emphasis moves to the search
for active leads, and the screening of new compounds uses automation and
computer control to assist this process. Normally a separate high-throughput
screening department will be established to screen large numbers of compounds,
with the purpose of identifying novel leads, using a high-throughput variation of
one of the in vitro assays. This requires major investment in equipment and specialist biologists trained in assay development, the application of automated
equipment and data management. This group is pivotal in ensuring success, as it

must liaise closely with high-throughput and medicinal chemists as well as with therapeutic area research biologists. At this interface it must take, develop and apply biologically relevant assays, provide high-quality feedback to guide the high-throughput chemistry campaign and help medicinal chemists in the selection of preferred lead compounds.

The Work of the Project Team

The term 'project team' has different meanings in different companies and is, in some cases, interchangeable with programme team. Where there is a genetics department this may effectively contain several teams charged with defining targets in specific therapeutic areas. In other cases project teams may not be formed until a therapeutic area discovery team feels that it has amassed sufficient evidence to support the proposal of a lead compound or therapy for development status. Until that point the discovery, or programme team fills the project team role.

The team's primary function is to evaluate and project manage targets/leads to, and through, the development phase. The engine which drives research forward in the search for a new drug is the collaborative interaction between medicinal chemists, who propose and synthesise new molecules, and biologists (pharmacologists, biochemists and cell biologists), who evaluate the biological properties of these molecules using a range of molecular, cellular, tissue and whole-animal assay procedures. Biological activities of compounds in these assays are measured quantitatively and structure–activity relationships (SARs) are defined by the medicinal chemists using molecular parameters measured or calculated by physical organic chemists who will also participate actively in the project team.

Other key members of the project team are likely to include:

- Molecular modellers (usually trained as organic or theoretical chemists) who will assist in understanding three-dimensional interactions of molecules;
- Biochemists or chemists with expertise in drug metabolism who will provide early assessment of the biotransformation and fate of selected compounds, both in vitro and in vivo.

In addition, depending on the nature of the research, the team may require crucial input from specialist biologists such as electrophysiologists, immunologists and microbiologists. Then, as research progresses, with compounds nearing exploratory development, the team will be expanded to involve representatives from process research, clinical research, analytical chemistry, pharmacy and toxicology.

Entry Requirements for a Career in Discovery Research

With a few exceptions a career in discovery research requires a graduate qualification. A small number of researchers join the industry after A-levels but, to progress, they should aspire to gaining a degree by part-time study, usually involving day release. A useful way to obtain research experience is via a sandwich degree course, which allows students to spend a year in industry as part of their training.

At graduate level, scientists will join research programmes as biologists or chemists and, through assignment to a particular discipline, will become medicinal chemists, high-throughput chemists, computational chemists, physical organic chemists, pharmacologists, geneticists, enzymologists, biochemists, etc.

In essence, there are career opportunities in almost every area of biological and chemical science in addition to those mentioned above. Thus tissue culture specialists may function within a service department or work in specific project teams. Drug metabolism and pharmacokinetics may contain specialists in HPLC, hepatocyte metabolism of drug candidates and autoradiography alongside enzymologists and biochemists. Medicinal chemists will generally have open access to analytical tools such as mass spectrometry, NMR and IR, but the department of physical organic chemistry will also provide specialist services in these areas amongst others.

Outside of scientific areas there are also numerous openings in support services that are essential to the discovery process. For example, statisticians liase with biologists on experimental design, mathematicians work in modelling within drug metabolism and distribution, and IT specialists are vital in general areas such as data management and specialist roles such as developing the 'in silica' laboratory for use by molecular graphics.

To progress to positions of scientific leadership a postgraduate research qualification (ideally to PhD level) is almost always required. Occasionally, companies will provide opportunities for outstanding graduates to undertake PhD training utilising results obtained from an in-house research project and collaborative help from an external supervisor and academic establishment.

Career Development

Within research

The pharmaceutical industry is generally considered to provide scientists in research with excellent opportunities for further training and personal development. For the bench scientist, budgets will usually allow for the purchase of state-of-the-art instrumentation and equipment and off-site training on specialised courses organised by academic centres. In addition, experienced scientists are encouraged to attend scientific conferences and present posters and papers. The publication of original research results is usually encouraged, although important inventions relating to the biological activities of new compounds will need to be patented before disclosure. These activities establish links with the outside research community and assist in building an independent scientific reputation.

In most progressive organisations researchers at all levels will be encouraged to develop as experimental scientists and research leaders, with emphasis on individual decision-making and creative input to the team effort. Once supervisory and strategic skills are evident the responsibility for managing a small team will usually follow.

Biologists are often employed initially, particularly at the post-doctoral level, because of their specific expertise. This specialisation may continue and, although it will encourage the development of in-depth expertise, it may lead to over-specialisation, such that difficulty can be experienced in switching from one therapeutic area or research programme to another. This limitation does not apply in new technology areas such as genomics or high-throughput screening where skills are transferable. Chemists, on the other hand, usually move more readily between research programmes since their skills and experience as synthetic and/or medicinal chemists are readily applied in different therapeutic areas.

Career development is usually linked either to leadership of a discipline team or a multidisciplinary project team. In some organisations a separate scientific ladder will exist to allow for the recognition of gifted creative scientists who may not necessarily wish to manage large resources. Undoubtedly, though, promotion to senior positions (department head, project leader, therapeutic area head) will require an established track record as a creative scientist and the ability to lead others and manage resources. Such positions might be attainable within a period of 10 years after joining the industry for outstanding individuals.

Discovery scientists often find attractive opportunities for career advancement within research by moving from one company to another. For example, a move from a large multinational to a smaller company (start-up, biotechnology or single-country institute) will offer the chance to utilise much valued expertise in a wider and more varied role. Increasingly, the flow is no longer one way, since the specialised expertise gained in a biotechnology company is often in demand in the major ethical pharmaceutical companies. Biotechnology companies, on the other hand, value the focus on 'the medicine in the bottle' engendered by the large pharmaceutical companies.

Careers leading on from discovery

For many scientists the opportunity to lead a small team and manage a laboratory, while staying closely in touch with science as a hands-on experimentalist, provides a supremely satisfying career. However, the increasing specialisation and inevitable focus of a research role of this type is often perceived as too narrow for other scientists, particularly in the longer term. It is appropriate, therefore, to consider the various alternative career options outside research for the discovery scientist.

Discovery usually provides excellent training and experience for a career move into other divisions within a pharmaceutical company, especially where the discipline overlap is significant. Thus, various options are available in development, particularly for those who are interested in seeing more tangible results of their work. Some examples include medicinal chemists moving to process research, physical organic chemists to analytical chemistry, biochemists and pharmacologists to clinical research, and chemists or biochemists to drug metabolism and pharmacokinetics. Regulatory affairs also offers a good career move for scientists from all disciplines. Major developments in Europe and moves towards international harmonisation between Europe, the USA and Japan make regulatory affairs a particularly interesting and important area of activity within the development sphere.

Project management is a growing and vital activity at the heart of the development process. Increasingly, companies are appointing professional full-time project managers who have broad experience and knowledge of project management in discovery or development, coupled with good organisational and communication skills.

Alternative opportunities exist outside R&D for the discovery scientist and should be considered seriously as career options. Thus, chemists who are interested in moving away from the bench are often able to move into the legal department as a patent agent. This will require obtaining further qualifications as a chartered patent agent (CPA) and European patent agent (EPA) in order to rise to senior positions. Trademarks are often handled by the same department and give an added dimension to the work.

Increasingly, scientists are finding that successful alternative careers can be pursued in the commercial arena. The usual route has been via an early move into a medical representative position and then promotion up the sales and marketing ladder. However, scientists are finding that business development or licensing can also offer both an alternative career option and pave the way to promotion to other senior positions in marketing and general management.

The Future

Scientific, regulatory and commercial pressures are leading to greater diversity and flexibility in the way research will be conducted in the future. There is also an inexorable process of mergers of pharmaceutical companies to form ever-larger corporations with subsequent 'rationalisation' which inevitably reduces total numbers of projects and employee numbers in research. Some large R&D groups may reduce their in-house staff and budgets but increase alliances with smaller companies, research institutes and universities which will, in turn, expand research opportunities.

Scientists now entering pharmaceutical industry R&D will do so at the sector's most exciting and dynamic time to date. They will, however, require a less risk-averse approach to career planning including the consideration of options outside research.

PART II

CAREERS IN PRE-CLINICAL AND CLINICAL RESEARCH

Careers with the Pharmaceutical Industry, Second edition. Edited by P. D. Stonier.
© 2003 John Wiley & Sons Ltd. ISBN 0 470 84328 4

4

A Career in Clinical Pharmacology

Roger Yates

Astra Zeneca Ltd, Macclesfield, UK

Introduction

Clinical pharmacology is the scientific study of the actions and modes of action of drugs in the human species and the actions and modes of action of human physiology and metabolism on drugs. Any individual with expertise in this area is of enormous potential value and can usefully fill a wide range of roles within the pharmaceutical industry.

This chapter will briefly describe some typical routes to a clinical pharmacology post within the pharmaceutical industry, the various roles the clinical pharmacologist can play in the industry, in approximately the order in which they occur during the various stages of drug development, and the further opportunities which may become open to the appropriately talented individual. The topics of continuing medical education (CME) and re-registration as applicable to clinical pharmacology will be addressed and a brief personal view of the future of clinical pharmacology in the pharmaceutical industry offered.

Qualifications

The ideal industrial clinical pharmacologist should be equally familiar with the worlds of medicine and of science. The first requirement is a medical degree supplemented by an intercalated BSc or BMedSci, ideally in pharmacology, or an equivalent introduction to scientific methodology. Ideally the candidate will have completed two or more years of research and earned an MD or PhD. An individual will enter industry only after completing sufficient clinical work and meeting the requirements for (Medical) General Professional Training. Ideally the individual will

Careers with the Pharmaceutical Industry, Second edition. Edited by P. D. Stonier.
© 2003 John Wiley & Sons Ltd. ISBN 0 470 84328 4

have obtained MRCP or equivalent (anaesthetics is particularly relevant). On this basis, in the UK, many entering industrial clinical pharmacology have joined at the stage in their careers equivalent to the current Specialist Registrar years. Rarely in the UK but more commonly in countries such as Sweden the move into industry is made from a more senior clinical or academic post—sometimes initially on a part-time basis.

Whatever their previous experience, few if any individuals recruited into an industrial clinical pharmacology job already have all the knowledge and skills required. Usually there is much to learn. Each individual will establish his or her existing skills and knowledge as necessary 'on the job'. The areas of expertise required will emerge during the following description of the various roles the clinical pharmacologist can fill. The formal frameworks into which such learning should fit are summarised towards the end of the chapter.

Personal Attributes and Roles in Clinical Pharmacology

The personal characteristics desirable in a physician who is considering a career in clinical pharmacology include curiosity, a desire to understand the patho-physiology of, and modes of drug action in, disease, and the ability to assimilate information from several different disciplines and reduce it to a few key questions which can be answered by focused research. The individual will be questioning and will instinctively think 'laterally'. He or she will need to feel confident in dealing with experts in other disciplines, such as chemists, pre-clinical biologists, pharma-cologists, toxicologists and statisticians, who may not fully appreciate the limitations of clinical research and particularly of testing novel substances in man for the first time.

Research and discovery

The clinical pharmacologist with a strong background in pre-clinical science (and no strong interest in developing clinical expertise) may join the research and discovery function and work alongside a pre-clinical research team. Here the clinical pharmacologist's potential contribution will be to assist in directing and focusing the research so that pre-clinical pharmacological activity can be readily tested in man. This would be a job at an extreme edge of the spectrum of roles for the industrial clinical pharmacologist.

Exploratory clinical pharmacology

The clinical pharmacologist is typically assumed to work somewhere in what is best described as 'exploratory clinical pharmacology'. This basically begins with pure research. It is immediately evident that for potential drugs with a new mode of action there will be no established methodology for detecting, let alone quantifying, that activity in man. It is therefore necessary to develop methodology to detect in man the novel pharmacology demonstrated in pre-clinical tests and predicted to be the basis for a new therapy. Once such methodology has been validated it can be used in a short series of studies, which are traditionally labelled as 'phase I'.

Phase I

This series will begin with a rising single dose tolerance study and at an early stage include a multiple dose tolerance study. In these studies preliminary pharmacokinetic data and perhaps pharmacodynamic data using the newly designed methodology will be generated. Subsequent studies will be designed to define the dose response for the desired pharmacology in man and provide initial data relevant to questions suggested by the available pre-clinical data. The clinical pharmacologist will have a critical role in the decision to initiate investigation in man, the doses to be evaluated, the precautions to be taken, the critical questions to be addressed and the design of the studies. The critical issues will differ from compound to compound and may include concerns around pharmacological efficacy or potency, pharmacokinetics such as extent of absorption or rate of elimination, or safety concerns such as therapeutic ratio with respect to possible adverse effects such as prolongation of QT interval or interaction with the P450 system.

Filling this role requires critical review of the available pre-clinical data so that the studies are safe for the subjects participating in them and, for successful developments, provide adequate data to select the doses to be evaluated in Phase II studies in patients.

The majority of compounds entering phase I, however, do not continue to become marketed products. Often it will be data from an early clinical pharmacology study which signals the unsuitability of a compound for further development; an obvious example being that for an antibiotic a plasma elimination half-life in man of less than three hours is incompatible with once-a-day dosing providing sustained plasma concentrations across the dose interval. In such circumstances the clinical pharmacologist must realise that his/her role is to limit exposure of volunteers and patients to compounds which will never reach the market and save the development budget for use on potentially more useful projects.

Providing data of this kind and pointing out their implications is important to the business—but will not always be popular with any colleagues who may have spent years developing the compound to reach phase I and assumed its development will be successful.

Regulatory clinical pharmacology

As clinical development proceeds the clinical pharmacologist will be the key player in what is best described as 'regulatory clinical pharmacology'—the package of studies necessary to generate the data required for a Marketing Authorisation Application (MAA in Europe) or New Drug Application (NDA in the USA) which will be the basis for much of the data sheet. These will include studies to define the compound's metabolism and pharmacokinetics, to identify any clinically significant difference in the compound's kinetics in special patient groups such as those with hepatic or renal impairment, or the elderly. There will also be studies to identify or address particular issues such as effects of food or absorption, to demonstrate absence of (or identify and perhaps quantify) drug interactions, and to characterise the pharmacokinetics of new formulations or routes of administration as they emerge during drug development. By this stage the compound will be in phase III safety and efficacy trials and the clinical pharmacologist will have a role in defining the schedule of sampling to allow a population pharmacokinetic analysis to supplement small formal pharmacokinetic studies.

Clinical pharmacology and commercial support

The clinical pharmacology contribution to a compound does not end as the compound becomes a licensed product in an increasing number of territories. At this stage of a product's life cycle the clinical pharmacologist is needed to provide 'commercial clinical pharmacology' support. This will comprise studies specifically designed to further define mode or range of action and/or to investigate reports of unexpected drug interactions. These studies may be the foundation of further research and increase the value of a product to both patients and the company. Inevitably such studies will generate publications for market support and may lead to modification of the prescribing information.

Transferable skills of the clinical pharmacologist

In all the phases of drug development the clinical pharmacologist will be a key member, and with enough experience, probably leader or chairman of a multi-disciplinary team definitely including pharmacokineticists, statisticians and data managers and perhaps also relevant biologists, toxicologists and other physicians. Interpersonal skills are important. The clinical pharmacologist must be expert in clinical trial design so that throughout a development essential data can be generated as quickly and cost-effectively as possible whilst providing the highest ethical, clinical and scientific standards for the healthy volunteers and patients who participate in the trials. Not infrequently this will require a careful balancing of the different opinions of other experts contributing to the study design. Good verbal and written communication skills are a considerable asset to the clinical pharmacologist. Data from all well-designed and conducted clinical pharmacology studies should be published or presented at an appropriate medical/scientific meeting.

Coordinating role in phase I clinical research

The majority of these studies for most compounds (the area of commonest exception being oncology) will be conducted in healthy volunteers. The clinical pharmacologist may only be required to contribute to the design and integration of the data from these studies if they are conducted by a contract research organisation (CRO), or in an academic unit. However, if the clinical pharmacologist's employing company has its own in-house clinical pharmacology unit the clinical pharmacologist will, for at least part of his/her career, serve as the clinician responsible for the conduct of the clinical phase of those studies conducted in-house. This role will include responsibility for selection and clinical care of the volunteers in the trials and obtaining ethics approval from the relevant independent research ethics committee.

The foregoing has summarised the clinical pharmacologist's role in design and conduct of individual studies. The clinical pharmacologist will also contribute to ensuring that the total package of studies is optimally designed to meet the needs of optimised drug development; this necessitates providing a sound basis for internal decision-making and then for registration of the product in as many markets as possible.

Regulatory activities

The clinical pharmacologist will be expected to play a major role in generating the clinical pharmacology sections of MAAs (and NDAs) and representing the company in presentations to and other interactions with drug regulatory authorities on clinical pharmacology topics. A typical topic requiring the clinical pharmacologist's input would be relative bioavailability, which can be particularly important in establishing acceptability of data generated with an early 'clinical trial' formulation as relevant to subsequent clinical use of a final 'sales' formulation. More recently using clinical pharmacology to establish the relevance of clinical data obtained in one ethnic group to another may facilitate obtaining marketing approval in a territory, such as Japan, with only a limited clinical trial programme having been conducted in that territory.

Multi-tasking and time management

Most clinical pharmacologists will find, even if they are part of a large team within a large research-based company, that they are required to contribute to several projects simultaneously. This demands real multi-tasking and time management skills. Advantages are varied job content and some protection against becoming too personally committed to any one development, which may come to an unexpected end!

Clinical pharmacology infrastructure

One might expect that there would be consensus on organisational structure for clinical pharmacologists working in the industry. It seems there isn't! Clinical pharmacology can be a single group or department within either of research or development functions. Alternatively there may be separate clinical pharmacology groups within larger organisational units defined by therapeutic area, phase of development or geography. A clinical pharmacology organisation group may be small and consist of only the single discipline or larger and include representatives of related disciplines such as pharmacokinetics, statistics or project management. During a career in industrial clinical pharmacology, even within a single organisation, the individual should expect to work within several of these managerial options.

The role of the individual clinical pharmacologist is not necessarily confined to the relatively narrow specialist input. The appropriately trained and skilled clinical pharmacologist can in addition function as either or both of project and personnel manager with the specialty.

Clinical pharmacology is a discipline from which an individual with the appropriate skills and aptitude can successfully move into any of a range of other functions within the industry. Drug safety assessment function can use both the scientific and clinical expertise of a clinical pharmacologist. On occasion the clinical pharmacologist may be a key member of a team reviewing technical aspects of options for licensing agreements. Whilst there will be a tendency for a clinical pharmacologist to remain within the technical, medical and development functions there is no barrier to transfer into and success in other areas including marketing.

Broader management responsibilities

An individual who has been successful as a people or project manager within clinical pharmacology can successfully become a project or personnel manager with a much wider area of responsibility—one or more research or therapeutic areas, one or more projects or products, or a functional department or site—any of which may be a large part of even a large company.

Career Development

The foregoing has summarised the roles in which the clinical pharmacologist may contribute within the industry as a whole. All these options will be available with a large multinational research-based company. However an individual working within a large company will almost certainly need to change departments, and perhaps locations and even countries, to obtain experience of working in all these areas.

At a particular site within a particular company the options open to the clinical pharmacologist may be restricted geographically and/or to a particular phase of development or a particular therapeutic area or even to a restricted role within the broader constraints. It is not unknown for 'HQ' to send out finalised protocols or other defined pieces of work for completion at a subsidiary site, giving little opportunity for the staff at that site to contribute to the design of the work, or analysis of the resultant data or evaluation of its importance to a wider research or development programme. Similarly, a clinical pharmacologist working within a CRO (particularly a specialised phase I unit) may be restricted to responsibility for conduct of studies without any major contribution to the design or subsequent data analysis or interpretation. Such roles will quickly become frustrating for an ambitious clinical pharmacologist but can provide a couple of years' excellent experience, particularly early in a career.

As in a larger company a clinical pharmacologist in a CRO can progress into management and become the unit director. A career in industrial clinical pharmacology may involve changing companies, perhaps several times, but there are real benefits to be gained from obtaining a broad experience—which can include working and living in more than one country. Some clinical pharmacologists may follow a 'poacher turned game-keeper' career path and transfer, perhaps temporarily, to working within a drug regulatory authority. Such opportunities will be attractive to some individuals, and the opposite to others!

A clinical pharmacologist, particularly one with clinical responsibility for subjects in clinical trials, is well advised to retain some active involvement in clinical practice, such as a clinical assistantship. Many, particularly outside the UK, may divide their time approximately equally between industry and practice in a clinical academic environment. More senior industrial clinical pharmacologists may become involved in work of the Faculty of Pharmaceutical Medicine, the Royal Colleges or other relevant academic institutions. Industrial clinical pharmacologists can and do make valuable contributions to both undergraduate and postgraduate teaching in both science and medicine.

Training and Continuing Education

Like all other physicians within the industry, the clinical pharmacologist will naturally continue his or her medical education by natural growth of experience, by attending specific internal and external training events and medical scientific conferences, and staying abreast of relevant paper and electronic literature. At least in the UK these activities will need to be documented as a basis for revalidation. More specifically in the first four years in industry the clinical pharmacologist will be well advised to study for and pass the exam currently affectionately known as the 'Dip Pharm Med' and then proceed to complete the curriculum for obtaining a Certificate of Completion of Specialist Training and registration as a specialist in pharmaceutical medicine. Clinical pharmacology is a significant part of this curriculum and in future many younger pharmaceutical physicians will work for a time (perhaps six months to two years) in one or more of the clinical pharmacology roles described above.

The Future

Within the industry the clinical pharmacologist has the opportunity and is often required to work with colleagues from almost the entire range of other disciplines represented there. This 'central' position reflects both the importance of clinical pharmacology in product development and the wide range of directions open to clinical pharmacologists as their skills, competences and careers develop. This seems unlikely to change in future although the knowledge and skills required will change in time with advances in clinical science, in medical practice and in processes of delivery of healthcare to the population.

The most obvious areas of predictable change are the consequences of political initiatives designed to maximise healthcare at minimum cost and the advent of new types of therapy derived from ever-increasing knowledge and understanding of the human genome. The design of appropriate pre-clinical and clinical development programmes for 'gene-based' therapies will be very different to those used in the past for 'traditional' drugs. The clinical pharmacologist should be one of those at the forefront of these scientific and medical advances.

It seems likely that clinical pharmacology will remain an essential discipline within the pharmaceutical industry as it continues the research and development of increasingly novel medicines for the first century of the new millennium.

5

Career Opportunities for Physicians in the Pharmaceutical Industry

Bert Spilker

Bert Spilker & Associates, Bethesda, USA

Introduction

The roles of physicians in the pharmaceutical industry are exciting ones but are not generally well understood by most physicians who work outside the industry. Reasons for this relate to a lack of knowledge about specific activities conducted by physicians working within the pharmaceutical industry and a lack of information about the processes and issues involved in drug discovery, development and marketing. Little information about potential careers in this industry is provided in medical schools, and most medical students do not have contact with industry physicians.

This chapter, which describes activities conducted by physicians within the pharmaceutical industry, is organised around a series of questions that physicians outside the industry might ask of physicians working within the industry.

Why do Physicians Join a Pharmaceutical Company?

More physicians are applying to the pharmaceutical industry for positions than ever before, because these careers offer meaningful challenges, and there is increasing competition for research grants and/or positions in patient care and in academia. There is also increased frustration about the administration demands of managed care, the inability to prescribe whichever drugs one wishes, and the pressure to see more patients per hour. The result of this situation is that the quality of physicians

Careers with the Pharmaceutical Industry, Second edition. Edited by P. D. Stonier.
© 2003 John Wiley & Sons Ltd. ISBN 0 470 84328 4

joining the pharmaceutical industry is increasing dramatically, as is the competition among physicians to obtain these positions.

The reasons for which a physician joins a pharmaceutical company are identical to the reasons for which a physician makes any career decision. Major ones include that the position seems challenging, offers opportunities for developing a meaningful career, does not have onerous administrative responsibilities, provides generally adequate financial security, and provides other benefits. These factors provide physicians and their families with the basis for a positive quality of life.

Numerous reasons for choosing a career within the pharmaceutical industry, as compared with other careers, relate to specific attributes of the position. These reasons often include the sense of personal satisfaction that evolves from participating in the development of important new drugs, and advancing public health. These drugs offer increased benefits to patients in terms of enhanced survival, decreased symptoms or risk factors, improved quality of life and a more productive life.

Another reason is that many physicians have opportunities to be managers. Even for physicians who have little interest in management, administrative support and technical services they usually have support available to help them perform their job efficiently. This allows physicians to focus more of their attention on activities that require medical training. Other reasons for physicians to choose a pharmaceutical career are opportunities to attend medical and scientific meetings, to function as a member of a team in planning and implementing clinical studies, to interpret data, and to trouble-shoot and solve health-related issues that arise.

Both clinical practice and academic life are viewed in a very positive way by the majority of physicians working in those areas. However, some individuals join the pharmaceutical industry because of negative aspects (in their view) of responsibilities and the atmosphere in these or other careers. Some of the negative responsibilities might include long and often irregular hours on call, direct interactions with patients, teaching and preparing grant proposals. Aspects of the negative atmosphere might relate to high malpractice insurance premiums, financial constraints on research, limited time available for research, or some responsibilities that are viewed in a negative light.

For some industry physicians, a great proportion of their time is spent addressing clinical and scientific challenges. Clinical and scientific responsibilities include designing new studies, writing protocols, initiating and monitoring studies, interpreting data, preparing medical reports, extrapolating results, developing a clinical strategy to bring a new drug or new indication forward, and directing co-workers to help in these activities. These and many other activities will be discussed in more detail.

Administrative responsibilities may or may not differ for physicians within a pharmaceutical company as compared with physicians in other positions in academia. At some companies there may be specialists to help physicians with administrative tasks or to perform them (e.g. write final medical reports based on the physician's evaluation).

Individuals in numerous departments are available to help physicians perform their jobs more efficiently, thus enabling physicians to spend a greater proportion of their time on activities that require medical training.

What do Physicians do in a Pharmaceutical Company?

Medical departments are the primary area in which physicians work. Companies organise medical departments in a variety of ways, and few positions exist that are standard among all companies. Positions with the same job title often vary from being highly focused to extremely broad. Focused positions may consist of a single role (e.g. set up clinical studies on drug A; consult on clinical studies in therapeutic area B). Broad positions usually consist of multiple roles, possibly involving multiple drugs. The majority of physicians in industry are closer to the multiple-role end of the spectrum, but for each position it depends to a large extent on the management, the personality of the physician, and whether they welcome or resist additional assignments and responsibilities. The nature and structure of the company also plays a role, since some companies are more likely than others to assign multiple responsibilities to physicians. Common types of roles, activities, interactions and collaborations are described later.

Roles

A number of roles assigned to physicians require medical training, while other roles require scientific training. Physicians are generally challenged most by and enjoy best those roles for which their training and experience have prepared them. Although a large number of roles are mentioned, physicians do not participate in all of them and most companies provide staff to help physicians conduct other roles.

The most common role of physicians in industry is to plan, initiate and monitor clinical studies (Spilker, 1991). After clinical studies are complete, some physicians edit data and supervise data processing. The next major step is to interpret the data. This process is either carried out directly (or is reviewed) by physicians.

An industry physician is also a consultant within their company. Instead of conducting the activities mentioned above themselves, physicians often advise others on the medical perspective that must be considered on various points.

The consultant's role may be informal or it may be the central focus and formal role assigned by the company. In this situation the physician might advise non-physicians in the same or a different therapeutic area, or may advise people in a different discipline, for example, marketing.

Many physicians are managers who direct people, resources and activities. They are part of the line management, that is vertical hierarchy of a company. Another aspect of a company's management refers to the matrix system, or horizontal organisation, in which each drug's development effort is referred to as a project. In a matrix management role, some physicians function as project leaders (Spilker, 1994). They are in charge of efforts to guide a drug's development from the pre-clinical stage to the stage of submitting one or more regulatory applications. To do this, they head a team of approximately six to 20 people from various research, medical, marketing and other departments that cuts across the organisation.

A physician also may collaborate with marketing staff to advise on design of appropriate market research studies, review advertising copy for appropriateness of medical content, and seek marketing product managers' views in designing marketing-orientated clinical studies or quality-of-life studies.

A number of the roles described in this section are listed in Table 5.1. Four categories are used in the table to list specific roles, for ease of presentation.

Interactions

Collaborations with statisticians are important to virtually all pharmaceutical physicians, and developing a good relationship with a competent statistician is an important goal for industry clinicians. Statisticians give advice on the number of patients required for a clinical study, provide randomisation schedules for clinical studies, review clinical study protocols for content, determine which statistical analyses will be applied to study results, review the interpretation of data, and help write combined statistical and medical reports. Nonetheless, it is the clinician's responsibility to determine the clinical importance of the statistical findings.

Interactions with personnel working in drug regulatory affairs occur frequently. Companies generally use their drug regulatory affairs department as a funnel to enable written and verbal interactions from many groups within the company to present a common front to national regulatory agencies. All correspondence is usually officially transmitted through this group. Each physician who interacts with a regulatory agency is usually briefed and may be rehearsed by regulatory personnel prior to these meetings. Rehearsals are held and anticipated questions discussed. If the physician is responsible for an investigational or marketed drug that has many regulatory issues associated with it, then a significant portion of his or her time may involve meetings with the regulatory agency and with other sections of the company.

Depending on the company, there may be a number of physicians within the regulatory affairs department. Even drugs with few regulatory issues involve various meetings, the preparation of applications, plus a number of data reviews (for example, at end of phase II meetings). A knowledge of pharmaceutical regulations is generally acquired on the job, rather than in a training programme taken before joining the industry. Some individuals within a company develop

Table 5.1 Selected roles of physicians in the pharmaceutical industry

Clinical research roles and functions
- Identify, meet, interview and persuade clinicians outside the company to conduct clinical trials. Many of these clinicians are the most well-known experts in their field
- Negotiate details of the protocol and budget with clinical investigators
- Plan and write the clinical trial protocol
- Lead round-table discussions with clinical investigators, monitors and consultants
- Initiate clinical trials
- Monitor clinical trials
- Maintain contact with clinical investigators and deal with any problems or issues that arise
- Assess adverse reactions that arise during clinical trials and discuss possible treatments with clinical investigators
- Edit data collection forms
- Interpret data obtained in clinical trials
- Extrapolate data to new situations and develop new clinical hypotheses to test
- Create clinical strategies for developing investigational drugs to the point of market approval
- Create clinical strategies for post-marketing surveillance studies and new indications of marketed drugs
- Collaborate with the medical team developing the drug
- Collaborate with the company's project team developing the drug
- Liaise with professionals in other divisions of the company as required
- Order bulk drug and clinical trial drug supplies
- Write periodic reports of project activities and other functions
- Interact with other physicians, statisticians, pre-clinical scientists, information specialists, computer specialists and many others on an ongoing basis
- Approve the supply of drug samples to outside academicians who wish to conduct animal studies. Approve the supply of formulated drug to outside clinicians who wish to conduct human studies
- Critique potential licensing opportunities

Marketing support roles and functions
- Review marketing advertisements and promotional materials
- Telephone healthcare professionals to discuss and answer their questions

Professional development and educational activities
- Teach university students
- Conduct research or collaborate in research projects at universities
- Lecture to different groups of company representatives
- Discuss the process of drug development with civic groups
- Attend seminars, courses and meetings within and outside the company. Present information when relevant
- Read medical literature to maintain current awareness and knowledge
- Advise company lawyers, marketers and non-medical scientists on medical perspectives
- Improve expertise in one's specific area
- Consult with other physicians

Regulatory activities
- Generate regulatory submissions through written reports, summaries or evaluations
- Report serious adverse reactions and deaths to regulatory authorities as prescribed by regulations or to regulatory personnel within the company
- Participate at meetings with regulatory authorities

interest and knowledge in regulations and transfer to the regulatory affairs department.

Physicians who head projects usually have a project coordinator or planner assigned to assist them. This individual provides many important services, such as planning the overall schedule and milestone dates for the group to achieve. This person also monitors the work being conducted in all departments to assess how well project members are adhering to their schedules. The coordinator acts to facilitate agreements and settle issues between departments, but does not get involved in issues within departments. This person often raises red flags for the project leader or others to address. Physicians may fulfil most or all of the support roles themselves in small or start-up companies. Interactions with other physicians occur not only within a company, but at professional meetings, investigator meetings and at professional society and professional association meetings of many types. These allow for professional and career growth for any motivated physician.

The scope of a physician's responsibilities is usually limited to either national or international activities. This factor may depend on the ownership of the company. It also depends on the organisational structure of the medical department. For instance, US-based pharmaceutical companies may have separate medical groups to conduct domestic and foreign studies. A number of companies are organised so that different medical groups conduct investigational drug studies and marketing-orientated studies. The latter group of physicians may report to either marketing or medical division managers.

What are the Other Areas in which Physicians Work?

Areas in which physicians work that are outside the formal medical department investigating new drugs are mentioned briefly to provide a broad view of other areas in which many physicians work.

Drug regulatory affairs. Develops regulatory strategies, assembles regulatory applications and interacts with regulatory agencies via letters and at meetings. Serves as an interface for others within the company who interact with regulatory agencies.

Drug information services. Interacts with health professionals to provide information on the company's drugs regarding adverse reactions, treatment of overdose, various publications or other topics.

Epidemiology. Assembles adverse reaction information on the company's drugs. Designs, conducts and evaluates post-marketing surveillance and other studies. May interact directly with regulatory agencies.

Statistics and data processing. Involves numerous steps of editing data, entering them into computers, ensuring their quality, tabulating them, analysing them and preparing reports of the results. Statisticians maintain frequent interactions with clinicians and regulatory agencies.

Pre-clinical sciences. Some physicians join pre-clinical departments (e.g. pharma-cology, microbiology, biochemistry, molecular biology) and conduct research relating to new drug discovery.

Medical services. This is a general term for a group that usually has a mixture of medical, marketing and administrative tasks. Its profile usually differs in each company, and may include arranging courses or programmes for physician training (e.g. Continuing Medical Education). Physicians who prefer administrative, marketing and promotional activities may enjoy a position in this type of department.

Project coordination. This group oversees the project system and the matrix arm of the investigational projects in a company's portfolio. Roles combine managerial and administrative responsibilities with scientific input through a wide variety of activities.

Other areas. These include patents, licensing, computers, education and training, commercial liaison and financial controller functions within the medical or R&D division. In addition, there are some physicians who become involved in pre-clinical sciences (e.g. pharmacology, biochemistry, toxicology) but these areas are not discussed in this chapter.

What are the Challenges and Opportunities for Advancement?

Challenges come both from without and within an individual. Those from outside the person are provided primarily by the company. Other external opportunities for challenges include committee assignments for trade associations, professional societies associated with the pharmaceutical industry, professional societies independent of the industry, hospital work, research activities or teaching assign-ments at a medical school. Challenges from within individuals motivate them to work hard and achieve their goals. Challenges to excel are the same in individuals who join the pharmaceutical industry as in those based in academia or clinical practice.

Most medium and large pharmaceutical companies have a wide variety of positions that are available to experienced physicians who have demonstrated managerial and technical skills within the industry. These positions are often described as a 'dual ladder'. This refers to the fact that advancement may progress along either an administrative/management or a clinical/scientific tract. Enlightened companies provide commensurate benefits to scientists and clinicians who become more experienced and interested in their assigned area but do not wish to give up their professional activities to take on purely administrative positions. Keeping creative scientists working in the laboratories and keeping productive clinicians working on developing drugs often provides greater benefits to a company than promoting these individuals outside their area of competence. Not all highly successful clinicians and scientists are competent and successful managers.

Specific positions that physicians may fill within the industry include:

- Assistant medical director;
- Associate medical director;
- Medical director;
- Medical division director;
- Drug information services director;
- Regulatory affairs director (plus assistant and associate directors);
- Director of development;
- Research and development director;
- Project coordination director.

Exact titles often vary among companies and the relative rank, level and responsibilities are more important in judging a position than is the title. For example, a company may have two or three vice-presidents within R&D, whereas another company of equal size may have 10–15 vice-presidents in the same area. Physicians with special interests in other areas, for example marketing or statistics, may seek and find positions in those areas. Also, depending on the company, numerous hybrid positions either exist or may be created to provide opportunities for physicians to develop their careers. The nature and responsibilities of these and other positions are described in more detail by Sampson (1984). Staff within medical departments may desire or be asked to focus their activities on one phase (or more) of clinical development.

What Types of Pharmaceutical Companies Exist?

This chapter primarily describes research-based companies that are attempting to discover new drugs of medical benefit to humans. For example, there are 40–60 such companies in the USA depending on how categories are defined and how companies are classified. Many small companies that are attempting to invent new drugs, particularly biotechnology companies, are not included in this category. A few biotechnology, medical device, diagnostic or genetic-orientated companies hire physicians to help with clinical development if they have products in (or near) the clinical research stage. On the other hand, many biotechnology companies either do not have drugs in clinical trials or they may have joint development or licensing arrangements with larger R&D companies. A few companies develop and then market drugs but do not seek to discover drugs. These companies also hire physicians. Companies that produce only generic drugs rarely hire physicians.

What Characteristics do Pharmaceutical Companies Seek in Physicians?

It is extremely beneficial, though not essential, for all physicians to have a period of clinical experience, after clinical training is complete, prior to joining a company. In the UK, for example, to undertake the Diploma in Pharmaceutical Medicine, to join the Higher Medical Training programme in the specialty of pharmaceutical medicine, or to apply for membership of the Faculty of Pharmaceutical Medicine a period of at least two years' post-registration general medical training is required.

A physician who joins a pharmaceutical company may well be trained and qualified (board certified) in the therapeutic area in which he or she will work. This usually involves internal medicine or one of its subspecialties, or another specialty (e.g. psychiatry, neurology, anaesthetics, ophthalmology, paediatrics), or general practice. Experience as a clinical investigator is extremely beneficial and worthwhile. Clinical pharmacology training and postdoctoral positions provide a good training for entering the industry. Physicians with training in a number of areas such as nuclear medicine or radiology may find that career opportunities are greater with diagnostic or medical device companies. On the other hand, pharmaceutical companies also hire many young physicians who are not specialists, but who have the personality to switch between fields, and are flexible in their approach. Therefore both medical specialists and generalists are desirable employees of a pharmaceutical company.

Two important characteristics that a company seeks in new physicians are a scientific orientation and the ability to work as a team player. Scientific ability is extremely important for physicians in industry because it is needed to design state-of-the-art clinical studies, develop clinical strategies, interpret data fully, prepare sound articles for publication, and develop drugs effectively and efficiently. A number of years ago most physicians who entered industry came from general practice. They generally had little or no training or experience in the science of medicine and were not orientated towards thinking as a scientist. Over the last 10–20 years there has been a steady increase in the number of physicians entering industry who have strong scientific backgrounds. In several cases, physicians have also earned PhD or MD degrees prior to joining the industry.

Being a team player means that one operates as part of a group and not as an independent star. Teamwork is a comforting feeling to most people, because everyone on the team shares important goals and wants their project to succeed. The advantages for the physician using this approach are that ideas are constantly being discussed and debated among several people, and it is hopeful that good ideas and approaches become better ideas and approaches. On the other hand, the team approach may not favour the development of novel or risky ideas. Teams can be a conservative force, especially if a consensus is needed to make decisions. Success is often defined as completing assignments on time and answering questions posed. Therefore, the team is judged on its ability to meet its goals, not on the outcome. Goals for a new drug should be to determine if it works, not to show that it works. Therefore, even if a new drug is found to be inactive or if unacceptable animal or human toxicity is found, the team would be judged successful if they determined that result rapidly and efficiently. Resources scheduled for use by the terminated drug project would become available for other projects. This enables the new projects receiving resources to move ahead more rapidly.

What Types of Physicians should not Consider Careers in the Pharmaceutical Industry?

Certain physicians, because of interests or temperament, probably should not seek a career in the pharmaceutical industry. The major characteristic that would raise a warning signal about entering the industry would be whether the physician enjoys clinical practice above all other professional activities. Other characteristics of those who would probably be unhappy in industry include wanting to be one's own boss, not particularly enjoying working with others on a collaborative team, or finding it difficult to be directed by non-physicians. Physicians who are not research oriented or do not enjoy research should not consider positions in clinical research, as scientific approaches to clinical research are a critical component of this position. Also, some physicians may have misgivings about ethical standards in industry. While physicians in industry almost entirely believe that ethical standards do not have to be compromised, anyone with concerns should discuss this matter openly with those in industry prior to reaching a decision to apply for a position.

Finally, some individuals do not like the idea that marketing considerations sometimes force compromises of clinical positions or even overrule clinical considerations. For example, a physician may believe it medically relevant and useful to test one of the company's drugs in a new indication, but marketing groups may state that the eventual commercial return would be too small to justify the proposed clinical studies. Some companies are more willing to test new drugs in less commercially attractive disease areas than others. Nonetheless, a physician who is unable to accept the commercial influence on drug development decisions should carefully consider whether a career in industry represents the most appropriate choice.

Conclusion

More and more physicians are finding that a career in the pharmaceutical industry is scientifically challenging, intellectually stimulating, and provides opportunities for personal and professional development that are outstanding. The wide variety of positions offers research, clinical, managerial and other focuses that are attracting an increasing number of physicians to the pharmaceutical industry.

References

Sampson, M. (1984) Career opportunities in industrial clinical research, in *The Clinical Research Process in the Pharmaceutical Industry* (ed. G. Matoren), Marcel Dekker, New York.

Spilker, B. (1991) *Guide to Clinical Trials*, Raven Press, New York.

Spilker, B. (1994) *Multinational Pharmaceutical Companies: Principles and Practices*, 2nd edn, Raven Press, New York.

6

The Clinical Research Associate

Gareth Hayes

nrg pathway, Cumbria, UK

Introduction

In the organisation, implementation, conduct and completion of clinical trials on medicines sponsored by the pharmaceutical industry, many people would agree that the Clinical Research Associate (CRA) is the person who wants to have a finger in every pie. This is not necessarily true, as the role has changed significantly over the last 10 years. They certainly have to be someone prepared to be a lynchpin, a major cog and binding ribbon with a degree of arrogance to want to be in the middle of things.

The role may have changed with the greater development of the 'clinical team' but the CRA still has to be the one who knows what is going on at every point during the clinical trial process. From protocol development to relationships with investigators, nurses and pharmacists, and a transferable skill of being a completer/finisher (i.e. not running away until the final statistical and clinical reports are complete), the CRA must understand and react to the internal politics and demands of a driven pharmaceutical company, or contract research organisation (CRO) which undertakes the clinical trial project on behalf of the sponsoring company.

Right from the start it is worthy of mention that it can be a stressful role with time pressures competing against standards of quality, but a role that can be immensely satisfying and rewarding.

Background

It could be true that the first CRA in the late 1960s was the first clinical scientist (and note I don't say physician) without a white coat. Following the typical structure of Introduction, Methods, Results and Conclusions we must not forget the scientific basis to which the CRA belongs.

Careers with the Pharmaceutical Industry, Second edition. Edited by P. D. Stonier.
© 2003 John Wiley & Sons Ltd. ISBN 0 470 84328 4

Throughout the 1970s the role of the CRA evolved alongside the growth of the company medical department. Books such as *Clinical Research For All* (Maxwell, 1973), with aligned training courses, meant that clinical research was no longer entirely within the domain of the physician.

At this time the industry formed the Association for Clinical Research in the Pharmaceutical Industry (ACRPI), primarily for CRAs alone, as the physicians had their own network of professional bodies. Originally numbering about 20 members this body has now grown to around 5000 members chiefly in the UK and mainland Europe. Through formal recognition of its value to education and quality, it has changed its name to the Institute of Clinical Research. The Institute has spread its wings in terms of membership too and while the majority still retain the function of a CRA (Smith and Tanner, 2001), other key research professionals are members. Subscription to the Institute is very reasonable and strongly advised.

In parallel to the Institute of Clinical Research, the USA began a similar body over 20 years ago and now the Association of Clinical Research Professionals (ACRP) has grown to have over 15 000 members. Whilst their emphasis is clearly with a state-side slant it should not be ignored by those seeking global options.

The CRA acronym itself is probably one of the most common in the industry yet it doesn't appear in many, if any, of the numerous clinical research dictionaries supporting research and development. We hear of GCP, we hear of ICH, we hear of SOPs and to the new graduates these in themselves are still new (but not for long!), but not of CRA. Winslade (1996) provides an excellent guide to the role and the adjacent roles (but practically the same) of CRE and CRS where E is Executive and S is Scientist. He even refers to Clinical Research Co-ordinator (but with no acronym) as a similar role. Gradually over time the title of CRA has evolved into the term Monitor or Site Monitor and not without some controversy. It may be obvious to have changed the title to Clinical Research Monitor but the acronym CRM already belongs to Clinical Research Manager! It is interesting to note that Winslade's dictionary refers to the non-acronymised Clinical Research Assistant as someone who may be called a Monitor. Monitor may be a more accurate term in relation to what an 'on the road' CRA actually does today with regard to their obser-vatory and vigilant role in looking at protocols, case record forms, data listings and reports, but it does not really cover the interpersonal skills and role of 'major cog' that are needed to be a successful CRA.

Whether CRA or Monitor there is certainly a growing trend for the CRA to be field-based and someone who works from home. This in many cases is a career benefit but may limit options for promotion that would typically involve a need to be office-based.

Job Description

It is in this description that we see that the role of a CRA can extend far beyond Site Monitor. Whilst numerically in terms of need for a rapid and effective conduct of the active phase of a clinical trial the Site Monitor function may be the commonest role, there are many other facets and features available in a CRA's job description. In some companies, particularly smaller pharmaceutical companies, the CRA will find him or herself doing all these functions. In larger companies the role may be limited to only one task, on only one study, at only one study site. It is important to keep your mind open to the variety of tasks undertaken and as your career develops to keep a record (via your CV) of your achievements under each category.

The Institute of Clinical Research (ICR, 2002) has produced a short booklet outlining CRA tasks, *To be a CRA*, and their summary list is an excellent overview of what the CRA can do within the conduct of a trial:

- Steering committee organisation and attendance/presentation at meetings;
- Protocol and case record form (CRF) development;
- Supervision and/or distribution of study supplies, including study drugs;
- Co-ordination of ethics committee and regulatory authority applications and approvals;
- Investigator identification and selection;
- Investigator meeting arrangement and presentation;
- Pre-study procedures including collation of necessary documentation;
- Initiation, monitoring and close-out of study centres;
- Archiving of study documentation and correspondence;
- Preparation of the final report.

All of these tasks can be developed to a greater or lesser extent depending on the nature of the project and the type of company running the study. For example, there can be a great deal of thought and effort required in putting together a successful ethics committee application and the writing of an understandable and appropriate subject consent form and information leaflet must not be underestimated.

Another good example involves preparation of the final report which can include a great deal of team effort with work alongside data management and statistical personnel or it may simply be a function that is taken on by experienced medical writers. The Site Monitor role is only really seen in 'initiation to close-out' above and for a more in-depth consideration of this task Illingworth (2001) is highly recommended. The tasks of a Monitor are qualified even further by the ICH Harmonised Tripartite Guideline of Good Clinical Practice (ICH, 1996) and European Clinical Trials Directive (EC, 2001) which illustrate what must be done to complement regulatory and legislative requirements.

Education and Qualifications

The same ICH Guidelines mentioned above give direction to the selection and qualification of Monitors: 'Monitors should be appropriately trained, and should have the scientific and/or clinical knowledge needed to monitor the trial adequately' which actually opens the door to people with a variety of disciplines and a wider level of education being able to enter the role. As described in the last section, the variability of tasks allows the open-minded manager to appoint the most suitable character for specific CRA positions knowing what needs to be done when, and by whom. That said, it is true that the most typical CRA will come with a scientific graduation from HND through BSc, MSc and/or PhD or nursing qualifications.

As other industry roles develop, for example the Clinical Trials Administrator (CTA), a stepping stone into a CRA role may be provided. However it is usual that companies will ask such applicants to take on further education to support their new ambitions. A supportive company may sponsor such education and allow it to continue as the individual 'dives' straight into the CRA role. In this situation it is highly likely that a special contract will be imposed between company and CRA and the CRA should be warned of the additional stresses and commitment this may involve.

The type of scientific qualification may be key to the CRA work available. For example, a graduate in microbiology may find opportunities to work for a company specialising in antibiotic studies. However, personality traits are important and the ability to show competence at a graduate level may be all that is needed. There are CRAs with geography degrees, so the positive aspect of the CRA role is that the keen, determined, ambitious individual has an opportunity to become a CRA if illustrating the right competency base.

Knowledge Base, Skills, Competencies

It is possible to have limited rounded pharmaceutical knowledge if assigned a specific single task as a CRA in for example a large multinational multicentre clinical trial. All one needs to know is the protocol, the CRF and perhaps an idea of timelines to work towards. Including of course a basic knowledge of Good Clinical Practice (GCP). This attitude would be unwise and would do you no favours in career development. In addition to basic study details it is advisable to obtain knowledge about the development of the product (and comparator if used); this includes the research programme to date, usually taken from the investigator's brochure, and plans for the future. Aligned to this is an understanding of the therapeutic area under research. You do not have to be an expert and certainly should not be expected nor try to illustrate a greater understanding than the investigator actually treating the patients. Be expected to be trained on both product and therapy by the company running the trial. If this is not done, demand it!

A broad knowledge of the company's history and range of products is also wise. Apart from a basic feeling of belonging and instinctive drive to succeed on behalf of yourself and the company, you can be made to look foolish if an enquiring doctor, pharmacist or anyone from the site staff repeatedly asks questions to which the answer is 'I don't know'. It also makes good sense to have a sound knowledge of the pharmaceutical industry itself. It goes without saying that by reading this book you are already collecting an advantage point. Thinking slightly out of the box by reading related publications will also benefit the ambitious CRA. Books for data management personnel (Rondel *et al.*, 1993), investigators (Bohaychuk and Ball, 1993) and/or pharmacists (Hutchinson, 1999) are good starting points.

Skills are important and something that can be brought to the job or learnt en route. Even as part of a team the CRA has to be highly self-motivated with strong organisational abilities for multi-tasking. Everyone has different interpersonal skills as they define their own individual characteristics and whilst you must have the ability to work with and motivate others, it is important to try and retain some individuality and not become a 'clone CRA'. Your individuality may be key to efficient study set-up, successful patient recruitment and/or rapid data analysis. Essential interpersonal skills include diplomacy, negotiation, problem solving and at the top of the pile, presentation skills. The latter will be used throughout the study from in-house meetings to one-on-one interactions with (difficult) clinicians.

Many companies will provide a list of competencies essential for the CRA role and essential for development of the ambitious. If not, it is advisable to make a list and track your own to add weight to your CV and proof that goals have been met. Listed competencies will naturally include the knowledge and skills mentioned above, but should also list in detail tasks performed. These tasks can often be linked to Standard Operating Procedures (SOPs) and as such these make suitable reference points. For example, once a site initiation has been performed (and performed competently) this can be recorded and cross-referenced to the relevant SOP. The CRA manager can even, and it is recommended that they should, sign or initial the record to confirm achievement of the activity.

In this manner a competency list can be built up over time illustrating experience. This system works for both the CRA and the company. The CRA puts himself in a greater bargaining position for career advancement (either in or out of the company) or demands for modification of a role, for example, a demand to do some phase IV work if this has not been part of his/her normal work portfolio. The company can see that proper methods are being employed to develop staff and provide evidence to outside bodies (auditors, inspectors) that study conduct is of a high standard. It will also highlight problem areas and offer an opportunity for rapid resolution.

Interactions

As the central cog there is no doubting that the CRA can have the most interactions to contend with during the conduct of a clinical trial. The clinical team or study team representing the sponsor company can involve anything from three or four personnel to up to 20 and the CRA must be coherent with all of them. Other roles are discussed in this book in more detail, but the CRA must be aware of the demands these roles take on and how best co-operation can be guaranteed. Key team players must be the clinical trial administrator, the clinical trial supplies pharmacist, the data management team (analyst, programmer, co-ordinator), the statistician, the medical writer and probably most importantly the peer group of CRAs either working on the study or, with careful management, those not working on the study. Much can be learnt from a cohesive team of CRAs where gold nuggets can be shared and problems solved so that wheels are not reinvented. Other internal relationships will include CRM, Project Management, Product Managers in Marketing and the Medical Director. If given budgetary control the CRA will also have to liaise with the finance department. If given man management responsibilities, a link to the human resources unit is also necessary.

If involved in a multinational study, the CRA needs to feel part of the international team of Monitors as well as the local operation. Knowledge of cultural discipline becomes essential as the relationships between different company subsidiaries may force a degree of competition, resentment and unnecessary dispute. It is important to recognise differences and make competition healthy.

The CRA should also consider themselves part of the on-site team, at the very least in their own minds. This will include the principal investigator, the sub- or co-investigators, the nursing staff (usually recognised as the Study Site Co-ordinator or SSC), the pharmacist responsible for clinical trials, personnel in other units such as X-ray and laboratory. This is all based on a single-site scenario. The CRA has to be the linking team member across investigators and key site personnel when the study is multicentre. If all of these teams work well together and across teams, it makes the CRA role very rewarding. This may be rare however and the CRA will find themselves in the 'thick of it'. This is why interpersonal and problem solving skills are so important.

Personality Attributes

This has already been highlighted as something that can make or break a successful CRA. The ability to get on with people of all disciplines and creeds is important, but strength of character is equally essential. A tough skin and an ability to stand your ground are good virtues. Leaving a problem for someone else to resolve will not win you any friends nor help the progress of the study. It is sure to have been mentioned elsewhere in this book, but is worthy of repeat: if you can't meet face to face, use the telephone. This applies to all the teams mentioned previously, locally, internationally and on-site. Remember, smile when you use the telephone, people on the other end can 'hear' your smile.

Versatility or flexibility has to be expected, as awareness of sudden reorganisation is common in industry. It will have been highlighted elsewhere in this book but the attitude of proactivity will reap greater rewards than that of straightforward reactivity.

Training

Training has at long last been recognised as one of the more important aspects of an individual's career. Much of it still has to be self-driven, but the good companies (whether direct pharmaceutical or contract research organisation) now have solid training programmes written into their company policies. This can be through the medical or clinical departments themselves where training is linked to roll-out of SOPs and aforementioned competencies, or from human resource units for the softer skills relating to interpersonal needs.

Many companies will have a ready-made induction programme ready for new starters of all experiences. You may find yourself on two induction programmes, one for company matters deriving from human resources (products, company history, etc.) and one for clinical matters from the medical department (trial conduct, GCP, SOPs, etc.). However, you may find yourself on no induction programme and be out doing the job on day one.

The CRA should spread their wings regarding training options and sources. The company will provide a programme to satisfy many needs but may be limited in others. Due consideration should be given to the expectations to be gained from a particular training course or event. The Institute of Clinical Research offers a fine prospectus specifically aimed at the development of the CRA. For example, Advanced Monitoring Skills, First Steps To Management. Even so, one should look closely at all options available from the smaller independent consultancies, e.g. Calcis Consultants, NRG (Training) Consultants, to the larger organisations, e.g. Rostrum Training, Health Care Education.

On the job training is often a quick way to gain experience and is often unavoidable if not desirable. A good CRM will support the novice CRA. Many companies offer a sponsor or mentor system to help bring new CRAs up to speed rapidly and efficiently. It takes a great deal of hard work to do this well. It is worthwhile to force a comparison to the sales force team at this point. A Regional Sales Manager only knows how his team is performing by watching them in action. This should be the case with the CRM/CRA relationship, but so often the budget and project management excuses prevent this happening on a regular and consistent basis. The CRA may be reluctant to have their CRM watch them at work, but as a solid career move to prove ambition and to 'know where you are' it is worthwhile to ask for an accompanied visit if they are not happening.

Continuing Education

A number of universities and academic institutions now offer the opportunity for further education to HND, Degree or Master's level. It is not compulsory at all companies, some offer it along with sponsorship. Others offer nothing. Currently Cardiff, Guildford and Liverpool offer courses. In years to come there are sure to be more places setting up programmes via their specialist schools related to medicine or pharmacy as the demand for CRAs being the Qualified Person (QP) of study conduct becomes more essential as legislative control sets in.

The Institute of Clinical Research has and is working on accreditation schemes which will naturally evolve over time. A set programme of values and competencies will make the role of the CRA easier to define and measure (Lyness, 2001).

Career Development and Opportunities

As mentioned before each and every company will give the CRA a different job title (Smith and Tanner, 2001) and it is important to recognise the CRA specifically as a role, even if the role also varies from company to company. Most companies will offer a scale of promotion opportunities within the CRA role from management of a single study site, through multiple sites, multiple studies to man management. Job titles, salaries and benefits will (usually) change accordingly.

The 'role and responsibility' document is key and can be used alongside regular appraisals and aforementioned competency records to challenge and push for a rise up the ladder. The usual highest goal to be achieved would be Clinical Research Manager which may be more than just managing a large team of CRAs but also the invaluable family of secretaries, administrators and other support staff. As with CRA the role of CRM will vary from company to company. In some it may lean totally towards man management, in others the leaning may involve less personnel issues and focus more on the product development programme and the studies themselves. This is closer in function to project management and is a route taken by many who perhaps want a challenge with greater risks and accountability.

The problems of being field-based and deserving career development have been touched on before. It is in the company's best interest to make sure that a career development programme exists for those who need to and are willing to remain in the field. The parallels with the sales force structure are becoming more and more apparent as the number of CRAs based at home increases.

Other routine opportunities for the career minded CRA are sideways steps or moves into functions that can take value from experience gained as a CRA. Opportunities lie in regulatory, information, drug safety and medical writing. Probably the most common move onto a different ladder lies in quality assurance and/or training.

Whether remaining a CRA or changing role one has to find the right job at the right time. A number of recruitment agencies and specialist contract research organisations (see Useful Websites for examples) will be able to help, but the self-driven CRA will make use of the numerous journal advertisements. The Institute of Clinical Research's journal *Clinical Research focus* (*CRfocus*) is issued eight times a year and along with ACRP's *The Monitor* (issued quarterly) should be the starting place for prospective opportunities. The weekly *New Scientist* features jobs across and out of the industry and often features articles specifically aimed at pharmaceuticals (New Scientist, 2001).

The Association for the British Pharmaceutical Industry (ABPI) offers advice on education and career pathways. Like the Institute of Clinical Research it has an excellent website and also very useful links pages.

Challenges and Opportunities for Career Advancement

The number of CRAs 'going independent' and becoming freelance or self-employed has complemented the growing number of field-based CRAs. The benefits of freedom of choice and perhaps, financial reward are challenged by insecurity and other pitfalls such as unsatisfied training needs (Glenny and Mullinger, 1998).

CRAs seeking a change of direction but wishing to remain in the industry may seek opportunities in sales and marketing or marketing research. The common structures and knowledge base allow a mutual exchange if desired. Other options may lie in more specific functions such as in clinical pharmacology (phase I) units or in departments of health economics. In all these cases one shouldn't be expected to start at the bottom, particularly if the competency record is appropriate and man or project management has been previously pursued.

New challenges to the industry appear all the time and in recent years we have seen expansion in areas such as medical devices and genetic research. The latter is certainly one to watch, as medical departments will be requiring experts to develop an understanding of the application of genetic and genomic research in relation to clinical research.

Leaving the industry doesn't necessarily mean leaving the discipline or experience gained. In the UK the National Health Service is continually evolving and creating new research posts as academia and industry work closer together. The same is true across Europe and throughout the world.

The Future

The CRA role provides one of the most fascinating and stimulating jobs in industry with something different every day (and long days too), the opportunity to travel the world, to meet a vast array of people working in different cultures and different therapeutic areas, to gain a feeling of giving something most concrete for the benefit of patients and healthcare in general.

Years ago in the UK there may have been some 20–30 CRAs. Today this figure approaches 4000, with some 30 000 CRAs worldwide. The necessity for legislative control to achieve safe, more efficacious products may mean greater headcounts (against the odds!) in medical and clinical teams, with increased costs and greater pressure on timelines, but it is clear that the CRA has a very distinct role to play. To the CRA, professionalism, integrity and versatility are key attributes to undertake an exciting and important role and make a worthwhile contribution to clinical research.

References

Bohaychuk, W. and Ball, G. (1993) *Standard Operating Procedures For Investigators*, 2nd edn, Good Clinical Research Practices.

EC (2001) 2001/20/EC of the European Parliament and of the Council of 4 April 2002 on the approximation of the laws, regulations and administrative provisions of the Member States relating to the implementation of good clinical practice in the conduct of clinical trials on medicinal products for human use. *Official Journal of the European Communities*, 1.5.2001.

Glenny, H. and Mullinger, B. (1998) *The Institute of Clinical Research Guide to Freelancing*, The Institute of Clinical Research Booklet.

Hutchinson, D. (1999) *10 Golden GCP Rules for Pharmacists*, Canary Publications.

ICH (1996) ICH Harmonised Tripartite Guideline for Good Clinical Practice, ICH Guideline: Good Clinical Practice—Consolidated Guideline, International Federation of Pharmaceutical Manufacturers Associations, Geneva (CPMP/ICH/135/95).

ICR (2002) *To be a CRA, Information on the Pharmaceutical Industry, Clinical Research and the Role of a Clinical Research Associate*, The Institute of Clinical Research Booklet.

Illingworth, J. (2001) Monitoring, in *Principles of Clinical Research* (eds I. Di Giovanna and G. Hayes), Wrightson Biomedical Publishing Ltd.

Lyness, V. (2001) Your career in your own hands? *Clin. Res. focus*, **12**(7), October.

Maxwell, C. (1973) *Clinical Research For All*, Cambridge Medical Publications Ltd.

New Scientist (2001) Keeping taking the pills. *New Scientist*, **2301**, July.

Rondel, R.K., Varley, S.A. and Webb, C.F. (1993) *Clinical Data Management*, John Wiley and Sons.

Smith, A. and Tanner, J. (2001) Who are we? A demographic overview of the Institute's members. *Clin. Res. focus*, **12**(8), December.

Winslade, J. (1996) *Dictionary of Drug Development*, ACiX SCiENTiFiC Publications.

Further Reading

Beyond What is Written, A Researcher's Guide to Good Clinical Practice, Cambridge Healthcare Research Ltd, 1998.

Di Giovanna, I. and Hayes, G. (eds) (2001) *Principles of Clinical Research*, Wrightson Biomedical Publishing Ltd.

Raven, A. (1997) *Consider It Pure Joy, An Introduction to Clinical Trials*, Cambridge Healthcare Research Ltd.

Useful Websites

www.instituteofclinicalresearch.org
www.axess.co.uk
www.arcpnet.org
www.abpi.org.uk
www.newscientistjobs.com
www.phlexglobal.com
www.ingenix.com

Useful Contacts

The Institute of Clinical Research
PO Box 1208
Maidenhead
Berkshire
SL6 3GD

Association for Clinical Research Professionals
1012 14th Street, N.W.
Suite 807
Washington, DC 20005

7

Clinical Trial Administrator and Study Site Co-ordinator— Key Roles in Clinical Research

Nicola Murgatroyd[1], Caroline Crockatt[2] and Gareth Hayes[3]

[1]*Phlexglobal Ltd, Chalfont St Peter, UK*
[2]*Intercern Ltd, Reigate, UK*
[3]*nrg pathway, Cumbria, UK*

Introduction

Drug regulatory requirements and global clinical research standards (e.g. EU Clinical Trials Directive, 2001 and International Conference on Harmonisation Guidelines for Good Clinical Practice—ICH GCP, 1996) have developed rapidly during recent years alongside the ever-expanding growth of information technology (IT). It has been essential that the roles and responsibilities of those individuals running clinical studies have developed and expanded accordingly.

The Clinical Research Associate (CRA) has been faced with stressful demands on time to conquer logistical issues and manage the burden of increasing paperwork. The role of the Clinical Trial Administrator (CTA) has evolved through need and requirement, primarily from the secretary and/or administrator associated with specific clinical studies taking on more responsibility in logistical and administrative duties. The importance of these duties makes it an absolute necessity that the CTA is very active in the clinical study team of the pharmaceutical sponsor company. In the past, the secretary and/or administrator based in the sponsor

Careers with the Pharmaceutical Industry, Second edition. Edited by P. D. Stonier.
© 2003 John Wiley & Sons Ltd. ISBN 0 470 84328 4

company medical department may have had only limited contact with the clinical study team.

The Study Site Co-ordinator (SSC) in the clinical trial setting has evolved significantly since its formal conception some 15 years ago. This may have been largely due to the changes brought about by the advent of ICH GCP and the EU Clinical Trials Directive, but the recognition of the value of the role has also had an impact.

Traditionally the SSC was defined by GCP as: 'an appropriately experienced person nominated by the Investigator to assist in administrating the trial at the investigational site'. This definition fell short of the common view of an SSC because the role is pivotal, rather than just to assist, and thereby can form by far the greatest individual workload. As with the CTA, ICH GCP does not define the SSC role.

Administration is thus only a fraction of the SSC's activities as a wide range of trial-related duties are performed. The role encompasses a broad spectrum of essential extended skills that need to be put to good use as the SSC often acts as the interface between the investigator, the subject and the sponsor company. The job description must reflect the role in practice and be adhered to, in order to maintain the highest possible clinical trial standards, which in turn will produce reliable, high-quality data.

The Clinical Trial Administrator and the Study Site Co-ordinator, like the Clinical Research Associate, are job titles dogged by pharmaceutical jargon. Unlike the CRA, however, the roles of CTA and SSC are more apparent from the job title itself. Both functions have similar duties, and duties that are often performed in parallel. The main difference is that while the CTA is usually confined to working within the pharmaceutical sponsor company, or contract organisation, the SSC is, more often than not, based directly at the clinical research site (hence the name).

The other major difference is that the SSC is the only one of the sponsoring pharmaceutical company's clinical research team that may be likely to actually see the trial subject or patient. With this in mind, it is understandable that a large proportion of SSCs come from a nursing background, and why their role is often taken as being distinctly outside that normally included amongst pharmaceutical industry options.

The SSC role has been in existence for nearly 20 years and this is illustrated by a strong network of support in building education and training programmes, quality expectancies and career status.

The CTA, on the other hand, is a relatively new role which has developed in parallel to the Clinical Project Assistant (CPA), which is a CRA trainee role, and both are now recognised as industry standards. The CTA is learning from the successes of the SSCs (and other research roles, such as the CRA and now the CPA) to build an effective educational prospectus and positive career pathway.

When running studies there are three fundamental areas of concern: timing, results and costs. Both the CTA and the SSC, in co-operation, can have the greatest impact on turning each outcome into one of success.

Clinical Trial Administrator

Role and responsibility

The role of the CTA can be summarised as follows: 'To administer, maintain and co-ordinate the logistical aspects of clinical trials according to Good Clinical (Research) Practice (GCP) and the sponsor company Standard Operating Procedure (SOP) for clinical research and related activities'. The level of responsibility is inherent in this description. Administration, maintenance and co-ordination of something as central as trial logistics cannot be done from an outlying point of the clinical study team; to be successful the position must be central (alongside the team leader, usually a CRA). With GCP and SOPs as performance guidelines the discipline must respect the high quality demands of the work and must expect due respect in return. The CTA must be empowered to help free monitor time and, thus, keep the project running smoothly and efficiently (Murgatroyd, 2000).

Job description

The number of functions a CTA can take on depends on experience and the structure of the clinical study team, but since the options and variety for these are vast, as a result the job can become all the more rewarding. Within the UK, where the role first evolved, a grading system for the CTA has been implemented; the most senior grade acts as a good template for an extensive job description.

Study documents, case report forms (CRFs) and the trial master file (TMF)

Track (produce, distribute, retrieve, archive) all study documents in a manner appropriate to GCP and sponsor company SOP; build and manage the TMF such that version control of protocol and other essential documents is open to scrutiny and available when required; ensure such administrative management is achieved in a timely manner before, during and after the active phase of the clinical trial. Whilst providing input into CRF design, based on previous logistical experiences, liaise with printing house (internal or external) for production, storage and distribution of CRFs to and from study sites and/or sponsor subsidiary offices.

Independent ethics committees (IECs)

Liaison with this external body is key to a prompt study start and effective study progress. Often the IEC does not have administrative support and the sponsor company CTA can assist all parties by proactive document preparation and subsequent collection. More significantly, the CTA can act as a full-time IEC coordinator building a relationship that can be utilised for future work as well as the current project.

Central/contract laboratory services

The CTA can enable links between central laboratory, study team and study site. This must be matched with a suitable (i.e. usable) tracking system and it is the CTA's role to develop and maintain such a system.

Investigational product/study drug

The logistics of study drug management is one of the most important elements of a successful study. Each and every tablet, bottle and trial pack must be reconciled at the end of the study against the amount first distributed. The CTA may be responsible for such administrative tracking, from company pharmacist, to study site, to patient, and back. Experienced CTAs will design such tracking systems.

Study site

As with IECs, the study site may not have sufficient administrative help and the CTA can be proactive in providing study site files, essential documentation and general assistance to the site. The CTA should be recognised as the main point of contact for all site staff (investigator, SSC, pharmacy, etc.) and be able to disseminate information to relevant parties as appropriate.

Meetings

Effective meetings are a rare jewel in the pharmaceutical industry. The CTA can ensure that all meetings arranged run smoothly by producing agenda—including timetable—minutes and action points. The CTA should also attend investigator meetings and perform the same tasks as for in-house study team meetings. There is no reason why a CTA should not be called on to present at such meetings to discuss document and trial supply management issues.

Study budget

Inevitably, and especially in large multinational corporate bodies, payment for trial-related tasks to outside individuals (investigator, pharmacy, laboratory, courier) can take time. The CTA may be called to manage the financial administration by timely raising and distribution of such fees. An experienced CTA may be expected to manage aspects of the study budget, providing reports to senior management.

SOPs

With so many document management and trial supply issues to design and control, there is no one better placed than the CTA to write or offer input into the production of the SOPs for such tasks. Corporate or departmental templates may exist for many tracking systems and if they are not responsible for the design in the first place, the user's comments must be sought.

Communication

It is clear from all the activities listed that positive communication will act as a perfect conduit for document distribution, completion and return. Not only effective for the documents themselves but for the information contained therein. The CTA must be the central point of contact for the complete study team and all external contacts.

Staff supervision

For large studies more than one CTA may be required, either based at the sponsor company headquarters or posted to subsidiary sites, and a CTA Manager role may be necessary. Likewise, for companies where the CTA role is the norm, a team of CTAs across studies and products using similar templates and methodologies may exist. In this case a manager of CTA experience is preferred if not essential.

Education and qualifications

At the moment there are no formal qualifications or entry requirements for the position of CTA. Graduates and non-graduates alike have the opportunity of choosing this career path, although evidence of supportive education, experience and training will be deemed an advantage. Different companies have different expectancies within the role (Smith and Tanner, 2001).

As the evolution of the CTA has progressed, it has been inevitable that a qualification opportunity has arisen. The Institute of Clinical Research in collaboration with John Moores University, Liverpool has developed a Postgraduate Certificate in Clinical Trial Administration. This is not, as yet, an essential requirement for obtaining a post (see continuing education below).

Knowledge base, skills, competencies

As with the CRA and other study team members, a limited rounded pharmaceutical knowledge is possible if the comparable tasks are also limited, e.g. in a large multinational multicentre clinical trial. Such an outcome would also limit the opportunities for development. Basic study details are obvious, but it is also recommended to obtain knowledge about the trial product and the research programme to date. If considered an active member of the clinical study team, which the CTA should be, training should be available. Training should also be given regarding GCP and SOP guidelines. Even though an experienced CTA may come in with a wealth of GCP knowledge, some companies will still insist on taking their own measure of GCP competence. A keen CTA may obtain an understanding of the therapeutic area under research, but this is usually not essential.

A top-level understanding of the sponsor company's background and product portfolio is something to be acquired or demanded. Speaking to external parties will certainly involve discussion on a wide range of subjects and ignorance on matters that should be known will hardly motivate the other party nor help reputation. A common knowledge of the industry itself completes the all-round picture and this includes knowing what is involved within the roles of the other team members.

Books covering the functions of CRAs (ICR, 2002a), data management personnel (Rondel et al., 1993), investigators (Bohaychuk and Ball, 1993) and/or pharmacists (Hutchinson, 1999) should satisfy the ambitious CTA.

Unlike many roles within the clinical study team, the CTA may have a vast experience of administration outside of the pharmaceutical industry and additional skills can often be brought to the job rather than learnt en route. Whilst it goes without saying that IT skills are an absolute requirement, advanced IT skills are welcomed. With form design and tracking systems paramount, appliance of database systems such as Microsoft Access® is very useful. Most companies today assign essential competencies to measure progress and compliance to the role. This is also a useful personal tool to collect achievements aligned to career aspirations.

Interactions

The CTA is an integral part of the clinical study team who must become involved in all aspects of the study, acting as a pivotal point for communication issues across the whole team and with external parties. The image of the team, the company and the study can depend on the 'public relations' of the CTA. This includes the ability to act as a fire fighter to situations outside the limits of the CTA role. The most important interaction may be with the study team leader or head CRA. However, this relationship may already be sound if the leader has been able to select his or her team. It is likely that the first position to be picked by the team leader, if the option is within their remit, will be that of the CTA, thus highlighting the importance of the role. Other team members include the clinical trial supplies pharmacist, the data management team (analyst, programmer, co-ordinator), the statistician, the medical writer and the CRA team (often field-based). When central to a multinational study, the CTA must bring together an international team of CRAs and local operatives and as such knowledge of different cultures and characters becomes a valuable asset.

The CTA will need to be fully aware of the activities of each external party, especially the study site team. Much of their administration will be remote to the CTA and yet, the final collation of related administrative matters will rest heavy on the CTA's shoulders.

Personality attributes

The team-playing CTA will need flexibility, versatility and even dexterity to cope with not only the document burden and layer upon layer of tracking systems, but also the frequent amendments thrust at short notice on protocols, CRFs and other formal documents. Strong organisational abilities for multi-tasking are fairly obvious as are welcoming, but firm, interpersonal skills. The nature of the position, as a communication centre, may result in a feeling of receiving more bad news than good as problem issues tend to be aired louder than solutions. A successful CTA should be able to turn this to his or her advantage. It may be a case of 'not what you know, but who you know'; prompt resolution of problems through a positive network will enable the CTA to gain shared credit and due respect, with a favour in hand, from the problem originator. Thus, generation of an image of enthusiasm and commitment is important and will come naturally to those suited to the role.

Training

Training for secretaries and administrators has, in the past, been limited to skills not necessarily directly related to clinical research. This training, such as IT skills or interpersonal skills, is still essential. Usually it is co-ordinated by the human resource (personnel) department or the medical department.

The evolution of the CTA role has caused significant demands on training within the pharmaceutical industry. Whether this remains as an internal training unit or is conducted through an external training organisation, the number of people requiring training has suddenly increased. ICH GCP requires that members of the clinical study team are appropriately trained on matters pertaining to the clinical research programme and this clearly infers knowledge of GCP and company SOPs. Sponsor company induction programmes may cover much of this, including subjects such as product portfolios and therapeutic areas. As part of the study team, specific training on the clinical study is a necessity and if performed in a group will boost team morale and performance potential. Indeed, the CTA will probably end up organising the training programmes for the team as well as being a participant.

Continuing education

The number of available courses at universities and academic institutions is still very limited for such a new role, but there is no doubt that more will be established as the role is recognised as integral to the clinical study team. It is still the case that many continuing education possibilities will be taken as a result of the persistence of the CTA rather than the forward thinking of their manager. The Institute of Clinical Research has been proactive in investigating formal qualifications for CTAs (Marron and Murgatroyd, 1998; Murgatroyd, 2001) and as a result 'The CTA Qualification' has been launched to an enthusiastic CTA audience. ICR and Liverpool John Moores University have developed a modular course with two options for certification, depending on academic needs, of either a Certificate of Professional Development or a Postgraduate Certificate in Clinical Trial Administration. Curricula include the topics of Clinical Trial Practices, Management and Organisation, Planning and Tracking, and Business Management.

Career development and opportunities

As with other clinical study team roles (e.g. CRA, CPA), CTAs may find themselves doing the CTA job but holding a different job title. The spectrum of tasks within the job role will also vary and it is important to be aware of the scope that exists across the industry. Networking with other CTAs (at groups such as the ICR's CTA Forum) allows insight into roles and responsibilities at different companies. Resource organisations are often the first to put in place a career structure for 'new' functions; from trainee CTA to Senior CTA Grade III a distinct career path is drawn up and agreed for the ambitious CTA, using competencies and experience as measures of advancement. Many CTAs may have ambitions for continuous improvement, yet wish to remain in the CTA position, whilst others set goals to use the CTA role as a stepping-stone to other related careers. A common aim is to join the CRA career pathway, but this is not the limit of opportunity for the CTA, and auditing, quality assurance, training and archiving are all possible options, as are switches to similar roles outside clinical research. Marketing, sales and project management units will all benefit from an experienced CTA joining their team.

The future

The enthusiasm with which the pharmaceutical industry has greeted the role of the CTA has been nothing short of remarkable, and there is now a general recognition that the role is here to stay. Recognition is fundamental to the CTA success story and today's CTAs have the luck and good fortune to be shaping their own world. Tomorrow's CTAs will spread their wings even further, geographically and academically, and the role will continue to develop in parallel with the rapid changes impacting on the field of clinical research in the pharmaceutical and other healthcare industries.

Study Site Co-ordinator

Role and responsibility

In the past clinical trials were generally conducted by single site physicians, perhaps with the help of a clinic nurse. Trial protocols were simpler and trial patients or subjects were often recruited, and investigated, during a clinic, without great change to the workload. Today's research is more complex as the demands on consistency and quality have become paramount. Documentation has increased and trial processes have become both broader and more intensive, thus requiring a significant and greater liaison between site investigator and sponsor company. Alongside these advances lie changing healthcare structures and services. Many hospitals and research facilities are now operated as cost-accountable units, so the investigating physician can no longer recruit and treat the trial patient in the typical clinic environment, using local staff for support.

Most investigators find the commitment of greater administration and organisation impossible to meet, and, whilst they remain ultimately responsible for the conduct of the trial, many of them now employ an SSC to undertake the burden of the work. The term Study Site Co-ordinator was adopted by the Institute of Clinical Research (formerly the Association for Clinical Research in the Pharmaceutical Industry—ACRPI) in the UK in 1994 and is now widely used within the pharmaceutical industry (Smith and Tannner, 2001). However, as most SSCs are nurses it is uncommon to use this title within the site environment, i.e. their own department, and many retain their nursing origins in their job title. Common examples include:

- Study Site Co-ordinator
- Research Nurse
- Clinical Research Nurse

- Clinical Trial Co-ordinator
- Clinical Trial Officer
- Research Co-ordinator

In the USA, the role is more established and is commonly known as the Clinical Research Co-ordinator. The typical location for the SSC is within the primary/ secondary care setting or in academic institutions performing the clinical research project. The position can be recruited directly by the research site or, as is a growing trend, by the sponsor company itself or a contract research organisation (CRO). In the latter case the SSC can be considered most definitely part of the dedicated clinical study team even though they will find themselves contracted to an investigational clinical research site.

Job description

Qualifications and experience can determine the duties expected of the SSC, as can the complexity of the research project. Not every trial will involve all the tasks listed below, but the proactive SSC can initiate such actions if they are experienced enough to recognise the need and comfortable as the vital link between investigative site and sponsor clinical study team.

Marketing the site

Under aspects of new business development, the SSC can network with sponsors for potential trials, or simply to maintain contact for the future and gain insight into all facets of clinical research, e.g. regulatory changes, cost structures, international variability. From the site point of view the SSC must maintain links with referral services for recruitment of clinical trials subjects.

Protocol feasibility

As they are often closer to the practical aspects of the study, the SSC should evaluate, review and assess protocols and amendments for feasibility and subject safety and welfare. They will be expected to understand the study methodology and thus determine subject population availability. The protocol will allow the SSC to determine availability of facilities and equipment availability at the site and calculate timelines for conducting and completing the trial in conjunction with the sponsor's expectations. Attendance and input into investigator and trial-related meetings is essential.

Study budget

The SSC may negotiate payment schedules with the sponsor company, having calculated anticipated trial-related costs. This includes negotiating fees for associated costs, for example, trial-specific advertising, laboratory and additional resources. This may also include matters of insurance such as processing the Letter of Indemnity.

Site preparation

Preparation for the site in readiness for site initiation and active study phase is a key part of the SSC role where they are responsible for scheduling and co-ordinating all trial-related activities on site. Examples are given below:

- Facilitate IEC submission;
- Write SSC SOPs;
- Prepare and submit regulatory documentation for site and sponsor;
- Approve suitability of patient/subject information and consent documents;
- Design and distribute subject recruitment advertisements;
- Manage local requirements for hospital R&D department;
- Prepare space for trial-related equipment and supplies;
- Prepare and provide trial-related information and documentation and disseminate to study site team;
- Identify and provide training to trial team and associated staff, e.g. pharmacy, laboratory;
- Present and provide clinical trial timelines to every member of the team;
- Co-ordinate the site initiation visit with sponsor.

Site co-ordination

The active phase of the trial is where SSCs come into their own. Forming the pivotal role between investigator and subject, and investigator and sponsor company, the SSC must exhibit a visionary outlook on trial progress. Ample preparation has been shown to be key and if done well, should allow the SSC to co-ordinate the running of the trial smoothly, allowing time to predict problems, focus on subject welfare and motivate the study team. That said, the number of tasks to be completed is still endless and, inevitably, will not be without trauma.

Some examples are given below.

Recruitment

Formatting clinic recruitment screening logs, identifying and pre-screening subjects' medical notes for eligibility, and then contacting potential subjects and scheduling for trial visits can be time consuming. However, the rewards are high when recruitment goes well. Administrative tasks include preparing referral letters, logging and monitoring enrolment, and recording screen failures for future trial databases. The SSC should recognise if recruitment strategies need to be modified and initiate appropriate action.

The screening procedure itself requires the SSC to apply their knowledge and skills regarding the relationship between the protocol and the subject. Eligibility criteria and demographics must be obtained via medical notes, referral documents or the trial subjects themselves. The SSC is responsible for scheduling trial visits in accordance with the trial protocol and co-ordinating these dates with site team and allied functions. The SSC–subject interaction continues with a considered discourse regarding all aspects of the trial and trial-related activities, the risks and benefits and other pertinent information. With due care, the SSC must ensure that the trial subject has as much time as they need to consent and, when in agreement to participate, that they (or their representative) have signed and dated all the relevant forms (Chatfield and Getting, 2001). Throughout the trial the SSC will support the investigative team by monitoring subject compliance and assess subject safety during the trial.

Case report forms and essential documentation

Document management tasks involve not only general administration for investigator, subject (for diary cards), IECs and other team members, but a concise review and completion of much of this documentation. Protocol inclusion and exclusion criteria must be checked alongside ongoing trial visit procedures and deviations recorded. In some cases, the SSC will be responsible for entering specific data in CRFs or electronic databases. It is usual for the SSC to audit CRFs for accuracy and transmit completed documents by fax, email or express delivery. The SSC will liaise with sponsor company personnel, either the CRA or CTA, regarding data queries and agree resolution points along with realistic timelines.

Maintenance of the Investigator Site File—ISF (the equivalent of the CTA's TMF) on an ongoing basis is essential to site housekeeping and will secure positive outcomes from CRA Source Documentation Verification and independent inspection. The SSC will be called upon to retain all historical documents, i.e. medical/pathology reports, maintain subject records, status reports and subject demographic logs, and document all written and verbal trial contacts.

Drug accountability and laboratory

Even if the hospital pharmacy has taken on all or part of the tasks regarding trial medication, the SSC must have a co-ordinating involvement. If the pharmacy were not involved, as in a single site or general practice study, the SSC would expect to receive all trial supplies, maintain shipment and dispensing records and be responsible for storage, i.e. all aspects of accountability.

If laboratory tests form part of the study the SSC would be responsible for the collecting, processing and storing (or arranging storage) of samples in accordance with the protocol instructions.

Administrative tasks include collating normal laboratory values, obtaining accreditation certificates and filing all relevant documentation in the ISF.

Adverse events

The SSC assists the investigator where possible to document adverse events and ensure that all adverse events are documented in the subject's medical notes and CRFs. In such cases the SSC needs to co-ordinate subject follow-up and ensure resolution activities, including appropriate documentation, are completed. In the event of Serious Adverse Events the SSC must act promptly and in accordance with given guidelines to ensure full completion of relevant forms and subsequent distribution to relevant parties, whilst also notifying the subject's doctor and taking action where appropriate.

Close-out visit

As with all sponsor personnel visits throughout the trial, the SSC co-ordinates and schedules the close-out visit (the last meeting) with the CRA, other sponsor personnel (e.g. auditor) and the site staff required in attendance. To complete the services for the sponsor company the SSC would return all unused documentation and trial supplies, following reconciliation, to the sponsor company.

On behalf of the site the SSC needs to audit and prepare all files for archive, ensuring essential documents are kept as required according to ICH GCP. It is recommended to prepare a local trial report and evaluate the team effort at site to recognise development areas and promote achievements in readiness for the next business development opportunity.

Knowledge base, skills, competencies

Most SSCs hold a nursing qualification and clearly with many of the role-related tasks in mind, especially contact with the subject, this may often be considered the most appropriate. However, because working practices tend to be varied, SSCs do also come from many different backgrounds. Typical examples include:

- Registered Nurse
- Science Degree

- Medical Degree
- Pharmacy Technician/Assistant
- Laboratory Technician/Assistant
- Administrator

As GCP guidelines are unclear about specific roles and responsibilities for the position they are open to interpretation by SSCs, the principal investigator, the site team, and the company sponsoring the study. Some SSC working practices are controversial, particularly those concerning the division of responsibility between the SSC and investigator.

In the absence of clear guidelines SSCs tend to fall back on those of their original professional body (if they have one), e.g. the Royal College of Nursing and the Nursing and Midwifery Council (NMC), formerly the United Kingdom Central Council for Nursing, Midwifery and Health Visiting (UKCC). These bodies are beginning to recognise the role of the SSC and formal recognition, with support from professional bodies like the Institute of Clinical Research, will enhance the importance of the role.

The interpersonal and organisational skills required by the SSC are similar to those mentioned in the previous CTA section and are summarised below. In addition, the SSC must know the logistical workings of their hospital or clinic environment:

- Communication (verbal and written);
- Organisation and delegation of tasks;
- Independence and team player;
- Maintenance of self-discipline and self-motivation;
- Versatility and adaptability to ever-changing trial environment;
- Effective at planning and prioritisation of workload;
- Ability to anticipate, initiate, negotiate and motivate.

Interactions

The SSC will find themselves interacting with nearly all the disciplines involved in the clinical trial, at site and sponsor company, but ultimately the SSC is the subjects' advocate in every trial-related aspect. The final skills listed above illustrate how the SSC must interact with all their contacts. A combination of anticipation, initiation, negotiation and motivation must be applied at all times as the SSC provides the study with a vital conduit linking the laboratory to the investigator, the laboratory to the sponsor company, the investigator to the sponsor company, the sponsor company to the pharmacy, and so on. At all times the welfare of the subject will be foremost in the mind of the SSC.

The SSC will feel, at times, through these interactions, that they are doing the job of other team members as well as their own. This highlights the importance of delegation or perceived delegation and a careful approach to interaction through observation and instruction.

Personality attributes

As has been stated already the SSC will find themselves in the 'thick of it' regarding all site-based activities and, if not, must put themselves in that situation. It is only with being in this position that they can offer any sort of control over the trial. As such, they should be dynamic, self-driven and determined with the ability to handle highly stressful situations. There is always the likelihood that other parties may have other agendas (e.g. different units will have their own priority lists) and the SSC may have to illustrate forcefulness and strength of character to influence such occurrences. The art of persuasion must not be devious and the SSC should be able to exhibit extreme loyalty to the trial and the individuals involved. This is particularly the case concerning ethical issues and areas of confidentiality where sensitivity is required. A successful SSC will exhibit natural enthusiasm combined with commitment and a high degree of perfectionism. These attributes will be repaid by team loyalty and mutual commitment with subsequent rewards enjoyed.

Training

The multi-skilled SSC will put high demands on training and development if they are to be proven and to be fully qualified and equipped for the role. The search for such training will take the SSC down many avenues and the SSC must be careful not to put 'too many eggs in their basket'. As with all other industry positions, training must be prioritised from essential to nice-to-have. With the prospect of having a conflict between nursing skills and clinical research skills, the SSC should remember that the SSC role generally requires a combination of both. For the purposes of this chapter clinical research training should be the focus.

Sadly many SSCs may find themselves stuck in the middle between investigator site and sponsor company with each party expecting the other to provide a suitable training programme. The nature of the good SSC is not to accept this and to utilise the best training opportunities from both parties. This may be reflected in funding, availability and time restraints. A number of courses exist as one-day seminars concentrating on single aspects of clinical research practices, e.g. ICR's Introduction to ICH GCP for Study Site Personnel. Time and cost constraints may make one-day courses the only option. However, in the long term, it may be more effective to consider longer courses. ICR run a number of intensive three-day events, e.g. Clinical Trial Management; Ethics and Regulations; and Introduction to Clinical Trials and Clinical Trial Practice the Industry Benchmark. Many other training organisations offer a wide range of related courses and many more delve into the softer, more transferable, competencies such as problem solving, negotiation and team skills. A broad understanding of IT is essential when working with one unit and many sponsor companies as different companies will without doubt have different approaches to IT usage.

Continuing education

Having recognised the role of SSC and the, sometime, difficulty encountered with role justification concerning its site-based location, the Institute of Clinical Research produced the Professional Portfolio for Study Site Personnel (1999). This allows SSCs to maintain a portfolio of their past and current skills alongside their accreditation, aspirations and plans for professional advancement. Supporting these aspirations is the Certificate in Clinical Research, a one-year course running over three separate three-day periods. The alliance between ICR and Liverpool John Moores University has a track record of success and covers basic human biochemistry, physiology and pharmacology; oral and written communication skills; legal and ethical aspects; handling of statistical data; as well as the execution of clinical trials.

Career development and opportunities

Networking is inevitable considering the number of interactions that are inherent with the job of the CTA. It is largely through these contacts that the SSC will discover other roles that may attract personal career aspirations. Many SSCs, with experience behind them, move to be based in the medical departments of pharmaceutical companies with posts such as auditor, CRA, CTA, drug safety officer, information pharmacist or training. The options are not limited to duties in medical departments and extend to marketing, market research and sales.

The nursing background of many SSCs is not forgotten and it is important to maintain links even if the role of SSC sees less day-to-day contact with subjects. The SSC subcommittee of ICR was set up in 1993 (ICR, 2002b) to serve the needs of the SSC and to promote the image amongst other functions. The subcommittee maintains collaborative links with the Royal College of Nursing (RCN) and is working with the RCN to gain recognition of the research nurse role in therapeutic clinical trials (ICR, 1998). The SSC membership within ICR has nearly 700 members across the UK and Europe (over 10% of the total membership) and the subcommittee always needs to help to maintain the high standards that the SSC represents.

The future

The variety of SSC working practices and clear lack of formal recognition in the past has led to a disparity in the SSC role. The ICR's SSC subcommittee is continually working to provide educational programmes and allied support (e.g. query resolution, trouble-shooting) to promote the benefits of the role and develop it further. This, in time, may help the major problem of the SSC today, namely the lack of secure funding. Many SSCs have temporary contracts, usually based solely on the trial to which they are responsible and within that, usually against renewable terms of a period of one year, six months or less. A significant number are likely to be employed on unsecured funding, typically raised against future trial payments, which can obviously fall short of the original estimate. The role does not sit in a risk-free environment and therefore may prove transitory for some. There is no doubt that the SSC function is exciting and stimulating, with high rewards. There is no doubt that the industry respects the need for the SSC and now that alliance partners, such as the RCN, are recognising how the SSC should be developed, a career with a definite structure and pathway is here to stay. Sitting in the middle of the trial may be considered a seat of strength and SSCs, new and old, have the capability to shape their own evolution.

Acknowledgement

The authors would like to thank Angie Major of the Institute of Clinical Research for assisting in the preparation of this chapter.

References

Bohaychuk, W. and Ball, G. (1993) *Standard Operating Procedures For Investigators*, 2nd edn, Good Clinical Research Practices.

Chatfield, D. and Getting, L. (2001) Informed consent to research: the role of the research nurse. *Clin. Res. focus*, **12**(7), October.

EC (2001) 2001/20/EC of the European Parliament and of the Council of 4 April 2002 on the approximation of the laws, regulations and administrative provisions of the Member States relating to the implementation of good clinical practice in the conduct of clinical trials on medicinal products for human use. *Official Journal of the European Communities*, 1.5.2001.

Hutchinson, D. (1999) *10 Golden GCP Rules for Pharmacists*, Canary Publications.

ICH (1996) Harmonised Tripartite Guideline for Good Clinical Practice: Good Clinical Practice—Consolidated Guideline, International Federation of Pharmaceutical Manufacturers Associations, Geneva (CPMP/ICH/135/95).

ICR (1998) The Clinical Nurse in NHS Trusts and GP Practices: Guidance for Nurses and their Employees, EB22/98.

ICR (2002a) To be a CRA, Information on the Pharmaceutical Industry, Clinical Research and the Role of a Clinical Research Associate, The Institute of Clinical Research Booklet.

ICR (2002b) Institute Profile: SSC sub-committee. *Clin. Res. focus*, **13**(2), March.

Marron, M. and Murgatroyd, N. (1998) Clinical trial administrators—the bright future ahead. *Clin. Res. focus*, **9**(7), November.

Murgatroyd, N. (2000) Recognising potential in study team members. *Appl. Clin. Trials*, **9**(5), May.

Murgatroyd, N. (2001) About PgCert in clinical trial administration. *Clin. Res. focus*, **12**(5), July.

Rondel, R.K., Varley, S.A. and Webb, C.F. (eds) (1993) *Clinical Data Management*, John Wiley.

Smith, A. and Tanner, J. (2001) Who are we? A demographic overview of the Institute's members. *Clin. Res. focus*, **12**(8), December.

Further Reading

Beyond What is Written, A Researcher's Guide to Good Clinical Practice, Cambridge Healthcare Research Ltd, 1998.

Clinical Trials Survival Kit (for study site personnel), Institute of Clinical Research, 2002.

Di Giovanna, I. and Hayes, G. (eds) (2001) *Principles of Clinical Research*, Wrightson Biomedical Publishing Ltd.

Kenkre, J.E. (1997) The role of the nurse in primary care research, in *Research Methods in Primary Care* (eds Y. Carter and C. Thomas), Radcliffe Medical Press.

Raven, A. (1997) *Consider It Pure Joy, An Introduction to Clinical Trials*, Cambridge Healthcare Research Ltd.

Tarling, M. and Crofts, L. (2002) *The Essential Researcher's Handbook*, 2nd edn (for nurses and healthcare professionals).

Useful Websites

www.instituteofclinicalresearch.org
www.arcpnet.org
www.abpi.org.uk
www.newscientistjobs.com
www.phlexglobal.com
www.livjm.ac.uk/research_and_graduate
www.rcn.org.uk

Useful Contacts

The Institute of Clinical Research
PO Box 1208
Maidenhead
Berkshire SL6 3GD

Association for Clinical Research Professionals
1012 14th Street, N.W.
Suite 807
Washington, DC 20005

Phlexglobal Ltd
Dairy House
Churchfield Road
Chalfont St Peter
Bucks SL9 9EW

Nursing and Midwifery Council
23 Portland Place
London W1B 1PZ

Royal College of Nurses
20 Cavendish Square
London W1G 0RN

8

Statisticians in the Pharmaceutical Industry

Christopher Hilton and Trevor Lewis

Pfizer Global Research and Development, Sandwich, UK

Introduction

The primary aim of a development project in the pharmaceutical industry is to produce a dossier of information which satisfies regulatory authorities that a particular medicinal product is suitable for marketing. The information in the dossier is derived from data which have arisen from experimental work in the laboratory and in the clinic. Thus the design of experiments capable of producing useful information and the analysis and interpretation of the resulting data are central to achieving this primary aim. Since the design, analysis and interpretation of experiments are areas of primary activity for the statistician, it follows that the statistician has an important and central role to play in the process of pharmaceutical R&D.

In the context of clinical research, this central role is clearly recognised by the regulatory authorities. The International Conference on Harmonisation (ICH), whose aim was to look at the technical requirements for registration of pharmaceuticals for human use, developed a number of guidelines which have been adopted by the regulatory bodies of the European Union, Japan and the USA. For example the ICH E6 guideline on Good Clinical Practice (ICH, 1996) requires that: 'The sponsor should utilise qualified individuals (e.g. biostatisticians, clinical pharmacologists and physicians) as appropriate, throughout all stages of the trial process, from designing the protocol and CRFs (Case Report Forms) and planning the analyses to analysing and preparing interim and final clinical trials reports'. Further guidance on statistical involvement is given in ICH E9 (ICH, 1998) which attempted to harmonise the principles of statistical methodology as applied to clinical trials. ICH E9 states that 'the role and responsibility of the trial statistician, in collaboration with other clinical trial professionals, is to ensure that statistical

Careers with the Pharmaceutical Industry, Second edition. Edited by P. D. Stonier.
© 2003 John Wiley & Sons Ltd. ISBN 0 470 84328 4

principles are applied appropriately in clinical trials supporting drug development'. The guideline is also explicit in requiring that 'the trial statistician should ensure that the protocol and any amendments cover all relevant statistical issues clearly and accurately'. Perhaps more importantly the emphasis of the ICH E9 guideline is around ensuring that the importance of the statistical contribution in the areas of experimental design, randomisation and blinding and statistical analysis and interpretation is recognised and that access to biostatistical expertise throughout the entire trial procedure from the design of the protocol to the final report is necessary.

It is this enlightened view of the regulators, exemplified by the adoption of the ICH topic guidelines by the regulatory bodies of the European Union, Japan and the USA that encouraged the pharmaceutical industry to become one of the major employers of statisticians. In the UK alone there are over 1000 qualified statisticians working in the industry, employed by a variety of companies from large multinational research-based organisations to smaller domestic manufacturers of generic products, and also contract research organisations which now play a significant and important role in providing statistical resource for clinical trial reporting.

The vast majority of these UK-based statisticians are members of PSI (Statisticians in the Pharmaceutical Industry), an independent association formed in 1977 to promote professional standards of statistics in matters pertinent to the pharmaceutical industry. In 1992, PSI and other similar associations in Europe collaborated to form the European Federation of Statisticians in the Pharmaceutical Industry (EFSPI). This body, representing over 2000 statisticians in Europe, provides a European perspective on statistical issues in the industry by exchange of information, promoting professional standards and providing collective expert input on statistical matters to national and international authorities and organisations.

In this chapter we will attempt to describe the range of methodological challenges facing the statistician working in the pharmaceutical industry, the skills required by the statistician to succeed in this environment and the potential scope of the statistician's role (see also PSI, 2000). Purely for convenience in this chapter we will refer to the statistician as 'he', although it should be recognised that approximately 50% of statisticians in the industry are female.

The Variety of Methodological Challenges

One of the fascinating aspects of statistics as a subject is that the most fundamental concepts are often the most difficult to grasp and explain. These concepts, such as the nature of variation and the role of randomisation and blocking, guide the approach to experimental design, whilst the meaning of hypothesis testing, interval estimates and p-values guide the interpretation of the results of statistical analyses.

Thus, the first challenge facing the statistician embarking on a career in the pharmaceutical industry, as indeed in any industry, is to convert his theoretical knowledge about these concepts into the practicalities of the experimental setting in which he finds himself. He then has to move quickly to a position where he can guide the scientist or physician to understand not only how these basic concepts influence their experimental work, but also how to interpret the results of more advanced techniques based on mathematical models. These models make further assumptions about normality, homogeneity of variance, proportional hazards, and the like. The mistake often made is to focus on explaining the intricacies of the mathematical models, rather than ensuring that the data are viewed and summarised appropriately, and that the fundamental concepts which enable one to extrapolate from sample to underlying population are well understood.

A further important adjustment that the statistician needs to make in order for his contribution to be relevant to the experimental work is to appreciate the experimental constraints within which he is working and the nature of the measurements that are being made. Thus many textbook criteria for optimal design and analysis will need to be adapted to the real-life situation. For example, although it may be theoretically optimal to design a study so that all sequences of the three treatments to be investigated are used (i.e. ABC, BCA, CAB, BAC, ACB, CBA), safety and ethical constraints may dictate that treatment B must occur before treatment C, and so only the sequences (ABC, BCA, BAC) can actually be administered. Additionally, study design optimality criteria, such as minimum variance and unbiasedness for estimates, in practice may take second place to robustness in the presence of missing observations or outlying values.

It is these considerations that make each experimental situation and each data set a unique challenge to the applied statistician, ensuring a stimulating and invigorating environment in which to work.

The pharmaceutical industry is of course a regulated industry, which places a further framework within which those involved in experimental design and analysis need to work. This framework of regulatory guidelines is sometimes seen as a further set of constraints which limit the scope of the statistician to use his technical insight to most appropriately extract information from the data. In fact this is becoming less of an issue, as with the adoption of the regulatory agencies of the ICH guidelines, and with their willingness to engage in dialogue around statistical issues the guidance given by the regulators on statistically related topics is becoming more mature. Rather than prescribing specific approaches to use, the guidelines now seek to outline principles to follow, define conventions to adopt (where the choice is otherwise arbitrary) and on the basis of the regulator's experience of previous licence applications, proscribe against using inappropriate approaches. Thus well-thought-out guidelines are proving helpful to the industry statistician, rather than constraining. Of course the guidelines are written from the regulator's perspective, and so are often cautionary, advocating approaches which may help the regulator confirm the robustness of the findings presented by the pharmaceutical company. As an example, the regulators may wish to see an intent-to-treat analysis derived from all the data collected on all the patients. We do not believe this is because the regulators feel that such an analysis is ideal, rather that they want to confirm the findings presented in the dossier are not dependent on some rather arbitrary criteria chosen by the pharmaceutical company for selecting analysable data and evaluable patients.

The Statistician in Drug Development

There is probably a common misconception that statisticians in the pharmaceutical industry are 'clinical statisticians' and therefore that the role is primarily around analysing data from clinical trials. This is clearly a role that statisticians perform but there are many other roles, the scope and variety of which reflect the intrinsic interest of the process by which new medicines are discovered, developed, manufactured and marketed. In our experience of working for three different pharmaceutical companies the range of areas where statisticians are involved covers the entire spectrum of pharmaceutical activities, including:

- Drug discovery
- Phase I, II, III studies
- Regulatory support
- Genetics
- Portfolio management
- Toxicology
- Compassionate use studies
- Post-marketing studies
- Publications
- Process improvement
- Pharmacy & production
- PK/PD modelling & simulation
- Outcomes research
- Marketing support

But within these activities what is the range of techniques used by the statistician working in the pharmaceutical industry?

The modern discovery chemist has access to a database of information on hundreds of thousands of compounds. In order to efficiently select from this database, multivariate techniques of classification, clustering and discrimination clearly have a role to play. Quantitative structure–activity relationships (QSARs) have been utilised by discovery scientists for many years as part of the process of linking chemical properties to biological activity. These relationships rely on multiple regression and a variety of multivariate techniques which still require considerable refinement to fully address the problems posed in this area of application.

The discovery biologist typically works with scarce experimental material (tissues or animals) in a well-controlled laboratory setting. It is in this area of work that principles of experimental design can accrue great benefit in terms of efficient (and hence ethical) use of resources and optimising the precision of treatment comparisons. Experiments range from primary screens which typically focus on one primary endpoint per experimental unit (tissue/animal) to more complex experiments on promising compounds, with extensive measurement over the time-course of treatment effect.

A part of the development process which is well regulated is that of animal toxicology, with regulatory authorities laying down the broad requirements of experimental design in order to determine the toxicological profile and therapeutic index for the compound in prescribed species of animals. Although designs may be standard, this area of work throws up interesting problems in the analysis of the time-course and distribution of events.

The production of the compound on a small scale to support the research effort, the development of a pure and stable formulation with appropriate release properties to support clinical research, and subsequent scale-up of production for the commercial formulation present the pharmaceutical scientist with many interesting challenges, some of which benefit from a statistical contribution. For example, response surface methodology assists in determining the optimum formulation, mathematical modelling is used to assess drug action (metabolism and pharmacokinetics), and sampling inspection and quality-control methods are applied to large-scale production to guarantee the quality of the pharmaceutical product.

Clinical research

It is in clinical research (phases I–III) where the majority of statisticians in the industry provide their contribution, dealing with trials carried out on healthy human volunteers and patients. This is a fascinating area of research owing to the range of experimental situations. At one extreme small, short-term, well-controlled trials are carried out in specialist clinics with intensive measurement of volunteers on a second-by-second basis. At the other extreme large multicentre multinational trials are carried out, treating hundreds of patients for several years with infrequent visits to the clinic to assess the progress of patients who are otherwise going about their normal daily life.

A clinical development programme may take around five years, during which the statistical challenges evolve as progress is made from exploratory trials to confirmatory trials, as appropriate measures of drug effect are developed, as the safety profile of the drug is understood, and as the advantages over existing therapies are confirmed. It is important to recognise that each clinical trial is not an isolated experiment, rather a contribution to a full clinical development programme. Thus the advice given by the statistician on experimental design and statistical analysis of a particular clinical trial needs to recognise the trial's role within the total programme, the specific objectives of the trial, the overall objectives of the programme and the regulatory drug label that is being considered.

The specific statistical methodology used in clinical research is obviously dependent on the disease area under study. Because of the nature of most clinical trials, being carried out on out-patients, designs need to be simple in terms of structure in order to ensure compliance with the protocol of assessments. Thus the main issues of design relate to the nature and timing of measurements in order to achieve the trial objectives.

The design of any one study may often be highly influenced by computer simulations of possible outcome, based upon mathematical or statistical models that attempt to capture the current knowledge about a potential new medicine. By combining information from multiple studies, such models may help to identify important subgroups of patients in whom the new medicine may have a tendency to work less well or who might be at greater risk of experiencing adverse events. The result of statistical modelling of existing data and of simulating possible designs of later trials should be an improved development programme that makes a safe and effective medicine available to patients more quickly. Further reduction in this time may be brought about by identifying simple-to-measure surrogate clinical endpoints or biomarkers. Although observed in a short-term clinical trial, these endpoints accurately predict the outcomes that would have been observed in a longer-term study, thus reducing development time. The evaluation and validation of biomarkers and surrogate endpoints needs careful statistical input if the potential benefits are to be realised in practice.

Clinical trials typically generate large quantities of data as the safety of the patient is carefully monitored throughout the trial, and as the patient's response to treatment is assessed over time. A major analysis challenge is therefore one of data reduction with the aim of deriving summary measures of effect for each patient which are clinically relevant and so can be analysed in order to give a meaningful comparison of the experimental drug and positive/negative controls. Additionally, in order that valid conclusions can be drawn from the trial, the analyses need to account for the effect of missing data, early withdrawals from the trial and patients who violate the protocol. It is these practical issues of data analysis that provide a similar level of intellectual challenge for the statistician working with clinical trials data, as do the methodological issues for the statistician working with data from laboratory experiments.

As well as including analyses of data from each individual clinical trial, the regulatory dossier will also contain meta-analyses, pooling data from several studies. Some of these analyses will be prospectively defined in the clinical development plan, others will be post hoc to address questions that have arisen during the course of the development programme or that have arisen from the review of the dossier by the regulatory authority.

Finally, once the drug is marketed further data are collected from clinical trials, post-marketing surveillance studies and market research. Here again statistical methods have a role to play in extracting information to support the effective commercialisation of the pharmaceutical product which has resulted from many man-years of research investment.

Skills and Knowledge Required by the Statistician

In the previous section we have outlined some of the technical statistical challenges that are presented to the pharmaceutical statistician. However, the ability to apply statistical methodology to well-formulated problems is only the foundation on which the statistician must build other skills and knowledge in order to develop a rewarding and influential career in the pharmaceutical industry. The broader set of attributes that we believe are required are summarised in Table 8.1, and discussed in more detail below.

Table 8.1 Skills and knowledge required by an effective pharmaceutical statistician

Technical foundation
- Problem formulation/solving
- Statistical methodology
- Statistical computing/packages

Knowledge of the context
- Scientific background
- Drug development process
- Regulatory guidelines/company SOPs

Communication skills
- Report writing
- Oral presentation

Consultancy

Project management skills
- Task/resource planning
- Process engineering
- Managing change

Technical foundation

The statistician is always working with someone else's data, whether it be assisting the biologist with an experimental design or analysing the results of a clinical trial. In either case, when the research scientist (i.e. the client) comes to the statistician for input the starting point is invariably for the statistician to understand the experimental situation and its objectives. This discussion, as a minimum, will lead to the formulation of the problem to be addressed in statistical terms, but more often than not will also refine, and make more specific, the client's view of what is required. It is this process of problem formulation which is fundamental to the impact that a statistician can make on the research project.

Having correctly formulated the problem, it is the application of statistical methodology, which is at the centre of the statistician's education, that will enable progress to be made towards solving the problem. Thus a thorough understanding of statistical principles and methods and the ability to develop and apply them to real-life situations is the basic technical contribution required of the statistician.

The application of methods is typically achieved through the use of statistical computer software. Packages are now available which facilitate the processing of large databases of information, the exploration of data sets, the presentation of summaries and the carrying out of formal inferential statistical analyses. Long gone are the days when limitations in the computer power and suitable software inhibited the statistician's ability to complete an appropriate data analysis. The challenge of today is to understand the structure and conventions of the clinical database, and maintain an awareness of the full scope of analysis and reporting functionality that is available in extensive software products such as SAS and S+.

Knowledge of the context

For the advice given by the statistician to be relevant to the work of the research scientist, the statistician needs to understand the context of the experimental work. This can be split into three main areas, namely the scientific background of the project, the drug development process, and the framework of regulatory guidelines and requirements.

The scientific background includes the disease area being addressed, the measurement of disease and therapeutic benefit, and the mode of action of both the experimental drug and existing marketed products. Knowledge of the drug development process helps position the current experimental situation and understand how the results will be used to aid management decision-making or establish claims for the profile of the drug. An understanding of regulatory guidelines, and their reflection in the form of company SOPs, clarifies the requirements for quality processes, the extent of the information expected by the regulators, and the format in which they expect it to be presented.

Most major pharmaceutical companies recognise the benefits of ensuring that employees have this knowledge and so are prepared to invest in developing a broad understanding in their staff through extensive training programmes. The aim is not, for example, to make the statistician an expert cardiologist, rather to ensure that in consultation the cardiologist and statistician can design experiments to most effectively and efficiently deliver information to answer well-defined, relevant questions.

Communication skills

This is an area in which most statisticians do not have a natural gift when starting a career in the pharmaceutical industry. This could be a reflection of the attributes of the type of person who has a flair for mathematical, logical and analytical subjects, or simply that communication skills are of paramount importance to the pharmaceutical statistician and need to be developed at an early stage of the statistician's career.

To emphasise this point we would like to take two quotes from an excellent paper (ASA Committee on Training of Statisticians for Industry, 1980) entitled 'Preparing statisticians for careers in industry'. Although over 20 years old, and not directed specifically at the pharmaceutical industry, much of what is covered in this paper is very relevant to the subject of this chapter. The quotes are as follows:

> 'Industrial statisticians gain *recognition* through the quantity, quality, timeliness and *impact* of their work: do it, do it well, *see that it is used*.'

> 'Statistical results are of little value if the client doesn't *understand* them and *put them to work*. The success of an industrial statistician is a direct function of the *impact* of his or her work on company business.'

The parts of the quotes in italics emphasise where communication skills come into play. The statistician cannot expect his contribution to be adopted simply because it is logically sound, he needs to be prepared to represent it through formal presentations (written or oral) and persuasive argument in informal discussions. It is through these skills that the statistician and his subject have the appropriate level of impact and influence on the projects in which he is working.

The comments made above about the value of communication skills are, of course, appropriate to colleagues of all disciplines working in a multidisciplinary research environment. The reason to emphasise their value for the statistician goes back to a previous point; namely that the statistician is always working with someone else's data. Thus inevitably the statistician is part of a customer–supplier chain, in which he is both customer (at the problem formulation stage) and supplier (when delivering the results of analyses). Acquisition of knowledge and understanding, and dissemination of information, are critical to the statistician's ability to make a useful contribution.

Consultancy

Statistical consultancy in the industry takes on a number of forms, depending on the individuals involved, the organisation of the company and the culture within the company. The latter two points are mentioned as they strongly influence the expectation of the role that the statistician should play. Inevitably that role is part of a matrix organisational structure with function and project forming the two dimensions.

Simplistically, the statistician's influence in the projects is easier to achieve in an organisation with a strong project emphasis which recognises the statistician as a key project team member. In many large pharmaceutical companies this is the case in clinical development project teams. However for the quality of the statistical contribution to be maintained at a high level, this strong project emphasis must be reinforced by a strong functional structure. The reason for this is that it is the latter which guarantees the career development of the staff and advances the nature and quality of the statistical contribution over time. This is particularly important during a period of growth in the organisation and rapid change resulting from technical advances and process improvements.

The consultancy role for the statistician falls into two broad categories: advisory (providing the client with statistical guidance) and collaborative (participating as a member of a multidisciplinary research team).

In the advisory role, strong communication skills are required to work with the client to define the problem in a manner which empathises with the client in addressing the practical constraints which inevitably influence his experimental work. Wherever possible, the aim should be to provide the client with his own statistical tools and the knowledge of how to use them. In the collaborative role, the statistician will not only bring his technical expertise to the work of the project team, but will also contribute to broader activities of the team, playing a part in processes of planning, problem-solving and decision-making. It is in these areas that the logical, objective and analytical skills often possessed by the statistician prove to be of considerable value.

Project management skills

As alluded to in the previous section, the experienced statistician can play a full part in the management of a multidisciplinary project team. For example, clinical development project teams for major phase III drug candidates are often quite large, and the data processing and reporting may involve several data managers and statisticians. The data managers are responsible for the preparation of the database from which the statisticians and data managers generate material for the final report which forms part of the regulatory dossier. The coordination of this activity falls to an experienced statistician and its efficient conduct is often critical to the timely preparation of the dossier. This intensive involvement in the end-game of putting together the dossier, and subsequently responding to regulatory questions prior to gaining approval to market the medicinal product, is both invigorating and challenging.

The pharmaceutical industry is becoming an increasingly competitive industry. One aspect of maintaining a competitive edge is to develop medicinal products in a shorter period of time, despite the increasing demands of the regulatory agencies. This is in part addressed by pharmaceutical companies refining the complex process of drug development and taking advantage of technological advances in the collection, processing and presentation of data. As contributors to this process, experienced statisticians will often take part in initiatives to re-engineer the process or introduce new technology to provide improvements in quality and timeliness.

Conclusion

In describing the skills and knowledge required by the statistician we have hopefully conveyed some idea of the scope of the statistician's role in the pharmaceutical industry. It is a role that is based on the technical foundation given by a statistical education, which has the potential to extend to a fulfilling and influential role, provided these technical skills are allied with an understanding of the pharmaceutical industry, the regulatory environment and the development of project management and communication skills. Excitingly for the statistician, the role is ever-changing, with new statistical methods and ideas being suggested and evaluated. Currently developing areas requiring significant statistical input include the evaluation and validation of surrogate endpoints, the optimisation of development programmes through the modelling of data and the simulation of clinical trials, the use of genomic/genetic data and the application of Bayesian methods.

We have now each worked in the industry for over 15 years and have found it an exciting and rewarding area in which to develop a career. This is in part because of the intrinsic interest of the drug development process, seeing your work turn into medicines that meet real patient needs, and also because of the continued growth and change that have taken place in the industry over the last decade. It is an industry that provides the statistician with a broad range of data analysis applications in which to bring alive the statistical methods he has been taught. We would strongly recommend the industry to anyone embarking on a career as an applied statistician, as the challenges of the next decade are likely to present even more opportunities than those of the past decade.

References

ASA Committee on Training of Statisticians for Industry (1980) Preparing statisticians for careers in industry: report of the ASA Section on Statistical Education Committee on Training of Statisticians for Industry. *Am. Statist.*, **34**(2), 65–75.

ICH (1996) E6—Good Clinical Practice. International Conference on Harmonisation.

ICH (1998) E9—Statistical Principles in Clinical Trials. International Conference on Harmonisation.

PSI (2000) Careers for Statisticians within the Pharmaceutical Industry. PSI, Resources for Business, South Park Road, Macclesfield, Cheshire, SK11 6SH.

9

Careers in Data Management

Sheila Varley

Quintiles Ltd, Bracknell, UK

Introduction

Over the last 25 years, data management has become increasingly important to clinical development. There has also been an increase in regulatory requirements for establishing the efficacy and safety of new drugs, and therefore corresponding increases in both the quantity and quality of the required supporting data. Increasing computerisation and improved technological support within the pharmaceutical industry over this time, not only in study analysis but also in the planning, implementation and operation of clinical studies, have enabled review and registration to occur within realistic time limits. In this regard data management has made a significant contribution.

Over the last decade much attention has been given to the use of EDC (Electronic Data Capture) but it has not as yet made a significant difference to the coordination of clinical trials. True process re-engineering is now happening and within the next three to five years the adoption of eClinical processes will see a marked change in the data manager's career paths.

Functions of Data Management

Data management is concerned with all aspects relating to data processing and analysis. Data management has a multifunctional role within the various stages of clinical development, including some if not all of the following.

Review

Data management plays a role in protocol review. Data management reviews tables and listings to assist in clearing the data together with assisting statistical groups to categorise the data and assess patient outcomes.

Careers with the Pharmaceutical Industry, Second edition. Edited by P. D. Stonier.
© 2003 John Wiley & Sons Ltd. ISBN 0 470 84328 4

In addition, data management plays an important role in review of the clinical study report, ensuring consistency and accuracy in study results and conclusions.

Design

Data management plays a key role in the design of the database and case record forms (CRFs) for the clinical study. In association with the quality assurance group, data management is responsible for ensuring consistency between the protocol and CRF, and confirming all matters relating to data format and entry. Data management may also be responsible for organisation of the final printed CRF, ensuring that this is attractive and in logical order for the investigator.

Data processing and analysis

All aspects relating to processing of the clinical study data are the province of data management. These include data coding, entry, validation and verification and transfer of data.

The database is the fundamental clinical data source for registration of a new drug. Therefore, a crucial role for data management is to establish and maintain accurate computer databases for clinical studies, essential to the preparation of final study reports and data summaries for regulatory purposes.

Project management

Project management attempts to minimise any conflict of interests and to achieve reporting of the clinical studies within realistic time limits. Data management plays a key role in coordinating the requirements and priorities of different projects within and between each therapeutic group, with the data management function.

Range of Careers

Data management offers a range of important roles in clinical development and, as a consequence, attracts people from varied backgrounds and with different levels of qualifications. Data management may also offer an attractive alternative for personnel with experience in research, clinical research, quality assurance and auditing, regulatory affairs and information technology who may be looking for a career change. The growing importance of data management within the research and development structure has encouraged movement of personnel with a range of backgrounds.

Careers may range from that of data entry clerk to head or director of a data management department. For the majority of positions some medical and/or computing experience is required; often a degree in life sciences, nursing qualifications or a B-TECH is prerequisite. In addition, the individual needs to show an aptitude for computer work, be very methodical and accurate, and be able to work well both on his or her own and as part of a team involving clinical and statistical personnel.

Considering the different levels at which individuals may become involved in data management gives some idea of the range of careers available. Of course, as with other disciplines within the industry, there is some variation between companies in the job descriptions and responsibilities associated with the different titles.

Individuals with data entry experience and some medical background, such as that provided by medical secretary type experience, and with proven initiative and attention to detail, may consider a position in data entry, as for example a data entry clerk. In this position, the individual would work on his or her own with minimum supervision, entering data rapidly and accurately via a keyboard onto the computer, checking the data and editing any errors.

Those who have achieved GCSEs and have an aptitude for creative design and computer work may consider a role in CRF design, as a CRF designer. Here, the individual would gain experience in desktop publishing software used to design CRF pages, developing a library of standard CRFs to streamline CRF production. The person would need to be able to prioritise work in line with project management decisions within data management. The CRF designer may also be responsible for preparation of the final printed CRFs via liaison with external personnel.

Individuals with a degree or equivalent qualification in the life sciences, or a nursing qualification and with an aptitude for computer work and attention to detail may consider a position as a clinical data coordinator/manager. In this position, the individual would be responsible for the creation, updating, maintenance and validation of clinical study databases and for the provision of computerised reports of these data. Thus the clinical data coordinator is a key member of the clinical project team, and should be able to prioritise work in line with project management decisions. Proven aptitude for this work may lead to career possibilities within clinical operations or within an IT group.

Finally, those with a degree or equivalent computing qualification may consider a position as a programmer. In this position, the individual would be responsible for setting up and maintaining a secure database, and for analysing and reporting the data to specific deadlines. As a prerequisite, the individual would need to be able to work well as part of a team involving both computing and non-computing specialists. An essential component of the majority of positions within data management is the ability to work effectively as part of a multidisciplinary team, involving liaison predominately between clinical operation and statistical personnel. The individual must be able to ensure that other members of the team are able to recognise realistic time constraints involved in his work and to plan for

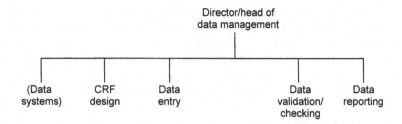

Figure 9.1 Reporting structure within data management: flat management structure

these within the different projects. Thus, communication and assertiveness form a very important characteristic for many of these positions.

Figures 9.1 and 9.2 indicate the interrelationships between these positions. Ultimately, all personnel working within data management will report to the

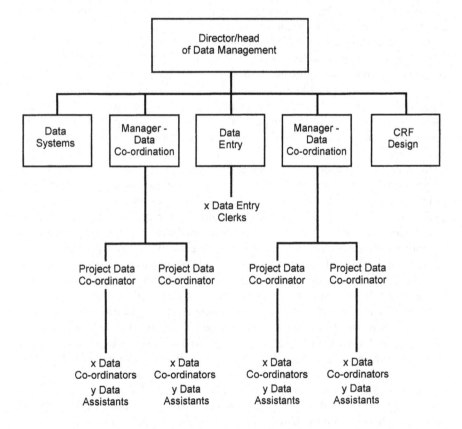

Figure 9.2 Reporting structure within data management: hierarchical management structure

director or head of data management. Depending on the size of the company or the contact research organisation (CRO), there may be either a flat management structure, in which each group reports directly to the head of data management (Figure 9.1), or a more hierarchical structure, in which personnel report to the manager for each group, who in turn reports to the head of data management (Figure 9.2), with the subgroups organised along project therapeutic lines.

Training

As with other disciplines within the industry, training is essential for any data management position. Training is needed to ensure consistency with standard operating procedures, to provide an appropriate understanding of the relevant therapeutic areas, and to provide education in new technologies and various aspects of data management.

Training is given on the job and in external and in-house seminars, courses and meetings. On-the-job training is an essential part of the training process. The individual needs to become familiar with internal operating procedures for coding, review and cleaning of data, and with the required software packages. It is usual for the clinical data coordinator or equivalent positions to play a key role in on-the-job training of new data management personnel.

The individual also needs to gain experience in a range of other subjects. All individuals require understanding of the different functions of data management and of clinical development as a whole entity. A basic understanding of Good Clinical (Research) Practice, the rules governing the conduct of clinical trials, and of quality assurance and audit are also required. In addition, for the majority of positions at least a basic understanding of the therapeutic areas is required. This training may be provided by external courses or by in-house seminars and workshops.

Furthermore, graduate staff may be offered training courses in personnel development, such as project and time management, presentation skills, problem solving and negotiation skills, to further career development.

Career Development

Experience in data management can offer a range of possibilities for career progression within the pharmaceutical industry.

Within data management, many companies offer, or are working towards, parallel career progression. A new graduate may work for two to five years as a data coordinator/monitor/analyst and then may take on additional project and management responsibilities for a number of staff. Training in management skills such as interviewing, counselling, coaching, delegation or people management would enable the individual to advance to a first-line management position at a relatively young age.

Alternatively, staff may decide to specialise in one of the many areas of data management, thereby progressing to a senior level as a sole contributor and being acknowledged for individual technological knowledge. However, progression within data management is not the only career option. Other possibilities include the following:

1. *Clinical research*. Transfer to clinical research, initially as a field monitor, is a popular option. An aptitude for attention to detail and previous nursing experience are very valuable attributes for such a career move. Prior experience of the problems associated with data collation are invaluable to this role. Additional key skills needed here are communication and interpersonal skills as this job involves day-to-day interaction with hospital staff, to track and monitor the recruitment of patients into the clinical study, and subsequent collection and review of the clinical data prior to submission to data management.
2. *Medical writing/regulatory*. Preparation of clinical reports, which involves good writing skills and the ability to interact with others in the team, may make medical writing an attractive option for data management staff. Alternatively, the qualities needed in data management would enable staff to work in a regulatory affairs group where attention to detail is vital.
3. *Quality assurance*. With changes in European regulations governing the conduct and reporting of clinical studies, quality assurance has become a rapidly growing area within the industry. Individuals, who have shown an aptitude for attention to detail within data management, may consider a move to quality assurance.

Characteristics necessary for positions in data management, i.e. an aptitude for attention to detail, accuracy, the ability to work as part of a team with varying experiences, assertiveness and the ability to organise work in accordance with various time schedules, are very much sought after in the range of disciplines within clinical development. Experience in data management therefore provides the individual with considerable flexibility in career progression.

The Future of Data Management

Data management has evolved as an integral and important part of the clinical development structure. Evidence of the dramatic growth in career development in data management is seen by the growth of the Association for Clinical Data Management (ACDM), which has expanded from a membership of 120 in its first year (1987) to over 1700 in 2001.

The growing importance of data management in clinical development has also been reflected in the changing patterns of reporting within companies. In the past data management had usually reported to the head of clinical research, in some cases via statistical groups. However, with recognition of the integral role of data management within clinical development, there has been a trend for a change in reporting structures to allow a direct reporting of the group to the medical director.

Today there is a considerable expansion of the role of data management in clinical development. Technological advances in computerisation, such as optical imaging, object-orientated databases, distributed databases, electronic data transfer from source, and voice and character recognition, mean that future prospects for careers in data management will be particularly bright and offer exciting opportunities.

The next decade will see the decrease of data managers as we know them today and over time the decline and eventual elimination of the data entry clerk role. This will be in line with the evolution of eClinical, where investigators will enter the data directly from their own hospital computer, and instantly perform online validation checks.

This will involve an interim period of data managers acting as advisors/trainers to their clinical counterparts to transfer their skill set to the field/site-based clinical monitors. It will also open up career opportunities for data managers to take on these roles if they wish to live and work near the sites, and have the language skills. New roles will emerge, as specialised data management staff will be needed (though in lesser numbers) to manage the assorted data streams (laboratory data, electronic ECGs, diary data) so that a complete database can be provided to the project statistician. The data manager today will also be well placed to manage data as we enter the genomics era, where we will see specific targeting of patients. This will necessitate the building and maintenance of large databases with sophisticated data mining techniques.

In summary a career in data management can offer the individual a range of benefits that other disciplines within the industry may not or cannot match. In addition, both medical research and technological advances in the coming decades will further enhance the need and future challenges for the data manager.

10
Working in a Contract Research Organisation

Jane Barrett

The Barrett Consultancy, Wokingham, UK

Introduction

Pharmaceutical companies are always under pressure to register and market their new drugs more quickly than their competitors. Changes in regulatory requirements seldom make the process easier or faster, and combinatorial chemistry, high-throughput screening and genomics continually widen the options for drug discovery. The technology of drug development, whilst improvement is sought, remains essentially the same, with an increasing need for manpower. Companies can therefore increase their permanent staff or choose to outsource certain functions of drug development. The original research is usually, though not always, kept firmly within the parent company, but development lends itself to being parcelled up and contracted out, sometimes to one contract research organisation (CRO), but more often to several for the different phases.

A CRO is a company that carries out scientific or medical research on behalf of client companies on a contract basis (other contract organisations provide manufacturing, filling and packing, but I shall not discuss them here). They are paid for the work usually on an item-by-item basis, although there is some evidence that payment by result is increasing, as I will discuss later in this chapter. A CRO may be working on similar drugs for different companies at any one time, and there need to be stringent safeguards to keep confidentiality between the projects and prevent conflict of interest. Because the choice for a pharmaceutical company is to do the work themselves or to outsource it, CROs must compete not only with each other for work but also with their clients, persuading them to give out the contract rather than do it themselves. In order to win this competition there has been much work done within CROs to streamline their processes in order to perfect and sell that elusive fast-track to registration. Whilst at first glance the cost of outsourcing

Careers with the Pharmaceutical Industry, Second edition. Edited by P. D. Stonier.
© 2003 John Wiley & Sons Ltd. ISBN 0 470 84328 4

a project to a CRO seems higher than doing it in-house, the true costs probably differ very little. CRO costing includes the 'invisible' costs of running a company that are never seen when a pharmaceutical company estimates their own costs. When the exercise is done to compare like with like, all observers agree that the cost differences are negligible.

CROs are a phenomenon of the mid-1980s and early 1990s. Many of them started as single consultants with a background of working within or consulting for the pharmaceutical industry. These innovators saw the need to provide additional resource to the industry and so recruited first a few, then many to help them provide it. The largest CROs today count their staff in tens of thousands, and are often larger than their client companies. Their growth in the mid-1990s was extraordinary, with the bigger companies acquiring their smaller, and sometimes not so small, competitors. Latest figures show nearly 23 000 staff in European clinical CROs and over 16 000 in pre-clinical. Equivalent figures for North America are 31 000 and 24 000 respectively (Hughes and O'Neill, 2001). There are currently over 400 clinical CROs in Europe and almost 300 in North America. The number in Japan, which has only relatively recently started using CROs, is much smaller but growing.

Today CROs can offer experience and capacity in every stage of drug development from pharmaceutical development to licensing. Some also offer sales and marketing capability, so a pharmaceutical company can effectively be 'virtual' using CROs. It is estimated that by 2002 the total expenditure on outsourcing work to CROs will be US$9.4bn, with 80% growth over 1997 figures predicted for clinical and regulatory (CMR International, 1999).

Roles and Responsibilities

Table 10.1 shows the distribution of some jobs in the CRO industry. Because the CRO provides resource to replace or enhance the functions of staff in a pharmaceutical company, the departments and roles within it will be similar. Some CROs specialise and have expertise in just one department; others have several or many.

Table 10.1 Staffing levels in clinical development

	Europe	North America
Phase I physicians	330	129
Phase II–IV physicians	594	1779
Full-time CRAs	2921	2636
Full-time statisticians	573	716
Full-time programmers	489	1492
Regulatory staff	1091	638
QA staff	652	624

Source: Adapted from Hughes and O'Neill (2001).

As a sweeping generalisation the more junior jobs will feel very much the same in a CRO or in a pharmaceutical company. In a CRO they will be protected from client interaction, so will work within their teams in an orthodox way. The more senior staff however have the added dimension of dealing with clients.

When the CRO phenomenon began, clients had little idea of how to outsource the work that they wanted done. They would choose a CRO and give them the outline of what needed to be achieved, but neither party understood at that time that a very detailed project plan was required. Too often assumptions were made that there was only one way to achieve the goal, which led to conflict when the CRO followed another route or even arrived at another goal altogether. Responsibilities were also sometimes not clearly defined, leading to a task being done by both parties or by neither. The introduction of departments of outsourcing professionals improved this situation beyond recognition, and although it adds considerably to the start-up time of an outsourced project, it has reduced even more considerably the scope for misunderstanding and conflict.

An important role for the more senior staff members of a CRO is the provision of advice to client companies. It is for this reason that I would not recommend a CRO as a first industry job for certain specialties, such as physicians. Customer companies often approach a CRO for expertise in drug development or licensing strategy on the assumption that the CRO will be able to provide someone with more knowledge on the subject than they have themselves. To be always slightly out of one's depth when giving advice is stressful and not helpful to anyone as wrong advice can have major implications of cost and time in drug development.

One of the greatest differences between CROs and pharmaceutical companies is the role of the full-time project manager. Within a CRO they are usually senior and experienced clinical research professionals, handling a project budget that is often more than the annual turnover of a small company. They have responsibility for the successful completion of the project in terms of time, cost and quality, be it a specific part of a study or a whole drug development. They therefore have significant power but are also at the forefront if anything goes badly. The project manager often has staff from several departments reporting to him or her, so-called matrix management. Matrix management, where staff report both within their own departments and across departments on a project is much loved by CROs, but nobody claims it is easy to handle as conflict of interest and priority continuously threaten it.

Education and Qualifications

Because there are so many different roles in the CRO industry, there is room for a huge variety of educational backgrounds. That said, the professional staff are often some of the best qualified in the industry, with PhDs and other postgraduate qualifications being very frequent. The most senior staff, in particular, who are usually recruited by direct approach rather than through advertisements, are some of the best qualified in terms of experience and credentials.

Skills and personal attributes

Having an employing client does add another dimension to working in the pharmaceutical industry. If the project is going well and on time, life in a CRO is smooth. But if problems arise, for example patient recruitment is slow or the data need more cleaning before analysis, then it can all too easily be seen as the fault of the CRO and a scapegoat is sought. These days one sees fewer of the unrealistic timeframes formerly insisted on by clients, and less too of the over-enthusiastic estimates of speed of delivery by CROs. However I would still count tact and diplomacy as essential skills for a successful player in the CRO industry. One of the biggest challenges is to reassure companies that they still 'own' the drug and that the CRO does not now know more about it than they do.

One element that is constant in the CRO industry is ambiguity. One can spend much time and effort, even to the extent of travelling half-way round the world, to 'pitch' for a project. The chances of being awarded any one project vary, but can be as little as 1 in 10. Clearly one cannot wait to hear if a particular project has been won before pitching for the next, so it is impossible to know whether the CRO will be fully busy, under-utilised or significantly over-stretched one or six months down the line. When the award is given, it is usually expected that work will begin at once, despite the fact that key staff may not have finished a previous project. For this reason I always warn interview candidates that if they have problems with handling ambiguity life in a CRO is not for them!

Having worked in pharmaceutical companies at different levels and in a large CRO at a time of rapid growth, I believe that the speed of working and the accompanying pressures are considerably greater in a CRO. The rewards though are proportionately higher, and by that I do not mean financial, as salaries tend to be lower in CROs too (British Association of Pharmaceutical Physicians, 2001). There are often less politics in a CRO, though naturally that will vary, but the sense that the whole company is working on clinical trials is very supportive. In a pharmaceutical company the clinical trials group is often seen as spending money but not producing income. It is accepted that research is necessary to obtain a product licence and to provide up-to-date material for the sales and marketing groups to use, but it does not contribute visibly to the bottom line and, in addition, appears to take forever!

Coupled with the less competitive salaries is a greater focus on internal costs. Most CROs do not subsidise the level of comfort in travel accepted as normal in a pharmaceutical company. For example, the company car policy may mean taking a smaller car if moving from a multinational pharmaceutical company. This is a combination of good housekeeping and perceptions: if a potential client sees the team from the CRO coming to pitch for work in cars better than their own, an inevitable conclusion is 'so that's where the huge fee goes'. This despite the evidence as discussed above that costs do not really differ whether work is done internally or outsourced.

Training

All CROs today take training very seriously, the bigger ones having training departments of significant size and even offer professional training to pharmaceutical companies. Some train staff for which they do not yet have work available and call them in when a project is awarded. Having worked in both pharmaceutical companies and a CRO I should have to say that the on-the-job training given by the pharmaceutical companies tends to be more easily paced and gently nurturing than that in a CRO, where there can be a faster expectation of the time it takes to get a new member of staff up and running. This style of learning suits many people better than the more leisurely parental style; those who wish to race ahead may find the pace of life in a CRO more suited to them.

Continuous training is very much endorsed by CROs as it is by pharmaceutical companies, but project deadlines are perhaps more strongly felt and are less avoidable in a CRO than in a pharmaceutical company. If the project manager is under pressure to complete recruitment or finish data entry and lock the database, he or she is less likely to be sympathetic to project staff disappearing on training courses, however long ago they were booked. This is unfortunately a fact of life in a CRO; training may be booked more than once before it is received.

Career Pathways

Because of the more dynamic and rapidly changing manner of life in a CRO, the chances for rapid advancement are also great. For example, a large CRO will have many opportunities for staff to change therapeutic area. Such a company will be conducting studies in many different therapeutic areas (true and absolute therapeutic specialisation is rare), giving a clinical research associate, for example, the opportunity to move into new areas. By contrast, in a pharmaceutical company the number of therapeutic areas will be limited and staff can get locked into just one narrow field. Much is dependent on the size of the CRO and its state of growth. To join at a time of rapid growth can also mean rapid personal growth: a company usually prefers to promote someone whose track record is known at such sensitive times.

CROs are perhaps less rigid about always matching background to job description. They tend to be more entrepreneurial than pharmaceutical companies, so are more likely to allow someone with a background, say, in data management to head up clinical operations if that person has the desired skills for the job. Project managers come from many different backgrounds, their common attributes being attention to detail and management skills. Therefore career development and choice of pathways can be much wider than in a pharmaceutical company. On the downside (or upside, depending on your view), those who do not pull their weight will always be identified faster in a CRO.

Many who have previously worked for a CRO have found roles in pharmaceutical companies working in outsourcing management groups, either deciding what to outsource, or to whom. Knowledge gained on one side of the fence can be very valuable to those on the other side—a variation on 'poacher turned gamekeeper'! Client companies are also often guilty of being poachers themselves and tempting away good staff who have worked on their projects. This is a recognised hazard for CROs and many therefore have a policy of applying a transfer fee like a football club. However, working with several different client companies also allows CRO staff to sample life in other companies and so draw up lists of those they would and would not like to work for in the future. So the benefit of 'trying before you buy' is available both to employer and employee.

The Future

CROs are beginning to be used not just as spare manpower in emergencies or as a deliberate policy to allow companies to resource with permanent staff only for the troughs of activity. Some of the larger CROs are entering into risk-sharing agreements with their clients. Thus payment is made by milestone rather than by task. If a milestone is reached early, the fee is larger, if late, then smaller. These contracts typically allow the CRO more leeway on process; the focus is on a goal, not on the route of achieving it. The CRO can then concentrate on improving process and developing innovative ideas such as remote data capture, while the client company focuses on discovery and develops outsourcing skills as a core competency. Observers of the field predict that the major CROs will carry out full drug development on some drugs with some clients, the relationship with whom will become more that of partners than master and servant.

Despite the growth of CROs, they are not a more secure workplace than a pharmaceutical company. Perhaps as a result of too rapid growth in the 1990s many companies of all sizes have been reducing staff numbers in recent years. The claim is usually that this is to rationalise staffing levels and represents improved and more efficient processes internally. The fact is that the days of a job for life are no longer with us; any employment in any sector (except perhaps the NHS) should be regarded as potentially under threat of redundancy. The CRO sector of the industry is probably no worse than any other, and indeed in 2000 increased the total numbers of its clinical staff in Europe by 11%, and pre-clinical staff by 27%. In North America, however, clinical numbers were static and pre-clinical numbers dropped by 7% (Hughes and O'Neill, 2001).

References

British Association of Pharmaceutical Physicians (2001) Salary survey 2001. *Pharmaceut. Physician*, **December**.

CMR International (1999) Outsourcing in operation: contracting out pharmaceutical R&D. *R&D Briefing*, **20**(February).

Hughes, R.G. and O'Neill, M. (2001) The worldwide CRO scene in 2001. *Eur. Pharmaceut. Contract.*, **February**.

Further Reading

Hughes, R.G. and Lumley, C.E. (eds) (2000) *Current Strategies and Future Prospects in Pharmaceutical Outsourcing*, Technomark Consulting Services & CMR International.

Useful Websites

Centre for Medicines Research International; www.cmr.org

European Pharmaceutical Contractor; www.samedanltd.com/publications/epc/epc.htm

Technomark Registers: find CROs who fulfil certain functions; www.technomarkregisters.com/technomark

PART III

CAREERS IN SALES AND MARKETING

Careers with the Pharmaceutical Industry, Second edition. Edited by P. D. Stonier.
© 2003 John Wiley & Sons Ltd. ISBN 0 470 84328 4

11
A Career in Product Management

Roy Carlisle
PharmaSolutions Ltd, Bourne End, UK

Introduction

What is marketing?

Well, to handle immediately one of the more common misunderstandings, marketing isn't just a slick word for selling (although selling can be described as the 'active arm of marketing'), backed up by the production of some selling brochures and a few advertisements. Marketing is really about the whole business, or in the words of the Chartered Institute of Marketing, 'Marketing is Business'. This definition helps to underscore the concept that marketing encompasses *all* the activities in the business, from research and development, clinical trials, manufacture, regulatory affairs, medical and business information, even supply chain management to the promotional activities and tools which some would traditionally call 'marketing'. Key to this is the integration of all these activities into a coherent strategy with a tactical implementation plan, which will be used to first launch and then grow a product, designed to achieve the company's commercial objectives.

Marketing's very multi-faceted nature does mean that a career in this area will be equally varied, interesting, absorbing, dynamic and a wonderful opportunity for career progression. As these activities need a focal point, the person to take responsibility plus accountability for their delivery and the ultimate achievement of commercial objectives is the pharma product or brand manager. By way of clarifying the nomenclature, the term 'brand manager' is often substituted for 'product' as the concept of brand development, which is widely used in consumer marketing, has come back into vogue in pharma marketing. This reflects, after Stephen King in *Developing New Brands,* that 'A product is something made in a factory, a brand is

---

Careers with the Pharmaceutical Industry, Second edition. Edited by P. D. Stonier.
© 2003 John Wiley & Sons Ltd. ISBN 0 470 84328 4

something that you buy'. Or in the words of Sergio Zyman in *The End of Marketing as We Know It*, 'The name, the expectation, the distinction—that's branding'.

The concept of buying a product because of its intrinsic value or what it contains and its extrinsic value or what it does, or what we think it does, comprises the 'brand value'. The application of these principles, despite an increasingly complex customer decision-making and buying process, is as true in the pharmaceutical market place as anywhere else. Hence, the trend to call those responsible for marketing 'brand manager' is more than a name change; it represents a different philosophy of business, one that it more market-orientated or market-aligned than perhaps some of the industry has been in the past.

So in summary, the brand manager is at the heart of a dynamic and exciting marketing process and is charged with making a significant contribution to the company's growth and commercial success. In essence, the brand manager has the responsibility, either individually or as part of a 'brand team', for everything to do with marketing and developing the brand and generating sales in the form of selling packs of pharmaceuticals, which are then dispensed to fill patient prescriptions.

The target audience is then, of course firstly, the traditional one of healthcare professionals such as doctors, pharmacists and nurses in both the primary and secondary care environment. Secondly, however, changes in healthcare structures in Europe and particularly in the UK mean that the buying/influence chain is more complex and the brand manager now has to be more sophisticated with a more diverse skill set than ever before. For instance, additional but crucially important customers at a higher level now have to be considered, including the government itself, the NHS at national and regional level, the Commission for Health Improvement, the National Institute for Clinical Excellence, the new Strategic Health Authorities, Primary Care Trusts, bodies representing healthcare professionals, patients and carers. All of these will have a major part to play in determining the future commercial success of existing and newly introduced drugs. It is fair to say that the modern brand manager has to be prepared for a challenge!

An essential skill is the ability to segment or split up the market to ensure that the most appropriate key brand messages reach these diverse groups in an integrated and consistent manner. We will see in the sections below how a brand management career can be secured, details of what the job can entail, how the role fits into the organisation, and finally how, once the brand manager has delivered on objectives, their career can be developed.

The key personal attributes required seem to vary from place to place but the most common include that the individual should be strategic, tactical, hard working, tenacious, tough, resolute, a good team worker, have good interpersonal skills, be able to prioritise, be analytical, creative, have a high sense of commercial awareness, be outgoing and demonstrate a high level of presentation skills. Without wishing to 'over-egg the pudding', it could be said that sometimes the frenetic pace of life as a brand manager can, in a stressed moment, make the job-holder wonder with all these expectations if the only requirement for the position should be the ability to don a red cape, wear your underwear outside a blue body suit, and rescue distressed people from burning buildings! But then, Clark Kent only did the Superman thing in his spare time; something the dedicated brand manager will find in short supply.

The Product/Brand Manager Career

How to get a job as a product/brand manager

So having outlined the positive side of brand management, the dynamic nature of being at the 'cutting edge' and the potential negative, for some, that this is most certainly not a '9 to 5' role, how can you get the job?

Most individuals move into brand/product management usually after a period, probably at least two to three years, in a number of senior sales roles, perhaps after having been a regional therapy specialist or having worked on some marketing projects. In most instances, having been identified through the company's appraisal/personal development process as a potential marketer, the aspiring brand manager will have to participate in an assessment centre. Having cleared this hurdle, they will be appointed as a brand manager or in some circumstances as an assistant brand/product manager or a marketing assistant/executive dependent on the opportunity or the marketing departmental structure which is in force at the time.

There is also the role of marketing trainee as well in some organisations, which is a junior position typically filled by those who have joined the company straight from university or on a company fast-track commercial trainee scheme. These individuals will then go out into the sales force, before coming back into the office as described above.

Occasionally, experienced brand marketers from outside the industry join at brand manager level but this does not tend to be that common, despite the fact that similar marketing tools are deployed. The prevailing view is that the appropriate restrictions on marketing such as the guidelines contained in the Pharmaceutical Industry Code of Practice and legislation such as the Medicines Act mean that it is better to have 'home-grown' marketers who understand the environment.

Alternative routes to brand management can be via first-line sales management, with a number of companies having policies of opening up opportunities for cross-fertilisation between marketing and sales. Indeed, this occasionally extends to providing marketing opportunities for suitable individuals from key accounts, NHS liaison or clinical liaison teams.

Finally, in terms of qualifications, it is likely that the brand manager will be a graduate, most probably in life sciences, although other disciplines are considered. As part of career planning en route to achieving the brand/product management position, it is worthwhile taking the Chartered Institute of Marketing Diploma in

Marketing, part time at a local university or college (although some pharmaceutical marketing-specific courses are currently being mooted). A Master of Business Administration (MBA), although beneficial for more senior roles, is probably 'overkill' for a first-line marketing role and best left until some marketing/business management experience has been gained.

The Details of the Brand/Product Manager Role

So we have outlined marketing, the brand manager role and how to secure the position. But what does the brand manager do on a day-to-day basis?

Although there are some opportunities to go to nice places and meet interesting people and customers, it is not all champagne and roses! At a strategic level there is a lot of hard graft analysing/segmenting markets to find out where the differential opportunities may be to ensure that 'the right message gets to the right target customer in the right place at the right time'. In other words, the brand manager has to be able to answer the questions, 'Are we aiming our brand offering to the customers who are most likely to need it, understand its benefits and then use it, via the most relevant (and sometimes creative) communication channels? Who or what else will have an influence?'

A key part of the brand manager's planning and desk market research will also involve competitor analysis to gain a firm handle on how our brand can be positioned more attractively through gaining an understanding of which attributes make competitor offerings successful in the market. Tracking market trends in terms of new product introductions and treatment or prescribing guidelines, which are produced by healthcare professional and government bodies and have a major influence, is a key part of the brand manager's remit. The objective is to ensure that brand strategy is market-aligned to maximise competitive advantage and that appropriate contingency plans are in place. This means that building detailed market models using the audits, primary and secondary research plus the assumptions of future trends and competitive analyses discussed above is the major plank of the brand manager's marketing plan. Other key components of the brand manager's plan will include developing the most suitable market positioning/platform for the brand in the therapeutic area plus working with clinical liaison/medical departments to ensure that the appropriate clinical trials needed to secure additional indications are in place.

Having written the short/medium/long-term plans, the last part of the strategic process is their presentation by the brand manager and his colleagues on the brand team, to the senior managers and directors on the company's board. This is the normal process by which senior management can scrutinise and approve the marketing plan. It has to be said that if there is one occasion in the brand manager's year that can have a significant impact on career development, it is this plan presentation! It can be akin to being 'Daniel in the lion's den', but clear analyses, strategic thinking and tactical recommendations in the plan will lead to a good impression which can only enhance career prospects. Needless to say, if the thinking, creativity and action plans do not 'hang together' logically, the reverse may be true!

Aside from strategic planning, an important part of the brand manager's role is to become the company expert, or part of a team of experts, in the therapeutic area in question, through developing a level of knowledge as good as the external key opinion leaders. The clear advantage of being an 'expert' brand manager is that by having such a high-level understanding of the clinical market drivers, better marketing practice and commercial success will result. Indeed, the best brand managers develop the ability to tailor their strategy, tactics, messages and communication vehicles in response to environmental changes without compromising core brand values.

Part of the ongoing strategic planning is working in partnership with the medical department to agree key claims for the drug to ensure that all marketing activity complies with promotional regulations. So having looked at the strategic responsibilities of the brand manager, let's look at the tactical side of the job. This includes the following activities:

- Writing the tactical promotional plan otherwise known as 'the campaign' and then managing every aspect of its implementation.
- Part of the ongoing work is continual liaison with a number of departments including sales force, medical, medical information, regulatory affairs, clinical development and business information.
- Furthermore, there may be a need to liaise with the factory to help production scheduling for the product and all its various presentations. The big picture issue here is that of ensuring that supply meets demand and that sufficient packs are available to meet the projected growth. The converse is that if too much product is produced, ultimately it will have to be written off and will be cross-charged to the product budget as a loss against sales.
- Without doubt, the brand manager may have to manage a large promotional budget to fund the campaign. The key requirement here will be to work with the finance department to ensure that the spending is tracked and stays within agreed levels. The key tactical consideration is to think about the phasing, or how quickly the money will be spent during the year. For example, ensuring that sufficient funds are available to support the launch of any new indications or presentations, or to maintain or raise 'noise levels' at times of competitor activity or environmental turbulence.
- The campaign's brand values should be consistent and must be reflected in any journal advertising for which the brand manager may be responsible. Liaison with media scheduling companies to ensure that any ad insertions are in the best positions in the most appropriate journals is another brand management task.
- A very important part of ensuring consistent communication of the brand message by the sales force is the production of sales force support materials such as sales aids, mailings, leave pieces, give aways, product monographs plus

formulary packs. An excellent relationship with the sales force is essential to show a brand team support for their activity.

- The brand manager should have open lines of communication to the sales team, including chairing representative feedback panels, to receive campaign feedback as well as planning several field visits with the sales team to observe customer reaction to the marketing effort first-hand.

- Presenting the ongoing brand campaign plans to the sales force at conference is another vital communication vehicle. Thus an ability in public speaking is helpful, and most companies do give coaching in this area.

- Good knowledge of the Pharmaceutical Industry Code of Practice guidelines is needed to ensure compliance and manage promotional materials smoothly through the company's internal copy approval process.

- Given the complexity of the campaign, the brand manager will often have to choose and then manage external specialist communication agencies such as those delivering advertising, public relations, medical education, government affairs, media scheduling and print. Regular review meetings with these suppliers are necessary to ensure that they understand the campaign objectives and can add value as part of the 'virtual brand team'. The brand manager will have to ensure that the work is delivered on time and within budget. Occasionally, a fresh approach may be merited and the brand manager will have to conduct a 'pitch process' for a new agency.

- As part of becoming the internal expert and maintaining a market and competitor awareness, there may be the need to attend key international symposia relating to the therapeutic/disease area. Often the global company will organise a 'satellite symposium', alongside the main meeting to raise awareness of the disease area and the clinical evidence for the company's products. The brand manager may have a more active role to play in that key opinion leaders or those who are trialists of the company's new drugs, and who are the brand manager's contacts, may be speaking at the meeting or may be sponsored via an educational grant. The brand manager may thus have customers to host at the meeting and play the role of company representative.

- Alongside the other aspects of the co-ordinated campaign, there may be responsibility for managing market development/market shaping projects with some specialist agencies. Again this is all about communication, in this instance usually focusing on new needs for treatment, presenting the positive clinical evidence for changing prescribing guidelines due to, for example, better regimens now being available.

- Dependent on the role, the size of company and the mix of brands within the portfolio, the brand manager can have responsibility for dealing with commercial deals for off-patent products, although this is usually specialised within a key accounts/commercial function in larger companies.

- Last but not least, the brand manager may also interact with patient and carer groups as well as following the traditional route of building up a personal network of key opinion leaders within the therapeutic area.

The brand manager's tactical success, as well as producing the appropriate strategic thinking mentioned above, will be measured on parameters such as hitting sales targets, growing market share, customer recall of key communication messages, strength and recall of the campaign, both internal and external, overall campaign co-ordination and feedback from the other teams with which the brand manager interacts.

The Brand/Product Manager's Fit in the Organisation

We have discussed the many facets of the brand manager's role, but the extent to which an individual will become involved in some specific issues will very much depend upon the size and structure of the company. For example in a small company, with one or two brands, the brand manager may well do everything in great depth, for both brands. In a larger company, with many brands and a diverse brand portfolio, the brand manager may have responsibility for specific tasks, for example, one particular brand in the portfolio or the primary care environment or hospital market within a bigger brand.

On average, the brand manager will be in a brand team of around four marketers, which can be as high as eight for some 'mega' brands. There is likely to be another brand manager perhaps with responsibility for say the secondary care market, or another brand plus a senior brand manager or brand team leader who has managerial responsibility for the brand managers, reporting into a marketing manager. Sometimes, there is a market development manager who specialises in the market-shaping activities mentioned above, by running market educational programmes, key opinion leader advisory boards and increasingly, NHS liaison for the area. Some companies have regional product specialists in the sales team who have a dotted line report into the brand manager. In larger companies, the marketing manager may have several teams reporting to him or her, in which case the brand manager may be part of a larger team covering all the brands in, say, the 'respiratory portfolio'.

Career Progression

Obviously the successful first-line brand manager will have a very rounded understanding of pharma marketing and the key drivers and processes at both a strategic and tactical level. Having developed the key elements of the skill set, the world really is the brand manager's oyster! The logical career development routes include moving to a brand manager on a bigger brand which has greater company-wide focus, and with it the potential for positive personal exposure. Clearly, promotion to a market development manager, senior product manager and then marketing manager are the next steps for those set on a full marketing career.

Alternatively, the brand manager may choose, and indeed many companies encourage, a spell back into the field as a first-line sales manager such as a regional business manager (RBM). This can be a very beneficial step, firstly as it develops the individual's understanding and experience of the pharma selling business management process and secondly as it provides the opportunity to develop the vital man-management skills needed for further career progression, for example, moving back into marketing in the role of brand team leader.

Other next moves from brand manager could be into 'key accounts' or NHS liaison as alternatives to the RBM role. A very attractive option may be a posting into international/global marketing, which would give a much wider experience of the business and could provide a broader base for the next career step. Sometimes assignments to overseas affiliates or to corporate headquarters become available, with obvious opportunities for career enhancement, although usually these tend to be filled more often than not by more senior personnel such as marketing managers.

Conclusion

Brand/product management is one of the most diverse roles in the industry. It can be stimulating, dynamic and interesting, but it can also carry a massive workload and the frustration of being the focal point for a number of activities and inter-departmental interfaces. So why would you want to do it?

Well apart from the obvious challenge, to make a significant contribution to the company's commercial success or to help your medicine make a real difference in the community, if you want a route to the top, there is hardly a general manager in the industry who hasn't moved up the corporate ladder via brand management in increasingly senior roles. And you can't say fairer than that!

References

King, S. (1973) *Developing New Brands*, Pitman.

Zyman, S. (1999) *The End of Marketing as We Know It*, HarperCollins Business.

12

A Career in Medical Sales and Medical Sales Management

Roy Carlisle

PharmaSolutions Ltd, Bourne End, UK

Introduction

In a properly integrated commercial operation, sales is the active arm of marketing, the 'coal face' where daily contact and interaction takes place between the company which is selling its products and the customers, often called the 'target audience', when they have been accurately profiled. This chapter concentrates on pharmaceutical selling, both at the level of the sales representative and the sales manager. But what is selling anyway?

Well, we all sell in everyday life when we try to promote our ideas or opinions, or when we try to persuade friends to go to, say, a particular restaurant or event. In the commercial setting, selling in its simplest form involves finding out what people or, in this case, customers want or need and then showing them how to fulfil those needs with the benefits associated with our product's offering. Good sales people use a framework for their discussions with customers, using one of a number of selling systems, each of which has broadly similar objectives. This involves directing the sales communication towards either fulfilling a need of which customers are already aware, or questioning them around their current usage or habits to present them with evidence that our product represents an improvement. The final step is to gain the customer's agreement to buy/use what we are selling, by 'closing', which means asking them for a commitment to buy the idea, brand or product.

So why do we need selling in the pharmaceutical industry, where the sales people, usually called medical representatives, are trying to communicate to healthcare professionals the benefits of ethical pharmaceutical products? After all, it is well known that appropriately prescribed drugs will positively affect the treatment of disease. Shouldn't good drugs, assuming that they have the relevant indications and fulfil the criteria of 'evidence-based medicine', including 'well-powered' clinical

Careers with the Pharmaceutical Industry, Second edition. Edited by P. D. Stonier.
© 2003 John Wiley & Sons Ltd. ISBN 0 470 84328 4

trials which demonstrate efficacy, low side effect profiles and robust pharmaco-economic arguments, sell themselves? Well, no not quite!

Clinical trials do provide the data to obtain the product licence and are then used in conjunction with marketing tools such as peer reviewed publications, advertising, mailing and medical education to build awareness of the product as a brand. However, it is the interaction of face-to-face sales calls which has the biggest impact by enabling the healthcare professional customer to discuss and then be convinced by the evidence for the brand's benefits. Taking an analogy, in today's environment, we all know people who have purchased a car over the Internet or have used third-party evidence or reviews in a journal to assist their choice. However, we can be pretty sure that a significant proportion of potential buyers will have gone to a car showroom to get a sales person to 'take them through it', whether or not they ultimately buy on-line or at the showroom.

In pharmaceutical selling, the same principles hold, even though both the offering, prescription medicines, and the primary target audience or healthcare professionals, doctors, pharmacists and nurses, are more sophisticated. Furthermore, with the largest companies having up to 1000 representatives, often supplemented with additional temporary sales teams provided by contract sales organisations at the time of product launch or high competitor activity, the sales force represents both a major investment and one of the key means to ensuring 'marketing muscle' behind major products.

With the commitment to such a large resource, it is important that the team is well led, motivated and managed towards consistent communication of brand messages, which is why there is a need for first, second, and even third-line levels of sales management, all of whom usually and indeed should have come through the sales force, although spells in product marketing in between are quite common.

Having outlined a definition of selling and its relevance as part of the pharmaceutical marketing mix, let's look at what it means to have a career as a medical sales representative and their bosses, the pharmaceutical sales managers. It is assumed that the reader is seeking a career within the UK, but the general principles hold in other markets.

The Medical Representative Career

How to get a job as a medical representative

Most new entrants into the role are usually life science graduates (although other disciplines such as social sciences are not unknown), or teachers, nurses and other paramedics, with the key criteria being an ability to absorb clinical and pharmaceutical information, in conjunction with the highly developed interpersonal skills and attributes needed to sell. Having said that, some companies place more emphasis on a sales track record than a university education, which provides another entry route, meaning that often those who have sold confectionery, groceries or even double glazing have, after the relevant clinical training, become successful medical representatives.

Overall, first impressions do count, especially in a selling environment, where you have to strike an immediate rapport with a total stranger and sell them your offering in a very short space of time. The first adage of selling is that 'If you can't sell yourself, you can't sell anything'. So the first hurdle to clear en route to a medical selling career will be the job interview. But how do you get that interview?

The best way to secure an interview with a pharmaceutical company is to register with one of the specialist sales recruitment agencies who, if in the UK, tend to advertise generally or on behalf of specific companies in the *Daily Telegraph*, or are listed in pharmaceutical trade magazines. Another approach could be to write to the companies directly. Yet another route is to register with some of the contract sales organisations (CSOs) that supply the contract sales teams to pharmaceutical companies to supplement in-house teams. CSOs can offer the opportunity to work on a number of projects for different companies and the advantage here is that the successful contract representative can often transfer into the company's team once the project is completed. Increasingly, some medical sales staff enjoy the variety and stay with the CSO.

But going back to the interview, a good tip is obviously to research the company, or the CSO, and its products. You could try to find a friendly medical representative, and see if you can spend a day with them to see the job at first hand. This tactic will certainly help you decide if medical selling is your best career choice and will enable you to talk with some knowledge about the job at interview. At the interview, you will need to demonstrate why the company should 'buy' you and also be prepared to take psychometric, verbal and numerical tests.

Assuming that you have successfully completed the interview process, which could involve several meetings, including a selection centre, you will be placed on an initial training programme. This can last up to six months with a mix of continuously assessed, in-house training on disease areas and products plus field training. You will also be required to take and pass the Association of the British Pharmaceutical Industry (ABPI) Medical Representative's Examination within two years of entering the industry. Most companies provide coaching and support for this mandatory industry qualification and if you put in the work, you will almost certainly be successful.

So we now have an idea of how to get the job and the training and qualifications needed. But what does it really entail?

The medical representative role

However it is dressed up, the key role of the medical sales representative is to sell. This means that the representative has to visit or 'call on' doctors at their place of work, whether at a general practice surgery or at a hospital. To avoid any doubt, it is worth stating what the job is *not* about.

It is not 'medical information' or 'clinical liaison', which are important roles provided by highly professional teams in other pharmaceutical company departments. Also, the term 'representative' can be a misnomer or even confusing, so let's be clear, this does not mean that you would be an agent or some sort of company spokesperson.

To reiterate, the core job responsibility is to sell the company's products using selling skills to communicate the core brand marketing messages to healthcare professionals including doctors, pharmacists, nurses and NHS managers. The key objective is growth in patient prescriptions from the initial, and then ongoing, baseline. While this may be obvious, it is important to state the requirement to be able to sell up-front, as the key measure of success of a medical sales representative is achieving, or even better surpassing, sales targets.

In essence, the medical sales representative is used to 'personalise the offering' by building on the doctor's knowledge or awareness of the drug, arising from the rest of the marketing mix such as advertising and medical education. In a call, the usual approach involves finding out the individual doctor's prescribing needs for his or her patients, selling the benefits of the drug in satisfying those needs, for example, by showing how there may be improvements such as increased efficacy or a lower side-effect profile over existing therapies, which normally includes presenting the clinical trial evidence for the drug's claims. The discussion may then involve handling any misunderstandings or objections that the doctor may have to the drug by clarifying the issues and then by offering more evidence on the spot, or by asking the company's medical information department to contact the doctor with more data, which then becomes the objective of a follow-up call. Once it appears that the doctor is interested and has perhaps given a 'buying signal', the final part of the process is 'closing' or asking for a commitment from the doctor to use the drug in appropriate (licensed) indications in future patients. Without the commitment, there is no business.

Hence, 'be for ever closing', or 'ask for the business' are the sales manager's adages when training sales personnel in the art of selling. The complication is that unlike consumer selling, medical representatives make the selling case within the ethical regulations of the Pharmaceutical Industry's Code of Practice, which is only right, as any information imparted could influence patient treatment, although this is almost universally to their benefit. So this makes the medical sales career much more ethical than selling in some other industries, where 'over-claiming' or overstating product benefits can be commonplace.

Specialist medical representatives increasingly have to make the financial case to the 'payers' who fund the use of the drugs, such as ultimately the NHS and its hospitals and Primary Care Trusts in the UK or insurance funds or healthcare benefit providers in other countries. Indeed, this is another reason why a higher level of intellect and integrity is required in the pharmaceutical representative and amongst the sales managers who are needed to lead, motivate and manage the sales teams towards the achievement of their sales targets.

The medical representative's commercial responsibility

Typically, the medical sales person will first work as a 'GP rep' having a geographical area called the 'territory', containing around 200 to 300 GPs and perhaps one or two hospitals, plus a number of retail chemists and wholesalers, although this traditional model is changing (see below). Dependent on company size, the representative may be co-promoting with a territory partner who may either have responsibility for selling one or more of the same drugs to maximise the 'noise level' or who may have different drugs to sell. The commercial responsibility can be that of growing sales on a base of hundreds of thousands of pounds of existing business.

In terms of customers, most of the doctors are seen by appointment, which may be running several months or (years) in advance, although a decreasing number will see representatives on a first-come, first-served or 'speculative' basis. Contact with difficult-to-see customers can be achieved at lunchtime or evening meetings, with a meeting expenses budget being allocated to and managed by the individual representative. Dependent on the specific role, there may be a requirement to call into local hospitals to sell the products discussed in primary care to the consultant-led teams and pharmacy. Larger teaching hospitals are usually handled by specialist, and more experienced, teams of hospital representatives who sell the more hospital-specific products such as those for oncology. Retail chemists are typically visited to check the current level of prescriptions being received for the company's brands and to ask for a commitment to maintain a stock of the products on promotion.

Clearly good diary management and matching activity to areas of highest sales potential are crucial. This is usually facilitated by the Electronic Territory Management System (ETMS), which is software contained on notebook PCs and enables activity and sales reports to be transmitted to the sales manager and to head office.

The medical representative's position in the organisation

Typically, the medical representative will report to a first-line sales manager, such as the regional business manager (RBM), and will be part of a team of between eight and 12 representatives. The RBM will either report to the regional director or national sales director, dependent on company size, who will head a team of around 100 sales professionals.

Career development within the medical representative role

Having focused on the entry point, the GP representative, it is worth pointing out that there are many roles within primary care, hospitals, key accounts and a number of other roles which are emerging as the healthcare environment continues to evolve. These provide excellent opportunities for career development. Indeed over the next few years, it is reasonable to predict that the balance will shift meaning that there will be fewer 'generalists' calling in a traditional way on GPs and more specialists, with remits more closely aligned to the newer customer structures. Currently, however, the successful GP representative's first promotion may be to the position of hospital representative.

The hospital representative often has the responsibility for both gaining sales of specialist hospital-only products into the hospital and other more widely used drugs which are being promoted by the primary care team. The objective in the latter case is firstly to secure the relatively small hospital use and secondly to secure the endorsement of the hospital doctors or opinion leaders whose scrutiny of the data and consequent support of the drug in appropriately licensed circumstances will then give confidence in its use to GPs in the surrounding area.

Hospital representatives may also have responsibility for ensuring that the New Drugs Panel or Formulary Committee receive a presentation, in a non-promotional setting, of all the necessary data, often in conjunction with the company's medical department, in order to consider the possible benefits of listing the company's products. In today's environment, it is usual for the hospital representative to meet regularly with the drug information pharmacist and indeed chief pharmacists to ensure that they are appraised of the clinical benefits of the drugs and any new indications or developments. This is key to ensuring both pharmacy support for and stocking of the drug in question.

In terms of other career developmental roles, the team may have a regional sales trainer, as the metamorphosis of the old-style sales management role into more of a business manager has meant that less RBM time is spent on field visits with representatives. The field trainer will conduct much of the regional training relating to selling skills as well as observing and accompanying representatives on calls to observe customer reaction to the selling messages. Furthermore, as the portfolios have become more complex, there may also be regional therapy area specialist(s), who in addition to working as sales representatives, will be the local expert in a particular therapy area, with responsibility for regional product training plus a dotted reporting line into the relevant head office marketing team.

As mentioned above, there may be NHS liaison specialists either formally in the team or posted to the team, if they are organised on a national basis. These NHS representatives will be senior, experienced personnel, probably of similar grading to regional managers, RBMs, who have the remit for managing key accounts such as Strategic Health Authorities and increasingly Primary Care Trusts (PCTs), which are now coming on-line as the main primary care management system.

The key to this type of role, which is probably going to be more suited to those with first-line management experience, is that contact with the PCTs must deal with the whole company portfolio and needs to focus on specific issues within local PCT agendas or National Service Frameworks such as care of the elderly.

Clearly part of the changing environment will be the emergence of PCT formularies, which will at best seek more evidence that a given drug will help the achievement of local targets, or will attempt to limit the range of drugs to be prescribed for any given condition, or in some worst cases will prohibit the use of individual drugs on grounds such as cost or lack of clinical evidence. In future it could well be that once the NHS liaison manager or team have secured a PCT formulary listing, GP representatives will make the case for the company's drug being the drug of choice from three or four alternatives indicated in the formulary.

Key accounts teams or in some instances NHS teams, who may be part of the regional team or part of a separate commercial function, may have the remit for negotiating regional contracts for the supply of certain high-volume products or high-value specialised products.

In summary, the medical representative, whose role may evolve into something completely different, will continue to be an essential part of the company/customer selling interface. The role itself can be the 'stepping stone' to further progression such as sales management, product management, sales training or key accounts management to name the more obvious routes to career development.

The Sales Management Role

How to get a job as a sales manager

In essence, this is quite straightforward. The main requirement is a successful and credible level of sales achievement over a number of years, as a representative, probably including some of the more senior roles. The advantage of the latter case is that it gives the opportunity, through taking control of projects, for some of the rudiments of leadership and man-management to be clearly demonstrated. Dependent on the individual, this can be sufficient experience to enable a sales management job to be secured once, of course, the individual has been successful in the relevant selection process. However, aiming at a sales management role via a spell in product management can only strengthen your credentials as well as providing an additional 'string to the bow' in terms of marketing and business knowledge.

The role of the sales manager

The role of the pharmaceutical sales manager, whether first- or second-line, regional, national or director level is probably one of the best management jobs in the business. Indeed, where else can you have early responsibility for a range of usually highly driven individuals with the opportunity to motivate them, using skills such as 'situation adapted leadership' to deliver the sales results which the company both needs and demands to enable ultimately shareholder expectations to be realised.

Whether or not an individual aspires to be a career sales manager/director or wishes to climb the corporate ladder, a spell in sales management is an excellent step towards becoming a completely rounded manager. The core function is, as already indicated, to lead a team of medical sales representatives at district, regional, national or even sales director level, the latter case being where there are multiple national teams. The sales manager's role is also becoming increasingly complex as the shape and roles of the sales teams are evolving to meet the new drug decision-making processes in the NHS discussed above.

The sales manager who is today managing a team of eight to 10 representatives at regional level may have some primary care representatives calling on GPs, retail chemists and practice nurses and selling the company's primary care products. In some larger companies the manager may have multiple teams working the same geography, either overlapping with certain products to maximise 'noise' or selling an entirely different GP portfolio. Additionally, there may be one or two hospital representatives with responsibility for selling in the specialist hospital products to consultants and their medical teams, including specialist nurses and the ever-important hospital pharmacist. As mentioned above, there may be other specialists in training, NHS liaison managers, key accounts managers and therapy area specialists to manage as well!

Unsurprisingly the objective is as before, to enable sales in the ultimate form of patient prescriptions to be generated, except in this case the sales responsibility is bigger, as the manager is required to motivate his representatives to achieve, both as individuals and as a team, the larger geographical business target. So the sales management role, in which achievement of both sales and people objectives is paramount, in conjunction with interaction with other departments, including marketing, training, medical information, business information, medical and human resources, is vital to the consistent delivery of the key marketing messages to the customers. Without a well-led, motivated and directed sales team, the deployment of the company's selling effort would be significantly less efficient.

It is crucial to maximise the return on the investment in the sales team, where it has been variously estimated that the 'real cost' of a representative on territory when all costs have been defrayed can be as high as £100k per annum. Therefore companies ensure that they take the time to have well-trained and competent sales managers in place, which illustrates the career development benefits of the sales management role. Above all the sales manager is increasingly a business manager, in many companies with a profit/loss account responsibility and the tactical flexibility to deploy budgets, representatives and other resources to those areas within his remit which are likely to have the highest potential and therefore likely to generate the fastest sales growth. The new environment and the differing specialisations within the team have led to the job becoming even more challenging and stimulating!

For instance, every new drug coming to market has to demonstrate a case for its clinical effectiveness or its use could be restricted. At national level, bodies such as the National Institute for Clinical Excellence (NICE) or the National Prescribing Centre for example may make recommendations for or against the usage of a drug based on their review, in the case of NICE, of clinical and cost-effectiveness, and thus of the strength of its clinical evidence. More importantly, the changing structure means that the case for usage has also to be made at local level. For example, although national endorsement and positive NICE guidance may have been given, Strategic Health Authorities and Primary Care Trusts may decide to restrict the use of 'highly priced' drugs such as those for oncology, for budgetary considerations.

It is now often the job of the local sales manager and his key accounts team to ensure that the case for the use of any drug is made for the usage of the company's drugs at local Primary Care Organisation level, often using economic as well as clinical evidence and specialist support from head office to attempt to persuade the decision-makers. But which processes need to be in place to manage a diverse sales team in such a turbulent environment?

Well, it has often been said, and this does hold even in today's more complex market place, that the secret to success in sales management at any level is to have 'your ducks in a row'. In other words agreeing the sales and activity parameters by which your team are going to be measured on a weekly, monthly, quarterly, annual basis, communicating them to everyone in the team, measuring performance against these criteria and then at the end of each reporting period, communicating your praise, criticism/support, development plans/next actions to improve performance and then repeating the process with the next set of sales/activity data at the end of the next period. It is important that everyone knows the expectation in terms of sales and activity, how they are being measured and 'what "good" looks like'. A good sales manager 'rewards and celebrates' or incentivises over-target performance to drive the business, but should avoid falling into the trap of incentivising 'on-target' delivery as this is why representatives are paid.

The sales manager also has the responsibility for managing his or her team's career development, although their direct reports should take individual responsibility for their career plans. This will involve ongoing individual performance management and feedback on achievement of sales and activity objectives, but also interpersonal style and participation in team dynamics.

As part of the ongoing discussion, the sales manager should expect, or in the appropriate circumstances ask for, feedback on his management style/ communication from his representatives. These informal discussions will lead into annual appraisals, which sales managers will be required to conduct for their team. Direct report career expectation should be managed positively but realistically. For instance, the new medical representative whose aspiration is to be general manager next year may need some guidance with time frames and career pathway planning! The representative who aspires to be a first-line manager could be given projects or assume certain responsibilities within the region as well as being placed on man-management courses whether internal or external. In terms of ongoing team management, the career representative who is successfully bringing in and growing the business year after year is a business asset and should be rewarded and nurtured.

Similarly, poor performance must be dealt with in a fair and supportive manner. Ultimately, poor individual performance detracts from the whole team and the sales manager may have to manage and support the representative towards improvement via action plans agreed with human resources.

Overall, the sales manager is responsible for engendering team spirit across the whole team and the best route to do this is by having a constructive environment in which open and honest, two-way communication can be encouraged. Importantly, the team objectives, including sales targets, must be clear and agreed with the team members. To enable this culture to flourish, the sales manager must continually check his time allocation to key business and sales tasks as well as for the team and the individual.

The well-known John Adair leadership model is still applicable to taking such a helicopter view of the management of a sales team:

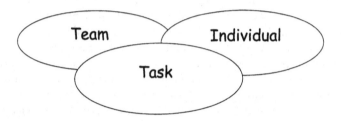

Source: After Adair (1988).

This model can help the sales manager perform an increasingly complex management role by considering the task, the team, and each member of the team. A well-motivated team, in which individuals have a high sense of their worth and fulfilment in conjunction with agreed and clearly communicated objectives, will indeed be a very effective contributor to the global marketing effort!

Other parts of the sales manager's multi-faceted job can include:

- Attending evening meetings with reps/managers, evening phone calls, management administration, etc.;
- Presenting at national sales conferences;
- Organising/running regional sales team meetings;
- Interaction at senior level with marketing teams;
- Membership of business unit teams;
- Interaction with business information/medical information;
- Human resource issues such as interviewing/selection/assessment centres/ appraisals;
- Hiring/firing/promoting;
- Participation in initial training programmes;
- ETMS project teams.

As such the sales manager's time must be carefully planned, but even the best planned sales manager would concede that this is not a 9 to 5 job!

Career development within the sales management role

The next step in career development could well be 'up the line' with promotion to a national or regional director level, or second-line sales management level, where typically there are six to eight first-line sales managers reporting into this function. The essence of the second-line sales manager role is to 'manage the managers', ensuring that the first-line managers are managing the local level implementation of sales strategy (or in some cases agreed variations to national strategy or indeed are setting regional strategy to satisfy local needs). The interfaces and key responsibilities are pretty similar to first-line sales management, although the more senior sales roles have a deeper involvement in setting company strategy.

Alternatively, the first-line sales manager may move into first-line product management or if they have done this already, they may well move into a second-line marketing management function. Occasionally, with the people management experience gained, sales managers even move into human resources!

In summary, unless the individual wishes to be a career sales director, it is desirable to have amassed other experience outside sales to enable further progression up the corporate career ladder. Overall, all sales functions with the training and development given, plus the business and interpersonal experience gained, represent excellent opportunities for personal growth and career development.

Reference

Adair, J. (1988) *Developing Leaders: The Ten Key Principles*, Higher Education.

PART IV

GENERAL CAREERS WITH THE PHARMACEUTICAL INDUSTRY

Careers with the Pharmaceutical Industry, Second edition. Edited by P. D. Stonier.
© 2003 John Wiley & Sons Ltd. ISBN 0 470 84328 4

13

The Role of the Pharmacist in Healthcare

David Jordan

Quintiles (Europe) Ltd, Edinburgh, UK

Introduction

One of many factors which contributes towards the special role of the pharmacist in healthcare generally and the development and supply of medicines in particular is pharmacy's multifaceted image. There is no single description of the role of the pharmacist. Syllabus topics in the pharmacy degree course cover many areas normally regarded as being pure subjects in themselves, for example, chemistry, biochemistry, radiochemistry, metabolism and pharmaceutical analysis. The graduate pharmacist might take on one of many roles in healthcare, industry or academia which could be deemed to be the domain of the specialist but to which he or she can contribute other impacting, yet relevant, sciences to achieve overall added value.

Job Description

Since the pharmacist, by definition, has a role involved with medicines at some point in their life cycle from creation to supply, it is relevant in this chapter to consider the jobs and career opportunities open to the graduate both outside and within the pharmaceutical industry.

Community pharmacy

The best-known role of the pharmacist is that of the community pharmacist, or in lay terms the 'high-street chemist'. In such a job, the pharmacist acts as patient

Careers with the Pharmaceutical Industry, Second edition. Edited by P. D. Stonier.
© 2003 John Wiley & Sons Ltd. ISBN 0 470 84328 4

counsellor as well as the supplier of a prescribed medicine, and as adviser on its best use and storage. He or she should be aware of the reasons for a particular medicine being prescribed and be able to counsel the patient on matters such as side-effects, drug or food interactions, and correct disposal route of any unused medication.

The community pharmacist role is more or less equivalent internationally, and the experienced traveller will have noticed a certain similarity in professional approach, counselling and advice. This central public service role is symbolised throughout the world by the shop sign, whether displayed as 'Pharmacy' or 'Apotheke'!

The responsibilities of community pharmacists extend to behind-the-scenes activities such as stock control, purchasing from wholesalers, communication with general practitioners, hospital doctors and dentists, and for the training of postgraduate pharmacists undertaking their one-year pre-registration experience in the UK prior to becoming members of the Royal Pharmaceutical Society. They will also liaise with other healthcare professionals, for example in health promotion on such community-related matters as smoking cessation, and thus make a contribution to the aims of national health strategy.

In a wider sense, a process has recently begun to integrate community pharmacy into local clinical governance arrangements insofar as community pharmacists with current and recent experience will be represented on clinical governance committees and be included in their plans from 2002/3 onwards.

Clinical governance is described by the Royal Pharmaceutical Society as a framework through which National Health Service (NHS) organisations are held accountable for continuously improving the quality of their services and safeguarding high standards of care, by creating an environment in which excellence in clinical care will flourish. The Department of Health is to provide funding of up to £2m per year to support clinical governance in community pharmacy.

Also of current interest, primary care trusts, which operate within the NHS, will have to provide schemes that are commercially positive or at least neutral and which can be used to enhance patients' perceptions of customer care in pharmacies, leading to customer retention. Further information on these topics may be obtained from the following Department of Health website: www.doh.gov.uk/clinicalgovernance/communitypharmacy.htm

Nowadays, links between the prescriber and the pharmacist are improved with the availability of computer-generated prescriptions which are associated with patient record software. This innovation has largely obviated the need for the pharmacist to double-check the sometimes indecipherable handwriting of the prescriber to avoid mistakes of confusion such as supplying Losec instead of Lasix, or Danol for Daonil.

The pharmacist increasingly has patient record software at his disposal in order to help check for consistency and regularity of medication supply, drug interactions as well as to computer-generate the label for the medication, again overcoming possible problems of illegible handwriting. Computers also aid in speeding up the process of dispensing, especially in a busy pharmacy. For similar reasons, the advent and growth of health centres, incorporating a GP surgery with possibly a dental practitioner, chiropodist and pharmacy to choose from, must be beneficial to the patient.

Hospital pharmacy

Since community pharmacy accounts for about 70% of all pharmacists in the UK, it is justifiable to have spent a little longer than average to describe their roles in pharmaceutical medicine. Some of the basic principles involved in the supply of medicines to the community also continue to apply in other areas of pharmacy too, namely in hospital pharmacy environments. Here, pharmacy services are organised into regions to provide a total drug supply function to hospitals, clinics and nursing homes in a given region, although the latter is more often the domain of community pharmacies.

Due to the greater complexity of this organisation compared with community pharmacy, career structures are involved, allowing pharmacists to progress through a multi-grade career pathway, up to Chief Pharmacist and District or Regional Pharmaceutical Managers. One added characteristic of hospital pharmacists (which differentiates them from other branches of pharmacy) is their proximity to hospital medical practitioners which, therefore, enables them to provide in situ advisory services in terms of drug information directly to the doctor. Over the years this has led to the concept of ward pharmacy, where pharmacists not only control the supply, storage and use of medicines, but can also advise doctors on specific drug matters, often on the spot during routine ward rounds or in emergency situations. A significant proportion (about 20%) of graduate pharmacists enter the hospital pharmacy service and the more senior or specialist roles (e.g. radiopharmaceuticals) are often held by those holding a doctorate (PhD).

Pharmaceutical industry

Last, but not least, approximately 5% of pharmacy graduates take up posts in the pharmaceutical industry, usually to work on the formulation or analytical development aspects of new drug compounds. Except when formulations are being prepared for clinical trials, the main activities of the industrial pharmacist do not involve any direct contact with members of the public, which differentiates this role from the majority of pharmacists working in healthcare.

During the drug development process, the pharmacist would be expected to become involved in the formulation of a wide variety of dosage forms and to carry out research into novel ways of delivering drugs, new or existing, to the body. They could also be expected to work on the development of stability-indicating analytical methods, leading ultimately to quality control tests, perform stability tests under simulated conditions of extreme climate, carry out quality reviews of existing products on the market, prepare clinical trial formulations and those suited to pre-clinical animal or human metabolism studies, scale up manufacturing procedures to production plant, and so on. The list and variety seem endless. Within most large pharmaceutical companies, there are even more opportunities for pharmacists to expand their knowledge base, and these possibilities will be explored later in this chapter.

Academic and other pharmacy careers

The remaining 5% of pharmacists opt for a career in academia or in other associated pharmaceutical activities, for example wholesaling or consulting. Academics generally, apart from their teaching commitments, would normally pioneer research into relevant areas of pharmaceutical science, including subjects such as drug targeting to receptors, improvement in bioavailability, timed release and the extension of the duration of effects of drugs (so reducing dose frequency). The more process-orientated choose to investigate such issues as tablet compression and coating, powder technology or capsule filling. Academics also perform original research into pharmacy practice issues, these days often along with their medical colleagues.

Whatever the chosen subject, there is no doubt that the newly graduated pharmacist has a wide choice of career directions and resultant job descriptions available, ranging from a community/business management orientation to the more scientific or academic. The ways in which these various options may be exploited by the individual will be discussed in detail in the remaining sections of this chapter.

Background to the Profession of Pharmacy

At present, there are more than 20 000 pharmacists practising in the UK, distributed among the various branches of the profession as indicated earlier. A more international figure is difficult to obtain but it may well be fair to assume that the same picture is reflected in other developed countries around the world.

In former times the pharmacist, known then as the apothecary, received an apprenticeship type of training from an experienced father figure or mentor. Such training would have included bizarre practices not associated with modern-day pharmacy, namely the production of concoctions according to folklore remedies, tooth extractions or even minor surgery.

Latterly, the rather more appropriately trained apprentice would be granted the status of Pharmaceutical Chemist (PhC), the forerunner to membership of the Pharmaceutical Society of Great Britain, now the Royal Pharmaceutical Society since 1991 (MRPhS).

Today pharmacists are trained in Schools of Pharmacy throughout England, Scotland, Ireland and Wales to degree level, with honours in many of these. Entry requirements are normally three or four 'A'-level passes in relevant subjects including chemistry, plus other science subjects such as physics, mathematics or biology, although this may vary between schools. Good standard pass grades would be expected. The subject matter contained in these four-year courses covers pharmaceutical chemistry (organic, inorganic and analytical), the science of the physicochemical properties of drugs along with processing methods for the preparation of medicines (pharmaceutics), the study of the action of drugs on the body (pharmacology), awareness of the potential of drugs from plants (pharmacognosy), and the law and practice relating to pharmacy. A modern approach in degree courses these days, in the more progressive universities, is a multidisciplined approach to teaching the overall concept of, for example, stability studies of drugs extracted from plants (e.g. digoxin), which would combine some pure chemistry, pharmaceutics, drug design and formulation, and analytical chemistry.

Pharmacy graduates almost invariably undertake an immediate postgraduate year of practical training (pre-registration) in order to gain membership of the Royal Pharmaceutical Society. This is only achieved after a taxing 12 months of working under the supervision of a qualified and experienced pharmacist tutor, gaining knowledge about a range of core and specialist subjects and successfully undertaking an examination paper at the end of the period, against stringent sets of pass criteria. The pre-registration year now includes a compulsory cross-sector experience, currently two weeks, projected to increase to four weeks working in an opposite sector, for example two weeks spent in a hospital pharmacy environment if the core training was undertaken in industry and community pharmacy.

Membership of the Society is a legal requirement for pharmacists working in contact with the public, which chiefly covers the community and hospital roles, although it is taken to be a very significant expression of professional commitment in other roles too, where patient contact is not so great, including those in the pharmaceutical industry. For this reason, the pre-registration year may be undertaken exclusively in a community pharmacy or hospital pharmacy department but is limited to a maximum of six months if undertaken in the pharmaceutical industry, regulatory agency (e.g. Medicines Control Agency) or university. Furthermore, within the European Union, reciprocation exists to enable the pharmacist to receive bona fide training in, for example, Germany or France.

It is felt that there is a need in the future for pharmacy qualifications to be more tailored to the chosen direction although, due to the fact that it would seem unfairly limiting to confine future pharmacists to only a narrow area of the profession from early on in their degree course, it is difficult to envisage how this could be implemented practically and satisfactorily.

Looking longer-term, continuing education, now replaced with continuing professional development (CPD), aims to embrace the process by which pharmacists continuously enhance their knowledge, skills and personal qualities throughout their professional careers. It covers clinical, community and evidence-based practice matters. We will almost definitely see an element of pharmacist prescribing being introduced as a result of this raised level of professional development and a parallel redefinition of the role of the pharmacist in clinical practice. Indeed, this is already underway in Scotland as part of 'The Right Medicine' initiative for pharmaceutical care, where pharmacists should be able to prescribe by 2003, to enable them to make dosage adjustments on repeat prescriptions as a result of, for example, therapeutic drug monitoring. Such moves are major objectives of medicines management in the UK.

Role and Responsibilities in Medicines Research and Development

In a publication dealing primarily with careers in pharmaceutical medicine or with the pharmaceutical industry, great emphasis must be placed on the opportunities for pharmacists working in research and development, in order to complete the chain of pharmacist involvement from creation to supply of medicines.

For this purpose, comments will be restricted to research and development (R&D) in the pharmaceutical industry, rather than in academic research. The commercial stimulus of such a role is often seen as the catalyst for the process of new product development and ultimate availability to the medical practitioner to prescribe to patients. A more realistic attraction is perhaps the general responsibility of medical scientists to identify new therapeutic areas of benefit to mankind through drug discovery and development activities initiated within the industry, followed by the complex and prolonged period (in the range of 5–15 years) of evaluating lead compound selection, and proving efficacy and safety, until sufficient evidence exists for a registration submission to the licensing body.

More often than not, however, the pharmacist will enter the pharmaceutical industry, and pursue a career in R&D in order to achieve scientific ambitions rather than community healthcare ones by people who believe their talents are best directed towards scientific challenges in order to benefit their profession and their customers, or patient populations, as a whole. Within this role, activities can be categorised under the headings of formulation design, pharmaceutical analysis and clinical trial supplies, each of which will be discussed separately.

Formulation design

Pharmacists working in this field must be highly innovative individuals, self-motivated and capable of high levels of problem-solving skills and creativity. Such people will utilise these skills to generate new product ideas, contribute to the development of new drug delivery systems and liaise closely with contracted university departments to achieve these goals. Although this may appear to many to be in the area of blue-sky research, it is often from such starting points that valuable and beneficial new products are born, in collaboration with other pharmaceutical scientists, pharmacokineticists, clinical pharmacologists, clinical research physicians and teams, and marketing executives.

From such beginnings, radical innovations such as transdermal patches, contraceptive implants, insulin pens and breath-activated aerosols for asthma have arisen. More routinely, however, such individuals will be involved in the task of formulating the dosage forms (e.g. tablets, capsules, injections, creams and suppositories) suitable for the dose level release kinetics and route of administration of new chemical entities. By optimising these activities with patient benefit in mind, it is normally possible to provide a convenient product for the market, to be used at a kinetically relevant dose interval; daily or twice daily might be regarded as convenient, whereas dosing seven times a day, for example, would be highly inconvenient to the patient.

A range of knowledge is required by the formulating pharmacist, from the microphysics of materials used in the product to ensure possibility of manufacture on a large scale and using high-speed production machinery, to the effects of the formulation on the shelf-life, availability, bioavailability and pharmacokinetics/dynamics of the drug in question.

More examples of problems in these areas spring to mind to emphasise the importance and influence of this activity in pharmaceutical development, not due to their alarming frequency but more because of their impact on personal pride and damaged ego! For example, cases where tranquillisers have been miraculously transformed into incredibly fast-acting hypnotics (hardly enough time to climb the stairs to bed before falling asleep!), improved hypoglycaemic products which produced impressive pharmacokinetics but no pharmacodynamic effects, and nasal products containing drug absorption enhancers capable of effectively encouraging the reverse transport of cerebrospinal fluid into the nasal cavity are all experiences which the formulator would prefer to be forgotten. Fortunately, there are many more examples of successful work in this field resulting in effective and convenient medication.

Pharmaceutical analysis

It is the role of a pharmacist, working in the area of pharmaceutical analysis, to ensure that developed formulations are stable, both physically and chemically, under a series of extreme temperature, light and humidity conditions. Resulting data, along with corresponding formulation details, form the core of the chemistry and pharmacy section of the regulatory submission, once combined with synthesis details of the drug substance itself. Far from being the domain of the pharmacist alone, the responsibilities of this role are very much shared, for example with analytical chemists, although the all-round experience of the pharmacist plays an important part in the overall product development objective.

Together, analysts generate official data for regulatory approval based on individual country requirements. There are still large differences in these requirements, the temperature/humidity conditions, number of batches to be tested, test duration and so on, and this whole issue is now an important part of the negotiations of the Expert Groups of the International Conference on Harmonisation (ICH) of regulatory requirements.

Apart from stability testing per se, the expertise of the graduate must first be directed to the establishment of suitable stability-indicating analytical methods, such that the appearance of degradation products of the drug can be mapped and quantified under real-time ambient or accelerated storage conditions. Similarly, the disappearance of the parent drug should be directly quantifiable. Such methods should use modern, fast techniques so that not only can they be used in the stability test programme, but also be translated into quick, efficient quality-control tests to release batches of the resultant medicine for sale once it is in full production. Whether an analytical or formulation pharmacist, both will work together as a team along with other life science graduates to ensure the smooth development of new medicines and their efficient transfer from the laboratory and clinic environment into the pharmaceutical 'factory' to supply the market continuously with effective, safe and high-quality products.

Clinical trial supplies

At the interface between pre-clinical and clinical development sits the clinical supplies pharmacist with a unique role in the organisation. To many people, this is seen as similar to a community pharmacist role, dispensing product against prescriptions, except that in the case of clinical trials the patients might be 2000–3000 in number (especially during the later phase III stages of clinical development) in 20–30 centres around the world and being supplied with often a complex programme of cross-over, randomised (sometimes active versus placebo or matched comparator drug) medication against a protocol agreed by an independent research ethics committee.

Like their other pharmacist colleagues, working in formulation, analysis or production, they work according to a code of practice known as Good Manufacturing Practice (GMP) and sometimes Good Laboratory Practice (GLP), where overlap with laboratory R&D areas such as toxicology or animal metabolism is necessary. Both codes provide guidelines and disciplines to steer scientists through the complicated array of activities such as good housekeeping, protocol generation and adherence, conducting experiments, report writing, training, record keeping, standard operating procedures, hygiene, stock control, labelling and archiving. Responsibility is therefore understandably very high in this role and could make the difference between a successful, informative and well-executed study and one which is inherently defective, inaccurate, expensive and potentially dangerous.

It is the one area of pharmaceutical R&D where the 'output' is actually directly administered to humans. In phase II, III and IV clinical trials this predominantly means people exhibiting the disease state for which that medicine has been designed whereas, at the earlier phase I clinical pharmacology stage, smaller numbers (12–24) of healthy volunteers are recruited into each trial, to have the medicine administered to them for the first time in humans. Such studies are designed specifically to research tolerance, dose ranges, drug or food interaction, or to study the pharmacokinetics resulting from the specific absorption, distribution, metabolism and elimination (ADME) characteristics of that drug, often using radiolabelled forms to aid identity and quantification of parent drug and metabolites.

Up to the present in the UK there have been no regulatory requirements for phase I work, although this is likely to change soon with the advent of the European Clinical Trials Directive translated into national law of member states. Meanwhile, the UK is seen as a fast-track, first-in-man environment for early clinical studies and, without question, pharmacists are very much involved in the provision of suitable formulations for this purpose. Whether this changes with the legal and regulatory implications of the Clinical Trials Directive for approval of phase I studies remains to be seen.

Career Pathways

Earlier in this chapter, emphasis was placed on the ways in which pharmacists could use their qualifications in the many directions which the profession offers and how this is reflected in the diverse ways in which the postgraduate, pre-registration training year may be structured.

Indeed, due to the understandable emphasis given to patient contact in the community, the suggestion has been made that the compulsory six-month minimum training in community pharmacy be extended to 12 months in order to underline the perceived importance of this aspect of the profession. Maybe then, rather like doctors working in the pharmaceutical industry, pharmacists ought to be encouraged to spend an agreed proportion of their time in public-related activities in order to maintain their professional community healthcare skills and image and avoid a too narrow sector of pharmacy generally. Stuart Anderson states: 'A single-minded approach in which we unambiguously train all pharmacy graduates to perform competently as community pharmacists, regardless of their future career aspirations may well prove to be the best investment the profession can make for its own future' (Anderson, 1993).

Healthcare professionals and history will have to wait to see whether this is prospective wise advice or cautious overkill.

Whatever the final details of pharmacy training turn out to be, resultant career structures vary enormously, from the pharmacist running a single community pharmacy all his or her working life, to the individual who progresses to a very senior position in the pharmaceutical industry.

Although not alone, the first two names which spring to mind in this latter respect are Professor Trevor Jones, Director General, Association of the British Pharmaceutical Industry (ABPI) and Sir David Jack, former Director of Glaxo plc. Within the scope of this range of career aspirations, and concentrating particularly on the pharmaceutical industry now, one still sees tremendous scope for interesting and varied careers for the ambitious pharmacist.

Earlier, it was stressed that a pharmacy graduate would probably enter the industry in a scientific role such as a pharmaceutical development scientist. Although typical, this would not deter a pharmacist from initiating his career in the industry as a registration officer, a medical information pharmacist or as a clinical research associate.

Within large pharmaceutical organisations, it is possible to see how the ambitions of the industrial pharmacist have been satisfied in many differing ways, either by choice or by encouragement, so that pharmacists are presently found working as registration executives, adverse drug reactions monitors, medical information officers, commercial directors, pharmaceutical representatives, clinical research associates and human resources officers, as well as the more traditionally accepted scientific roles within drug development. It is because of their rather special broad skills that the industrial pharmacist has the ability to cross scientific and managerial boundaries with comparative ease and confidence.

Within the scientific community of the industry, however, a typical pharmacist would hold the basic pharmacist role, for example as a formulator, for a relatively short time, perhaps three to four years. During this period, he would receive on-the-job scientific training and off-the-job management/personal training to be equipped as appropriate for future advancement. Due to the relatively small size of laboratory hierarchies, normal progression to section head/leader is sometimes long awaited and the graduate may prefer to fill vacancies in other companies in order to speed up the process. This is often the case especially for ambitious characters, anxious to achieve their career maxima as quickly as possible, and results in a justifiably long curriculum vitae for future employers to ponder over regarding logical approach, common sense and evidence of real advancement, as opposed to merely job-hopping.

As a section head, the pharmacist would lead a small team of graduates and technicians occupied in task-orientated scientific work such as formulation, manufacturing or analytical development, and the job itself would offer a mixture of scientific and management activity and responsibility.

Such a role naturally paves the way towards running an entire department, comprising typically three to four sections, along with a consequent increase in responsibilities to an even greater management and financial level. Scientific involvement would still remain very much in evidence, except that the individual would take on a more project administration task rather than benchwork, and would be known for his or her scientific philosophies and opinions nationally and often internationally, usually by virtue of publications, presentations and involvement in professional or industry bodies, for example Chemical Industries Association (CIA), ABPI, or Royal Pharmaceutical Society of Great Britain, including UKCAPS, Industrial Pharmacists Group, Pharmaceutical Analysis Group, etc.

The career pathway to department head would typically be expected to take 10–15 years, by which time the graduate would have reached his or her mid-thirties in age. Thereafter, armed hopefully with an impressive portfolio of qualifications, all-round scientific ability, successful track record and management skills, he or she could take any one of a number of career moves in the industry. From there on, these may have little direct relevance to pharmacy, being of a more general scientific or management nature, for example R&D director, or be in a totally different direction as previously mentioned. In large multinational companies, the prospect of transferring completely into another division such as fine chemicals, polymers or agrochemicals could also be a likelihood, based mainly on the management skills of the individual, whilst retaining some basic scientific links.

The Future

Finally, a word about the future of the pharmacist's role in industrial healthcare. For those pharmacists working in companies where the chief activity is that of drug discovery, the formulation and analytical skills of the pharmacist could unfairly be regarded as cosmetic and secondary to the perceived main job of designing new drug compounds.

However, in more enlightened companies where the true potential of the pharmacist is fully recognised, and his or her broad knowledge base combined with specialist scientific skill is fully utilised, then tremendous added value can be gained from the natural synergies that pharmacists have with other science professionals in optimising drug development for the patient and maximising its value for the company.

It is likely that pharmacy will continue to be used as a productive seed-bed for future industrial managers and, additionally, as the rate of attrition after 'Proof of Concept' increases, and the corresponding rate of discovery of new drug compounds perhaps inevitably and predictably falls, the importance of the pharmacist as an innovator, creator and problem-solver will increase still further to help meet the very latest challenges in the business of pharmaceutical medicine.

Reference

Anderson, S. (1993) *Pharm. J.*, **251**, 210.

14

Careers for Nurses with the Pharmaceutical Industry

Joyce E. Kenkre

University of Glamorgan, Pontypridd, UK

Introduction

It has long been acknowledged that the quality of clinical therapeutic trials (CTTs) is much improved when nurses are involved at the investigator site (Barnes, 1981). However, nurses are increasingly using their experience and knowledge to diversify their career options to include employment directly with a pharmaceutical company or contract research organisation (CRO). As nurses are newer to the research arena than their medical colleagues, their roles within the drug development process are still being evaluated and refined.

Nurses involved in clinical therapeutic trials have two distinctive career pathways to follow: study site co-ordinator (SSC)/clinical research nurse (CRN) (Kenkre and Foxcroft, 2001a), employed by a site monitoring organisation (SMO) on behalf of the study site(s) or by a pharmaceutical company or CRO on behalf of research sponsors and clinical research associate (CRA) employed by a pharmaceutical company or CRO (Kenkre and Foxcroft, 2001b). Nurses are also applying for positions as medical representatives and drug safety monitors amongst others within the pharmaceutical industry, and similar posts within the related healthcare industries.

A third distinctive career pathway for nurses which involves the pharmaceutical industry is as a nurse adviser, involved principally with field-based therapeutic audits (Ryan, 2002). The nurse adviser as part of his/her role undertakes clinical audits of patient records often in light of National Service Framework clinical guidelines for primary or secondary care. Since the pharmaceutical industry directly or indirectly sponsors many of these projects, the nurse is employed by a third-party organisation in order to maintain professional independence.

Careers with the Pharmaceutical Industry, Second edition. Edited by P. D. Stonier.
© 2003 John Wiley & Sons Ltd. ISBN 0 470 84328 4

Clinical Research Nurse/Study Site Co-ordinator

Background

There are many papers emerging from the 1980s onwards on the role of nurses in the conduct of CTTs (Barnes, 1981; Hubbard, 1982; Bersani et al., 1983; Johnson, 1986). Many of these cite nurses working as co-ordinators for CTTs, where the skills needed were reliability, organisation, communication, motivation, self-discipline and critical thought. The tasks completed by nurses in these studies were wide ranging, from the collection of data, the recruitment of patients, screening patients, randomisation of drugs and follow-up of patients to the standardisation of staff training. Unfortunately, clinical research nurses (CRNs) were frequently considered by their peers as mere data collectors, but that was often stated in ignorance of the true extent of their role. This appears to be changing following the publication of an employment brief for CRNs by the Royal College of Nursing (RCN, 1998), which details information on their role, knowledge, skills, expertise with appropriate grade and remuneration assigned. Indeed, nurses at the study site are now given the opportunity of roles as co-investigator or even lead investigator.

Role and responsibilities

The role of the clinical research nurse is to conduct a CTT to recognised international standards and regulations as laid down by governing bodies both nationally and internationally (ICH, 1995; Department of Health, 2001; The Scottish Executive, 2001; Wales Office of Research and Development, 2001; Northern Ireland Research Governance, 2002). This ensures scientific, ethical and safe practice. For the nurse to fulfil this role in the first instance there is an essential need to be able to read and assess a research protocol, to understand the methodology and its practical application within the trial.

The clinical research nurse on adhering to the protocol has to undertake the practical organisation and management of patients, administration of information and other members of the research team. This includes liaising with members of departments at the investigator site who are involved in the conduct of required trial procedures, analysis of samples and the dispensing of the trial medication. In the organisation of the trial the clinical research nurse will also liaise with personnel from the sponsoring company about the ethical, organisational, management and financial aspects of the trial.

The CRN will work in conjunction with the site investigator in the identification and screening of potential trial participants. In this role the CRN will take part in the process of gaining and continuing informed consent of the trial participant, prior to carrying out procedures and treatments as agreed within the trial protocol.

These diverse roles and responsibilities of the CRN may cause the nurse to experience a conflict of interest. This may be through loyalty to the investigator to enrol patients into the trial until completion, loyalty to the sponsoring company that the trial is completed to the required standard within the set timescale, and the responsibility as the primary advocate for the trial participant. The CRN as the participants' advocate has the primary responsibility to inform and protect the patients' interests. However, the investigator needs to depend on the CRN to adhere strictly to the trial protocol. Deviance from the protocol can make the participant unevaluable, resulting in a waste of time for both participant and research team.

Clinical research unit nurse

A specific role of the CRN is as a research nurse within a clinical research unit. Clinical research units, either within a pharmaceutical company or run independently, conduct exploratory clinical studies on new medicines. These studies are the first human studies and are usually conducted on healthy subjects (phase I studies), except in certain cases such as the administration of cytotoxic drugs as these can only be given to patients with known conditions.

The nurse within a clinical research unit works with physicians and scientists from the development of the protocol through to the completion of the studies of new compounds.

The emphasis in a phase I clinical trial is on safety so monitoring of the study subjects and adherence to the protocol are paramount. Nurses within this environment have a regular update on resuscitation training with a check for competency. Other competencies required include intravenous administration, reconstitution of drugs, administration of drugs and ensuring an adequate supply of drugs. At this early stage of drug development the reporting of adverse events and serious adverse events is an essential part of the role.

Career pathway

The first step along this career pathway is as a junior level research nurse who has qualified as a registered nurse with some post-registration experience. However, the remuneration for this post will be at a higher level than the clinical equivalent due to the research knowledge and eventual expertise required for this position, even though the CRN will be supervised either by a senior nurse or the trial investigator. At this junior level the CRN would be: identifying and screening potential participants, organising and managing procedures and intervention treatments to a predetermined protocol and recording the resulting information. The CRN should ensure that the informed consent process is ongoing throughout a trial as study subject adherence is central to this process.

Knowledge of the specialty field being researched is often required of the CRN. As the nurse will be new into this research position it is important that they are given a sound knowledge of the regulations and principles of practice laid down by the governing bodies within and outside the institution in which they are employed (ICH, 1995; Department of Health, 2001; The Scottish Executive, 2001; Wales Office of Research and Development, 2001; Northern Ireland Research Governance, 2002). It is also important that the CRN is capable of adhering to a predetermined protocol, is numerate and has IT skills, as increasingly data are being transferred electronically. They should be able to communicate with research colleagues at all levels and have excellent time and project management skills.

The next step for the CRN is as a specialist within their field of practice. The nurse would have a research, educational and developmental role within the research projects. They should be considering undertaking post-registration education in clinical research at certificate level with progression to master's level. As the CRN gains more experience s/he will be expected to work with a degree of autonomy, frequently conducting concurrent multicentre studies. However, this increased experience and expertise does not preclude them from undertaking elements of the junior role. The CRN would be expected to co-ordinate activities between the sponsoring companies, other departments involved in the research (such as pharmacy, laboratory staff and technicians) as well as the immediate multi-disciplinary research teams within the department. The CRN should have a sound knowledge of research design, methodology and understanding of the analytical process. The CRN would have an active role in ethical requirements including ethics committee submissions, the informed consent process and patient support. This may be especially pertinent, as they may frequently be the only nurse involved in the research. The developed skills should include project management, protocol development and experience at writing for publication. Working at this level of clinical and research expertise should be reflected in a higher clinical grading.

As they progress up the career ladder nurses should be developing their leadership skills. Hence, the next step is a lead role in the development, assessment and supervision of research projects. The management and organisation of human and financial resources, including the negotiation of financial contracts with the sponsoring companies and the negotiation of contracts for members of the research team, are important elements of the position. The person in this position should have a clear overview and strategy for the development of research programmes. As the nursing lead and a specialist in the field of practice the CRN is accountable for the nursing elements within the research projects, for the maintenance of ethical standards and other matters, for example, the dissemination and publication of research findings. They should have obtained or be considering undertaking a postgraduate degree at master's level. However, many nurses in this role have been leaders in their chosen field, resulting in numerous peer-reviewed publications, which may equate to a higher level of education.

There are many research units that are managed or led by nurses. These nurses have key responsibilities, which include: the management of large multidisciplinary teams of healthcare professionals in the conduct of international trials, capacity building and infrastructure, actively developing and promoting the research agenda for their institution, and leading by example in terms of research activity and publications. These nurses have a wealth of experience; however, a higher academic degree is desirable either in clinical research, research methods and/or business administration. At this level it is important to consider the development of all staff within the specialty and supervision of multidisciplinary postgraduate staff should be considered as an integral part of that development.

Personality attributes and fit for role

Although nursing does not assume primacy over other professions in the co-ordination of research at a study site, it is known that the majority of study site co-ordinators have nursing as their primary qualification (Scott, 1993). The CRN is recognised as a professional person by patients, volunteers and colleagues within primary and secondary care settings. The nurse as a professional person acknowledges their limitations and adherence to the code of professional practice, which includes safeguarding and promoting the interests of individuals, exercising accountability and the maintenance of high standards (NMC, 2002).

The nurse through experience develops management and organisational skills, which will assist them to be more efficient and effective for assigning or undertaking tasks. They have the theoretical background of the disease process with the ability to assess and evaluate tasks performed and their subsequent outcome. The CRN as a specialist practitioner should disseminate research findings to educate other healthcare professionals within the field of expertise to enable evidence-based practice.

Communication skills are an important element of the job in order to relate information to patients, healthcare colleagues and to the sponsoring company. The ability to pick up verbal and non-verbal communication to ensure all participants are comfortable and safe is equally important.

Training and qualifications

There are many courses for the CRN to attend organised by the sponsoring company, networks for CRNs, the Institute of Clinical Research and universities. Each offers the CRN different aspects of training. The sponsoring company offers training which will include specific information relating to their proposed future CTT to ensure investigators and their research teams are appropriately trained. The networks respond to the needs of the membership by offering the opportunity for nurses to meet on a regular basis to discuss aspects of their role and listen to speakers addressing issues of their choice. The Institute of Clinical Research also offers a wide selection of training days in response to its members' requirements.

All these groups usually supply a certificate of attendance that the nurse can insert into his/her portfolio. The nurse should be able to demonstrate that update in practice has been maintained by presentation of a portfolio to their regulatory body every three years (UKCC, 1996).

Postgraduate university education may be undertaken, which can be either research-specific or specialty-specific, as it is the standard of the level of study that is important. Within a postgraduate master's programme a nurse may decide at what level they want to complete the course, which may be at certificate or diploma level. However, within the field of research an individual may decide to conduct a research project and write it up to present as a master's by thesis. There are also various options to attain a PhD qualification, which can be by taught course, research, portfolio or publication.

Changing course

There are now a variety of career options for nurses to take after starting their research career as a CRN, as the discipline required in their conduct of CTT gives the nurse excellent training for all research. This includes a career in academia, clinical practice or research support, as a clinical research associate, nurse adviser or drug safety monitor in a pharmaceutical company/CRO or freelance as an auditor or medical writer.

The future

The establishment of this role has enabled CRNs to demonstrate an array of competencies and capabilities that are constantly being developed to enhance the quality of clinical therapeutic trials and the benefits to the general population.

Clinical Research Associate

Nurses who have been trained in the conduct of research at investigator sites frequently decide to change their career pathway to become a clinical research associate within a pharmaceutical company or CRO. This position would be to organise and monitor multicentre clinical therapeutic trials. Nurses often change their career pathway due to a feeling of lack of value in their present employment, of more promising career prospects, the opportunity to travel and financial reward.

Role and responsibilities

Within the first 12 weeks in the industry to monitor research nurses are employed as trainee clinical research associates. In this role the CRA is trained to perform monitoring visits at investigator sites with an assigned mentor. During this time they are trained to develop their skills to ensure complete accurate data can be retrieved from the investigator sites from initiation to the archiving of the trial master file. Both the pharmaceutical industry staff and the site personnel work to predefined standard operating procedures (SOPs) for their company or institution to ensure that the research is conducted to international standards of good clinical practice (GCP).

The more senior CRAs have the added responsibility of leading teams, which monitor programmes of research. As with any field team structure, communication and dissemination of information are an important part of their role. Another element of their role is the development of research protocols and study-specific documentation, which can be used internationally. Strategic planning for programmes of clinical research is within the remit of the more senior positions in the pharmaceutical company. This will include the resourcing of research programmes at an international level. The project manager will be appropriately remunerated for the responsibility of the position.

Career pathway

Many who decide to take this career route have a science degree or a nursing qualification and/or a postgraduate degree (Scott, 1993). The initial training period, mentioned above in relation to monitoring training, is under the close supervision of training the individual 'on the job'. It will include knowledge of good clinical practice, the company and the pharmaceutical industry. It is important that the supervisor ensures that the trainee is numerate, computer literate and able to communicate at all levels with research staff and company representatives. It is essential that the trainee is able to adhere to a predetermined protocol, check and obtain corrections of site clinical trial data to enable the comprehensive management of the CTT.

After training the CRA is assigned to a set of investigator sites to monitor and ensure that data standards are met. These sites may be within one country, but since clinical trials are today often multicentre, even multinational, studies, and clinical study programmes are co-ordinated in many countries, CRAs must expect to travel in the course of their work. Companies often employ CRAs in their subsidiaries in each country or through CROs in order to ensure the quality of local monitoring through an understanding of local practices, and also to reduce the amount of travelling and maximise resource allocation to the task of study monitoring. It is becoming increasingly common that within a single country, CRAs work from home in different regions, as much as being attached to a central head office or research department.

The experience of answering queries from the investigator for each trial, organising and monitoring the clinical therapeutic trials to the regulatory guidelines prepares the CRA for the next stage of their career development.

The senior clinical associate still monitors but has the added responsibility of leading research teams. The experience gained through monitoring trials in practice assists the senior CRA in the development of future trial protocols, documentation and organisation. As staff are monitoring studies in countries around the world it is important to have good communication, organisation and managerial skills.

A project manager or clinical research officer is involved in strategic planning at a global level but also needs to consider minutia of detail at country and site level. This includes the international financial management and negotiation of contracts. Knowledge of the required research evidence, documentation and mechanisms of licensing of products within each country is an essential component of the job.

Personality attributes and fit for role

Good verbal and written communication skills are an essential component of the role but working knowledge of another language would be beneficial. The CRA must be prepared to travel and make use of time while waiting for transport. Therefore good organisational skills including self-discipline and time management are required to be able to work effectively and efficiently. The clinical researcher must be pedantic when checking the detail of research documentation and be alert to the possibility of errors, which may be instigated by the study subject or the investigator site personnel. Although a relatively rare occurrence, the CRA must also be alert to and be prepared to report any suspicion of research misconduct, including the possibility of fraud, as these will have serious implications for the research findings.

Training and qualifications

It is not unknown for people to come into this role from a science/laboratory background with a PhD (Scott, 1993). But nurses tend to come into this role post-registration with clinical and research experience and expertise. Although the nurse may have attended relevant educational days it is beneficial for career progression to initially take a postgraduate research course to certificate or diploma level in clinical research, however, it would be beneficial to complete to master's level.

As the job entails presentations of the research design and findings, training for investigator sites and team member presentation skills is advantageous. It is frequently assumed that the more experienced within a job a person is, the more likely it is that he or she will be able to lead a team, but this is often an ill-founded assumption, and therefore leadership training is an excellent developmental experience.

As all of the above are essential it is necessary for pharmaceutical staff at all levels to be conversant with changes to research as a result of the International Conference on Harmonisation Good Clinical Practice (ICH GCP) guidelines (ICH, 1995),

European directives (notably the European Clinical Trial Directive, 2001, which will be implemented nationally from 2004), changes in legislation and ethical issues to conduct research to the highest of standards.

Changing course

It is often assumed that it is CRNs that decide to become CRAs, however, it is sometimes the other way round in that CRAs decide to become CRNs as they miss the clinical component and patient contact as a result of working at the investigator site.

Another job option to consider is as an auditor, meticulously checking that the CTT has been conducted to the standards outlined in ICH GCP, ensuring that all the research documentation is correct. Another course that the nurse may take is as a medical writer. This role involves writing protocols, research reports, manuscripts, patient information and other information required by the research sponsor (e.g. pharmaceutical company). In these roles, too, the nurse is often based entirely at home, but without the support of an office or site-based team. Working from home may be considered advantageous to many people but requires self-discipline.

The future

Research studies on new gene therapy treatments are really still embryonic but exciting and the pharmaceutical industry has an important role in the control of future developments. However, ethical dilemmas on these future developments will need serious consideration.

Nurse Adviser

The nurse adviser as part of his/her role undertakes clinical audits of patient records often in light of National Service Framework clinical guidelines for primary or secondary care (Ryan, 2002). Whilst these projects are often sponsored by pharmaceutical companies, the nurse advisers are employed by a third-party organisation to ensure that they remain independent practitioners. This innovative career pathway has been developed over recent years whereby advisers have enjoyed various job titles including Clinical Audit Facilitator, Clinical Resource Nurse and Therapy Review Specialist. The focus of the present government is on the health improvement of the population; however, this has put a requirement on the clinical team to perform additional data collection tasks relating, for example, to clinical audit and drug utilisation. Thus the nurse adviser can assist without incurring extra cost to the NHS Trust or clinical staff being assigned to conduct this extra work.

Role and responsibilities

The purpose of the nurse adviser auditing patients' records is to improve patient care. There are no commercial activities associated with this venture, and although it may be considered supporting a marketing function, it is strictly and entirely non-promotional. The nurse's regulatory body, the Nursing and Midwifery Council (NMC), considers that there is no conflict of interest provided the nurse is in a supportive role and can demonstrate that s/he has always acted in the best interest of the patient. The benefit to the sponsoring company is the enhancement of their reputation with the staff within the NHS Trust and use of the aggregated information from the audit (e.g. on the side-effect profiles of medicines within a therapeutic area). Many nurse advisers are allowed patient contact and run clinics within their specialist area as part of the process, as well as running educational sessions for patients and clinical colleagues.

Following the audit, a report is prepared for key clinicians only. As stated before, the sponsoring company has access only to the aggregated information. The report is fed back to the clinical teams, sometimes in a workshop format either for a full or half day. These are often organised by the lead clinician, the nurse adviser and the medical representative, again enhancing this supportive position. After the presentation of the audit results, the attendees are often split up into small groups to discuss the results, the implications of these and to develop action points. The ultimate aim of this process is to improve patient outcomes.

In the ideal situation the patients' records should be re-audited in 12–18 months to evaluate the impact of any intervention. A byproduct of this process is the building up of relationships between the nurse advisers, the medical representatives and the clinicians. The medical representative from the company may use the results and work in conjunction with the pharmacist to develop information leaflets for patients.

Another role of the nurse adviser is to provide a monitoring service for some drugs that have been proved as an excellent treatment for a condition but may have toxic side effects. The nurse would ensure that the patient has had the required blood tests, advise the clinicians on the results and recall the patient as required.

Career pathway

The normal career pathway for a nurse adviser is to start conducting audits in clinical placements and developing expertise and knowledge within their specialist area. When the nurse is more experienced, aspects of the role will involve training junior members of the team. Promotion is to senior nurse adviser. The position of field manager supervises national teams of nurse advisers. They also liaise with the members of the client institution to consider the progress of an audit, and the possible extension or closure of a project. The nurse manager or manager of nursing services is frequently office-based and is instrumental in the development of nurse adviser business plans, recruitment of staff and the formation of the nurse adviser teams.

The size of each team will depend on the size of the project within either primary or secondary care. The teams will have regular meetings at six to 12-weekly intervals. A field manager facilitates regional meetings.

Personality attributes and fit for role

The nurse adviser needs to be a conscientious practitioner as s/he works autonomously so needs to keep abreast of current evidence-based knowledge within their specialist area. The nurse adviser represents both the sponsoring pharmaceutical company and their own employing company, working in different healthcare settings, and therefore needs excellent communication skills, confident in their own knowledge and ability. In this nurse specialist role they have to be self-disciplined, outgoing and professional in their attitude. However, they also need to be self-motivated, meticulous in the quality of their work and the management of their audit documentation.

Training and qualifications

The nurse adviser is a registered nurse (e.g. RGN or RMN); usually with at least two years' post-registration experience. Nurse advisers usually hold relevant post-registration qualifications in their therapeutic area, and many have a teaching qualification. They are also given presentation skills, as part of their role is to educate healthcare workers and patients about current treatments and to present findings from their audits. They are often given basic assertiveness training and facilitation skills training to support them in this role.

The pharmaceutical companies that sponsor projects which deploy nurse advisers ensure that they receive a comprehensive ongoing education to support them in their requirements for Post Registration Education Professional Practice (PREPP) (UKCC, 2001) with an associated budget. Also, most sponsor companies have an initial training course for new advisers, which includes an update on the disease area that the adviser will be working in, an update of the products of the sponsoring company and those of companies with products within that specific area. On a more practical level the nurse advisers are given training in the use of paper and electronic record systems.

New advisers are often assigned a mentor; however, they are appraised by the line management of their employing organisation or agency, usually every six months.

At this time objectives are set that are specific to the project, to personal development and to time management.

Changing course

As the nurse adviser works in conjunction with the medical representative from the pharmaceutical company this may be considered an obvious job option. However, as the role of the nurse adviser is auditing patient records, advising on treatment and monitoring the effect, a worthwhile career within a pharmaceutical company would be as a drug safety monitor. But the nurse adviser may find client contact more enjoyable and opt to become a CRN.

The future

As the government continues to impose on the NHS Trusts the need to be able to demonstrate that they are achieving targets set in the National Service Frameworks, clinical governance and other directives, with an associated lack of funding to execute these tasks, the nurse adviser role appears to be addressing an integral need to complete the audit cycle.

Conclusion

Nurses are now realising their potential and progressing in these career pathways in clinical drug research, development and monitoring with the pharmaceutical industry due to the knowledge, skills, expertise and abilities they offer their employers. The experience and discipline gained through their involvement in medicines' development, and particularly clinical therapeutic trials, are invaluable to them when transferring to other research areas.

The nurse as a healthcare professional has tremendous potential to develop a research career in a number of areas. Nevertheless, it has to be remembered that the ultimate reason for the conduct of research is to improve patient care.

References

Barnes, G. (1981) The nurse's contribution to the Medical Research Council's trial on mild hypertension. *Nursing Times*, 1240–1245.

Bersani, G., Sheenan, A. and Murray, M. (1983) Innovations in cancer nursing and the role of the nurse in clinical trials. *Progr. Clin. Biol. Res.*, **121**, 87–92.

Department of Health (2001) Research Governance Framework for Health and Social Care, Department of Health, London.

EC (2001) Directive of the European Parliament and of the Council on the approximation of the laws, regulations and administrative provisions of the Member States relating to implementation of Good Clinical Practice in the conduct of clinical trials on medicinal products for human use. European Union Directive on GCP in Clinical Trials 2001/20/EC. *Official Journal of the European Communities.*

Hubbard, S.M. (1982) Cancer treatment research: the role of the nurse in cancer trials of cancer therapy. *Nursing Clinics North Am.*, **17**(4), 763–783.

ICH (1995) International Conference of Harmonisation of Technical Requirements for Registration of Pharmaceuticals for Human Use. Good Clinical Practice: Consolidated Guideline, CPMP/ICH/135/95.

Johnson, J.M. (1986) Clinical trials: new responsibilities and roles for nurses. *Nursing Outlook*, **34**(3), 149–153.

Kenkre, J.E. and Foxcroft, D.R. (2001a) Career pathways in research: clinical research. *Nursing Standard*, **16**(5), 41–44.

Kenkre, J.E. and Foxcroft, D.R. (2001b) Career pathways in research: pharmaceutical. *Nursing Standard*, **16**(4), 36–39.

NMC (2002) Nursing and Midwifery Council. Code of Professional Conduct, April.

Northern Ireland Research Governance (2002) http://www.rdo.csa.n-i.nhs.uk/rdo/resg/index.shtml

RCN (1998) The Clinical Research Nurse in NHS Trusts and GP Practices: Guidance for Nurses and their Employers. Employment Brief 2/98, Royal College of Nursing, London.

Ryan, K. (2002) Nurses in the Pharmaceutical Industry. Part 1: Unravelling the Role of the Nurse Advisor. http://www.pharmiweb.com/news/features/feature.asp?FeatID=108

Scott, G. (1993) SSC survey. *Clin. Res. focus*, **4**(8), 14–21.

The Scottish Executive (2001) Research Governance Framework for Health and Community Care, October.

UKCC (1996) United Kingdom Central Council for Nursing, Midwifery and Health Visiting. Guidelines for Professional Practice, UKCC, London.

UKCC (2001) United Kingdom Council for Nursing, Midwifery and Health Visiting. The PREP Handbook, UKCC, London.

Wales Office of Research and Development (2001) Research Framework for Health and Social Care in Wales. National Assembly for Wales, Wales Office of Research and Development for Health and Social Care in Wales.

Useful Websites

Royal College of Nursing Research Co-ordinating Centre
http://www.man.ac.uk/rcn

Royal College of Nursing Library
http://www.rcn.org.uk/home/home.html

Primary Care Nursing Research Network
http://PrimaryCareNursingResearchNetwork@yahoogroups.com

CHAIN—Contact.Help.Advice.Information.Network
http://www.doh.gov.uk/ntrd/chain/chain.htm

National Cancer Research Network
http://www.ncrn.org.uk

Institute of Clinical Research
http://acrpi.com

Register of Controlled Trials
http://www.controled-trials.com

Useful Addresses and Information

Look up pharmaceutical company websites for detailed information about their research and research governance.

15

The Toxicologist in Pharmaceutical Medicine

Geoffrey Diggle*

Formerly Department of Health, London, UK

Introduction

Interest in toxicology often starts at school. Those who study chemistry soon appreciate, during laboratory sessions, that chemical substances can have unpleasant effects. A drop of sodium hydroxide solution on the skin is enough to draw attention to cutaneous irritancy. The rule that some reactions must only be conducted in the fume cupboard is readily accepted when the noxious nature of some evolved gases is appreciated.

In practical biology classes it is realised that the acute lethality of some chemicals enables them to be used to immobilise protozoa prior to microscopic study, and to kill metazoan animals humanely and efficiently before dissection.

While chemistry and biology are the foundation sciences underlying modern toxicology, the field has no fixed definition. Toxicology is developing and expanding, and is perhaps best described in terms of what those who call themselves toxicologists actually do. Even this pragmatic approach has its difficulties, however. First, the problem of inconsistency: some of those who do not regard themselves as toxicologists carry out work and follow approaches indistinguishable from those who do. Second, there have been profound changes in the activities of toxicologists over time. However, there is general agreement about the role of modern toxicologists who work with pharmaceutical products, who are in fact the inheritors of an ancient tradition. It was appreciated in classical times that medicines and toxins had much in common, and that many substances had the

---

* The views expressed in this chapter are those of the author, and do not commit the Department of Health in any way.

Careers with the Pharmaceutical Industry, Second edition. Edited by P. D. Stonier.
© 2003 John Wiley & Sons Ltd. ISBN 0 470 84328 4

qualities of both, although it was left to the great Paracelsus (1493–1541) to remind Western science of this. For the Greeks, both drugs and poisons were denoted by pharmakon (+apzaxor), which also translates as dye, spell and a concealed thing used to bring about certain effects. The archer's bow was toxon (TOtOV) and these two words were combined to give the term for arrow poison, toxicon pharmakon (rotFxov fapyaxov). The English toxicology is in turn derived from this.

The earliest men knew of and used the toxic effects of animal venoms and poisonous plants, such as *Aconitum* spp. The knowledge of these early toxicologists was of value in hunting, in warfare and for getting rid of enemies. Some therapeutic properties of plant substances, such as the analgesic and euphoriant effects of opium from *Papaver somniferum*, were appreciated in the ancient world. In classical times, the poisoner was well established and there is much literature on the subject from the period. By 399 BC (the date of Socrates' death, allegedly following the administration of *Conium maculatum*) poisoning had become an official method of execution. By the Roman period, poisoners such as Locusta had become specialists in preparing and advising on the use of lethal substances, and their skills were much used by the imperial families, among others. Toxicology, in this sense, continued to develop through the Middle Ages, when specialists such as Catherine de Medici and Lucretia Borgia earned their reputations. The most infamous case on record is that of a professional poisoner known as La Voisine (The Neighbour), who was found guilty of poisoning many people, including 2000 children.

Today, however, most recognised toxicologists are concerned with the safety aspects of the subject, although a small minority deal with chemical weapons, riot control agents, etc. The main focus of toxicological safety is on the individual and on human populations, although this includes environmental effects mediated through the actions of toxic chemicals on plants and animals. All medicines are capable of producing adverse effects. For a pharmaceutical product, the key question is whether its toxicological effects are outweighed by its therapeutic benefits. The role of the toxicologist working in this area is, ultimately, to make the best possible prediction of what those effects will be.

The Work of the Toxicologist

The role of the toxicologist is of particular importance in research-based pharmaceutical companies in a number of areas, and especially in the testing of new active substances, in animals and in vitro to ensure eventual safety in use. The standard and thoroughness of pharmaceutical toxicology have been developed greatly since 1961, when the thalidomide tragedy came to light. In addition to the toxicological testing of candidate new drugs, the toxicologist may also be concerned with the correlation of animal and human pharmacology, the selection of compounds for exploratory human investigation and the planning of the developmental work required before initial human exposure can occur.

The toxicologist also requires an adequate understanding of the issues involved in the identification of promising candidate compounds; these include factors related to therapeutic indications and efficacy endpoints, as well as safety aspects.

In toxicity testing, the fundamental differences (and similarities) between the toxicology of compounds in animals and in man must be explored and assessed, by qualitative and quantitative methods. The comparative toxicity of metabolites, as well as parent compounds, must also be studied. The pharmacological differences, as between test species and humans, must be examined.

New candidate drugs are subjected to a wide range of toxicological studies, many of which are carried out in laboratory animals, such as rats, mice and dogs. The studies are designed to investigate the drug's potential to cause harm to any organ or physiological process. Short-term tests (e.g. 14-day tests) aim to identify the target organ(s) in which damage occurs, and assist in selecting dose levels for longer-term studies. A range of special studies are used to investigate the potential for damage to any part of the reproductive cycle. Lifetime studies in rodents are used to assess carcinogenic potential. Expertise in the choice of testing methods and a full understanding of their predictive value are needed. Information about the absorption, distribution, metabolism and excretion of the test compound in the species studied is very relevant to the toxicological assessment, and must be considered alongside similar data from human subjects before early dose-ranging in man is undertaken, prior to the first clinical trials.

In many toxicological studies in animals, the expertise of the pathologist is essential. A pathologist must carry out, or at least supervise closely, the histological examinations required at the conclusion of such studies, although much of the routine work of general post-mortem examination may be carried out by expert toxicology technicians, with the guidance of the pathologist as necessary. If the study director (i.e. the toxicologist responsible for the study) is not a qualified pathologist, then suitable arrangements will have to be made to obtain the services of a pathologist, perhaps someone on the company's staff or an independent expert on a consultancy basis. The pathologists who undertake this work include veterinary surgeons, doctors and graduates in other sciences who have obtained appropriate specialist qualifications in pathology. The toxicologist must possess the qualities needed to establish and maintain effective collaboration with pathologists and specialists in other fields.

Toxicological programmes must be managed strategically in order to ensure that they fit smoothly with clinical and other lines of development, that unnecessary delays are avoided and that timely planning allows for the unexpected. This requires a clear grasp of the regulatory requirements laid down by government agencies for clinical trials and eventual marketing approval, including the preparation and submission of marketing applications, and the approval and appeal processes in the relevant countries.

The development of a new medicine requires an integrated approach at corporate and, often, at international level. The toxicologist must be fully aware of the operational issues involved, including those concerned with the medical aspects of product development, and especially the production of the toxicological and toxicokinetic supporting information needed before the first studies in man can take place. In this context, it is advantageous if the toxicologist has some general appreciation of such matters as the arrangements for compensation of healthy volunteers and patients in pre-marketing studies, the consent procedures employed in volunteer work and clinical trials, and issues of confidentiality. Some awareness of the arrangements for indemnifying companies and investigators, the ethical review process, as well as problems of patenting and the contractual arrangements with external consultants, clinical investigators and contract research organisations can also be useful, although these matters are generally outside the domain of the toxicologist.

The development of new pharmaceutical products is not the only area in which the company may put the knowledge of the toxicologist to work. Employers must assess the risks, including the toxicological risks, to which their own employees are exposed and the availability of in-house toxicological expertise may be particularly advantageous in risk assessment in relation, for example, to production workers in the pharmaceutical industry. Similarly, the advice of company toxicologists may be sought occasionally on questions about the environmental impact of chemical effluents from production plants, etc., although these are properly questions for ecotoxicologists.

Even the most well-established medicines are monitored for their safety in use. Toxicological expertise may be crucial in interpreting reports of adverse reactions, overdosage and interactions with other drugs. The advice of the toxicologist may be sought on mechanisms, the feasibility of re-challenge, predisposing factors and methods for assessing adverse reactions.

Senior toxicologists frequently undertake staff management responsibilities, and may act as line managers of other toxicologists and toxicology technicians. Staff may require further training and their needs may be met, for example, by means of day-release courses, as well as by on-the-job training. Animal technicians, however, generally work under veterinary supervision. Animal technicians carry out important, labour-intensive tasks such as ensuring the welfare and accurate dosing of animals, and this work is not of course restricted to normal working hours. Veterinary supervision must ensure that the standard of animal care is high and that the animal technicians are properly trained in matters of animal welfare and husbandry.

The toxicologist who acts as the study director for a particular test is responsible for its planning, preparation of the protocol, overall conduct and preparation of the report which will be submitted eventually to the regulatory agency as part of the application for clinical trial or marketing approval. Many of the study director's functions are coordinating ones, involving liaison with specialist sections of the company such as the laboratories responsible for carrying out the haematological and biochemical analyses of blood samples taken from the animals under test, and the pharmacy charged with providing adequate and timely amounts of the test substance. Supervision of the toxicology technicians who obtain blood and urine samples from the test animals and monitor their clinical condition, all in compliance with Good Laboratory Practice (GLP), is a particular responsibility of the study director.

The study director must be a competent and resourceful scientist who is able, for example, to respond quickly and appropriately when untoward or unexpected findings emerge which call for additional investigations. It may be necessary to devise special experiments to follow up adverse findings in animal studies and assess whether they are predictive for a risk to humans.

Good documentation ensures that the unpredictable events which may always occur in the course of studies do not lead to subsequent difficulties and queries. While a protocol may be amended formally to take account of significant changes in the course of a study, undocumented, informal alterations following the emergence of adverse effects are subject to possible misinterpretations in the future, and must not be permitted.

Suppose, for example, that a protocol specifies that blood sampling is to be carried out at the seventh week, from a group of animals in a long-term study, with the work scheduled for a Monday and Tuesday: because of unforeseen staffing problems, the samples are all taken on Tuesday. The competent study director will ensure that a file note of this departure from the protocol, and the reason for it, is made. Adequate records of this kind can be of great importance when the results of reports of studies are eventually considered by regulatory assessors and GLP inspectors. When, for instance, a technical mishap, such as equipment breakdown, makes it necessary to abandon part of a study and start again, a clear note in the record is all that is needed to avert any future misunderstanding of what happened.

All experienced toxicologists are aware of the need to minimise the distress suffered by animals, and the conscientious professional will be at pains to ensure that unnecessary suffering is avoided, consistent with the need to establish the safety of medicines for human use. Occasionally there is a need to take difficult decisions in this area, although this is often best done in consultation with the appropriate regulatory agency. Suppose, for example, that a new substance is being developed for use as a general anaesthetic or as a muscle relaxant for use during surgical operations. If it is to be effective, it must be capable of inducing deep anaesthesia, or of paralysing the muscles, including those which are used to breathe. Safety must of course be assessed before use in man can be contemplated, and this would normally be achieved by means of studies in animals, including repeated-dose studies and evaluations in pregnant animals, at various dose levels well above the intended human dose. Examples of this kind illustrate the difficulty of the problems which may on occasion confront the toxicologist.

In addition to the need, for humane reasons, to minimise the numbers of living animals used in toxicity testing there are also economically important reasons. Some methods, such as those used to assess carcinogenic potential, are extremely expensive because of the numbers of animals which must be used if reliable information is to be obtained. In most areas of toxicology the development of alternative methods using fewer animals has been slow, although a notable advance is a new test for acute (single-dose) toxicity known as the fixed dose procedure, as an alternative to the traditional LD50 method. Another approach is the attempt to develop in vitro techniques employing cultured cells or tissues, or very small metazoan animals such as Hydra. Impressive development of in vitro approaches has taken place in genetic toxicology, in contrast to other specialised areas. Testing for genetic toxicity has been revolutionised by the development of standardised in vitro mutagenicity tests for detecting gene mutations caused by test substances in bacteria and in the cultured cells of higher organisms; reliable methods for revealing chromosome damage in cultured cells have also been achieved. The in vitro approach has made little headway in general toxicology because so many possible mechanisms of damage exist (unlike genetic toxicology, where there is a single underlying mechanism: damage to DNA). In vitro methods sometimes have a place in the further exploration of specific effects revealed by the general toxicity studies carried out in whole animals. Localised effects, such as cutaneous and ocular irritancy, also lend themselves to in vitro assays.

The Qualities and Abilities Needed

It is possible to identify a number of personal qualities which are desirable, and some of them indispensable, in the toxicologist working in today's pharmaceutical industry. The ability to work well with other specialists, both within and outside line management relationships, is essential. A thorough grasp of biology, of experimental methods and of regulatory guidelines is of course a *sine qua non*. Although this seems obvious, testing is sometimes carried out with an apparent disregard for biological common sense. One still sees bacterial tests for point mutation carried out on compounds having inhibitory properties which prevent the use of adequate dose levels, for example. It is essential that a check-list approach to implementation of guidelines be avoided.

The toxicologist must be comfortable with the meticulous approach needed when carrying out studies which meet the standards demanded by modern GLP. There can be no return to the working methods which necessitated the creation of the international GLP system. Nevertheless, the ability to carry out work meticulously is not the same as obsessionalism and rigidity; a flexible approach is needed when interpreting guidelines and deciding the programme of studies to be carried out. The toxicologist must be able to respond to guidelines as guidelines, when deciding which studies will be appropriate and when designing experimental protocols.

Allied to this is the ability to write clearly. For example, commentaries on the tests undertaken must be clear and unambiguous. If there are, for good scientific reasons, departures from regulatory guidelines, then the underlying thinking should be explained clearly and the assessors in the regulatory agencies who must eventually evaluate the data should be left in no doubt about the scientific reasons and reasoning involved. Pre-clinical reports are sometimes put together in final submissions by staff who are not fully conversant with the science, and the toxicologist's ability to write in such a way that the likelihood of misunderstanding is minimised is invaluable.

Investigative ability is an important quality, and of course this often requires intuition based on experience, as well as deduction. When a study suggests that there is an adverse effect which calls for an explanation, both time and money are saved when the toxicologist is able to distinguish promptly between experimental error, for example errors of measurement, allocation of animals to test groups, dosing, etc., and genuine findings.

Such a situation might arise when, for example, a test for fertility and general reproductive performance seems to show reduced fertility in terms of numbers of offspring. The ability to confirm that a real effect is occurring, perhaps by recognising and focusing on the relevant part of the reproductive cycle, is clearly important. The same investigative ability is required in the elucidation of genuine but unexplained findings. When, for example, a compound has shown no DNA-damaging potential in the standard mutagenicity tests, but has produced tumours at a single site in a lifespan rodent bioassay, much skill may be needed to establish without undue delay that the substance is really non-genotoxic and that the mechanism of tumorigenesis poses no hazard for patients.

Planning ability is of particular importance. Toxicological studies must be so planned that bottlenecks in the drug development process are avoided. Planning must also ensure that the requirements of different regulatory agencies are satisfied, if appropriate, without undue duplication of work. Of course, this in turn calls for the ability to work harmoniously with other departments concerned with the product, such as the medical and regulatory affairs departments. An understanding of methods such as critical path analysis may be important in setting the timing of toxicological work, to ensure that it does not hold up other essential streams of interrelated activity. Carcinogenicity studies, for example, are lengthy and the results which they produce are not always conclusive; they are also extremely expensive. Once it has become clear that they will be needed, ample time for them must be allowed, in order to ensure that they do not delay eventual marketing authorisation.

Of all personal qualities, sound judgement is perhaps the most important to the toxicologist, and above all in the area of risk assessment. There is an extraordinary amount of public confusion about the safety of drugs and other chemical products, such as food additives and pesticides.

Chemophobia is encouraged by irresponsible, alarmist media coverage, especially in the UK, and by the activities of certain interest groups, some politicians and members of the legal profession, especially in the USA. At the same time, there is relatively much less concern about agents, for example tobacco smoke, which are associated with real, substantial health risks. The balanced judgements of the professional toxicologist are indispensable in this atmosphere of misinformation and flawed perceptions. Toxicological risk assessment calls for the application of objective judgement and common sense to the question: how likely is it that the toxicological effect concerned could occur in patients receiving the medicine at the intended maximum dosage? In approaching this question, the toxicologist is at pains to establish the target organ toxicity for the compound under test in animals, as well as the maximum dose levels at which these effects cannot be observed. These levels are then compared with the proposed maximum therapeutic dose for patients, in order to judge whether the margins of safety are adequate. (The corresponding blood levels are often compared as well.) This judgement is essentially qualitative, although it is informed by much quantitative information. It must take into account many factors, including the toxicokinetics of the compound in the test species and in man. It must give due weight, for example, to interspecies differences in absorption, metabolism, etc.

To illustrate this by means of a somewhat simplified example, consider a new active substance intended for eventual marketing as a non-steroidal anti-inflammatory product. Among its toxicological effects it is found to cause gastric mucosal erosions and renal papillary necrosis in laboratory animals, in routine medium-term studies. The most sensitive species for the effect on the kidney is found to be the dog, in which this effect is still seen at doses which are too low to produce other toxicological effects. Further work establishes that the maximum level to which the dose can be raised without affecting the dog kidney is one-hundredth of the intended maximum dose for the treatment of patients with arthritis: the question at issue, then, is whether there is any significant risk of renal damage in patients. Clearly, much experience is needed in making reliable assessments of this kind; the ability to arrive at sound judgements and give reliable, informed advice in areas such as these is the hallmark of the professional toxicologist.

Training and Careers in Toxicology

The educational routes leading to toxicology as a profession are varied, and each has merits and disadvantages. In many cases, a first degree in a biological science is followed by some form of specialised training. For the graduate seeking introductory or part-time training in toxicology, suitable courses now exist in many countries. First degrees in toxicology are being introduced slowly. Postgraduate courses are also available for science graduates wishing to obtain higher and more specialised degrees, such as the MSc in toxicology, or in combinations of subjects which embody a toxicological component.

Suitably qualified scientists having at least five years' relevant experience may enter for the UK Diploma of the Institute of Biology (DIBT) and, in certain circumstances, membership of the Royal College of Pathologists (MRCPath) can sometimes be obtained by non-medical graduates. Similar qualifications conferred by professional bodies are available in some other countries.

Various career outlets are available to trained toxicologists interested in pharmaceutical work. In addition to the companies which develop and market medicinal products, contract research laboratories and government regulatory agencies also employ such specialists. For those whose interests extend to other, non-pharmaceutical products, similar posts both in industry and regulatory work are available in relation to agrochemicals including pesticides, consumer products including cosmetics, industrial chemicals and other groups. Career moves between these areas are not unusual, sometimes within the same large company.

A company toxicologist sometimes undertakes a complete career change within the same organisation, moving for example to the department responsible for dealing with regulatory agencies. There is also some movement between 'product-based' and other forms of toxicology, including forensic toxicology, ecotoxicology, clinical toxicology, occupational toxicology and, of course, academic work.

16

A Career in Clinical Quality Assurance

Rita Hattemer-Apostel

Verdandi AG, Zurich, Switzerland

Introduction

The ultimate task of quality assurance (QA) in clinical research is to ensure that the clinical trial participants are protected and that the data collected in clinical trials are valid and allow reliable conclusions to be drawn regarding the use of a drug.

Clinical quality assurance (CQA) auditors engage in auditing clinical trial documentation, investigator sites and processes; they provide training and consulting services and they manage the Standard Operating Procedures (SOPs). Usually, they are the 'driving forces' for managing the quality of clinical studies and for identifying areas of improvement. CQA auditors must be firmly grounded in clinical research and should be equipped with reliable knowledge of the international regulatory environment. Working in QA is a challenge, requiring a mature personality and seasoned communication skills.

Do you possess the analytical skills of Sherlock Holmes, the detached view of a pilot, the diplomacy of a politician and are you fond of travelling? Then you may consider a career in QA!

Quality assurance is a relatively young discipline in the pharmaceutical industry, and particularly in clinical research and development. However, the need for QA professionals is confirmed throughout the industry and the majority of pharmaceutical companies and contract research organisations (CROs) have established QA units. The backgrounds of QA specialists are diverse, and the training and education of QA auditors is still largely undefined.

Definitions for key terms related to QA in pharmaceutical development are noted in Table 16.1. Knowledge of the terminology helps in understanding the scope of QA tasks and responsibilities.

Careers with the Pharmaceutical Industry, Second edition. Edited by P. D. Stonier.
© 2003 John Wiley & Sons Ltd. ISBN 0 470 84328 4

Table 16.1 Definitions related to quality, according to ISO 9000:2000 (ISO, 2000) and the International Conference on Harmonisation (ICH) Good Clinical Practice (GCP) Guideline (ICH, 1997)

Applicable Regulatory Requirement(s)	ICH GCP 1.4: Any law(s) and regulation(s) addressing the conduct of clinical trials of investigational products.
Audit	ISO 9000:2000: A systematic, independent and documented process for obtaining audit evidence and evaluating it objectively to determine the extent to which audit criteria are fulfilled. ICH GCP 1.6: A systematic and independent examination of trial-related activities and documents to determine whether the evaluated trial-related activities were conducted, and the data were recorded, analysed and accurately reported according to the protocol, SOPs, GCP and the applicable regulatory requirement(s).
Audit Certificate	ICH GCP 1.7: A declaration of confirmation by the auditor that an audit has taken place.
Audit Report	ICH GCP 1.8: A written evaluation by the auditor of the results of the audit.
Audit Trail	ICH GCP 1.9: Documentation that allows reconstruction of the course of events.
Compliance	ICH GCP 1.15: Adherence to all the trial-related requirements, GCP requirements and the applicable regulatory requirements.
Good Clinical Practice (GCP)	ICH GCP 1.24: A standard for the design, conduct, performance, monitoring, auditing, recording, analyses and reporting of clinical trials that provides assurance that the data and reported results are credible and accurate, and that the rights, integrity and confidentiality of trial subjects are protected.
Quality	ISO 9000:2000: The degree to which a set of inherent characteristics fulfils needs or expectations that are stated, generally implied or obligatory.
Quality Assurance (QA)	ISO 9000:2000: The part of quality management focused on providing confidence that quality requirements will be fulfilled. ICH GCP 1.46: All those planned and systematic actions that are established to ensure that the trial is performed and the data are generated, documented (recorded) and reported in compliance with GCP and the applicable regulatory requirement(s).
Quality Control (QC)	ISO 9000:2000: The part of quality management focused on fulfilling quality requirements. ICH GCP 1.47: The operational techniques and activities undertaken within the quality assurance system to verify that the requirements for quality of the trial-related activities have been fulfilled.
Quality Management (QM)	ISO 9000:2000: The coordinated activities to direct and control an organisation with regard to quality.
Standard Operating Procedures (SOPs)	ICH GCP 1.55: Detailed, written instructions to achieve uniformity of the performance of a specific function.
Total Quality Management (TQM)	The total organisation using quality principles for the management of its processes (http://www.mazur.net/tqm/default.htm)

Background

Quality assurance or, in a broader sense, quality management (QM) activities are of central importance in the pharmaceutical industry. The goal of the entire process chain of pharmaceutical research, development and production is to provide safe and effective pharmaceutical products of high quality.

To help achieve this goal, a legal and regulatory framework exists for pre-clinical (laboratory) and clinical research and development as well as for the manufacturing processes of drugs. The regulations are known as Good Laboratory Practice (GLP), Good Clinical Practice (GCP) and Good Manufacturing Practice (GMP). The GLP, GCP and GMP regulations are sometimes referred to as 'GXP', summarising the quality standards in these areas.

Over the last five decades, the pharmaceutical industry has become more international and is constantly seeking new global markets. Although national regulatory systems for drug registration were based on similar fundamental obligations to assess the quality, safety and efficacy of the substances, the specific requirements differed to such an extent that unnecessary duplication of studies was necessary in order to market new products internationally.

Harmonisation of regulatory requirements became necessary and, in 1989, the International Conference on Harmonisation (ICH) initiated the process of developing international guidelines for the quality, safety and efficacy of pharmaceutical products. These guidelines are now the basis internationally for evaluating new substances before their registration.

The origins of modern quality management go back to the time when the product quality was evaluated at the end of the production process. Figure 16.1 displays the different development stages of quality management (from left to right):

1. Finished products were assessed to determine whether they fulfilled pre-established criteria: this process was only focused on quality control (QC). Quality improvements were achieved by narrowing the product specifications.
2. With the capability of evaluating large amounts of data, statistical methods were introduced to monitor the quality of the manufacturing process. Systematic analyses of data highlighted areas prone to errors. These evaluations, together with a growing awareness of how processes are connected, were the basis for extending the QA activities to the product development departments. Error prevention was now the primary resource for quality improvements.
3. Increasingly, quality was an attribute that could be managed—in a double sense. On one hand, the quality of products or services was manageable as long as the processes followed to produce the product or to provide the service could be controlled. On the other hand, quality was considered a task of management, and specialists in development and manufacturing were no longer solely responsible for the quality of the end product.
4. Further development of QM led to the conviction that all processes, areas and staff members contribute to achieve quality products or services. QM means

management of the entire business processes of an organisation or a company; and quality can only be improved by improving these business processes. The era of total quality management (TQM) is characterised by a strong focus on processes and customer satisfaction. No area in an organisation remains untouched when implementing TQM.

Quality management in the pharmaceutical industry developed in a similar way where initially government inspections were conducted for the manufacturing of drug substances. The purpose of these inspections was to verify the production processes and methods against the written pre-established standards to ensure that products were of defined and consistent quality. Following the development of GMP regulations for production, guidelines were established for pharmaceutical research and development: GLP regulations were developed to specify the requirements for conducting pre-clinical studies in laboratory animals, and GCP regulations were implemented to outline the standards for the conduct of clinical trials in humans.

Quality Requirements in Clinical Research

It is relatively easy to explain the quality concepts in production processes for products, e.g. for bicycles or mobile phones, whereas the concepts are more diffuse in the area of research and development. What is the final product of research and how can its quality be measured (Aschenbrenner, 2000)?

In general, the end product of research is information on the efficacy and safety of a new substance, summarised in a final study report. Based on this information, and provided the research results demonstrate that the therapeutic benefits exceed possible risks, regulatory authorities provide marketing authorisation for new drugs/devices, which, subsequently, are given to patients. However, valid risk–benefit assessments can only be performed based on reliable research results.

Quality requirements for clinical trials are therefore that data collected in clinical studies and the results of clinical trials should be reliable and should allow valid and meaningful conclusions to be drawn regarding the use of a drug/device.

As clinical trials are conducted with human subjects, either with healthy subjects or with patients suffering from the disease under investigation, further quality requirements are related to the performance of clinical studies. The participants' welfare and their right of self-determination must be guaranteed in clinical trials.

Hence, the quality requirements for clinical trials are:

1. Protection of the trial participants

   - Informed consent prior to study start.
   - Review of the trial by an Independent Ethics Committee (IEC)/Institutional Review Board (IRB).

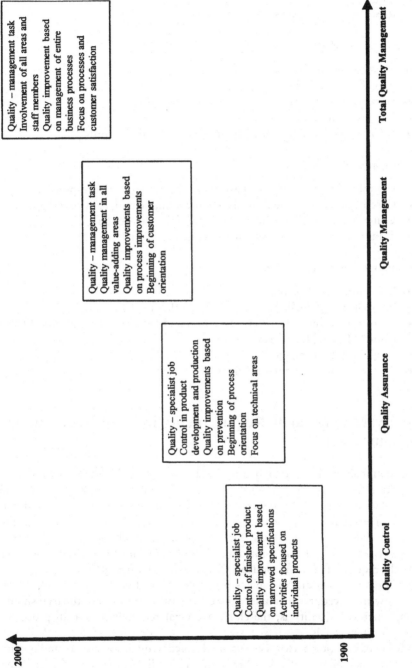

Figure 16.1 Development of quality management activities

- Compliance with the trial protocol, ethical guidelines and regulatory requirements.
- Reporting of adverse events.

2. Quality of the data

- Valid and credible.
- Representative and reproducible.
- Traceable and attributable to specific trial subjects.
- Timely recorded.
- Substantiated, e.g. by source documents or original records.

3. Transparency of conduct

- Contracts between involved parties outline the respective responsibilities.
- Careful planning of the clinical trial, including scientifically sound protocol.
- Complete and accurate documentation of the trial conduct.
- Transparency in data collection, processing and analysis.

4. Compliance with regulations and guidelines

- Declaration of Helsinki.
- International guidelines (e.g. ICH GCP, other ICH guidelines).
- Country-specific regulations (e.g. Food and Drug Administration's (FDA's) Code of Federal Regulations (CFR)).
- Standard Operating Procedures (SOPs).
- Any additional relevant guidelines.

Quality Management Requirements in GCP Regulations and Guidelines

The first hint about the need for quality checks was included in the FDA 'New Drug Application (NDA) rewrite' (21 CFR 314) in 1985. Sponsors were asked to indicate in the NDA submission documentation whether the clinical data submitted had been verified against source data during monitoring or audits. In 1991, the European Union (EU) GCP Guideline was published and one complete section was devoted to QA. ICH GCP, introduced in 1997, included more hints than ever about the requirements to introduce a QM system including QC and QA.

Quality is noted as one of the key principles of ICH GCP (2.13) (ICH, 1997): 'Systems with procedures that assure the quality of every aspect of the trial should be implemented'. Quality is, therefore, a crucial requirement for all processes related to clinical trials.

In ICH GCP chapter 5, two sections are devoted to quality assurance and quality control (5.1) and audit (5.19). Another paragraph outlines procedures for handling non-compliance by investigators (5.20). In addition, in ICH GCP sections 5.5.3 and 5.5.4, quality requirements are specified for handling and processing of electronic data.

Despite the numerous sections in ICH GCP addressing QM requirements in the various areas of trial planning, conduct and reporting, the guideline does not exactly outline which individual activities should be undertaken by an organisation to assure the quality of clinical trials. It is the responsibility of each organisation to establish their own QM system, which is tailored to specific needs and the organisational environment.

Role and Responsibility of Clinical Quality Assurance

The QM function in clinical research is often referred to as clinical quality assurance. The primary responsibility of CQA is to ensure that all processes contributing to the performance of a clinical trial are conducted in accordance with GCP regulations and related guidelines. To that end, the activities which are undertaken by an organisation should be identified, and rules and procedures (also called SOPs) for conducting these activities must be specified. Compliance with these SOPs should ensure that GCP requirements are met.

The purpose of SOPs is to:

- Ensure compliance with quality (GCP) requirements.
- Determine the internal standards for clinical trials.
- Ensure that all necessary activities are undertaken when they are required.
- Clarify who is responsible for conducting the different activities.
- Determine the interfaces and interactions between different persons and functional groups involved in performing the clinical trial (Aschenbrenner, 2000).

When the foundation for quality work has been prepared and the SOPs are available, it is the task of CQA to establish a QM system to ensure that all processes contributing to the clinical trial—from the design of the clinical trial to the preparation of the final trial report—are conducted in compliance with the pre-established SOPs.

The QM systems should comprise in-process QC steps performed by the functional groups as well as independent audits performed by the CQA unit. QC and QA are vital components for a QM system to be effective.

Quality control must be integrated in all processes so that the process owners are able to control the quality of the service (or product) provided. QC activities are performed as an integral part of each process. An example of a typical QC activity is the internal review of key documents in clinical research, such as the trial protocol or the study report. QC steps are performed by representatives of operational groups who are checking the compliance with SOPs and GCP requirements on a continuous basis, as a routine part of the day-to-day activities.

In contrast, CQA's role is to assess the processes and trial documents in order to provide an unbiased statement about the level of compliance with regulations and guidelines. To that end, CQA must be independent of operations, i.e. separate from those functional groups that are actually involved in designing, planning, conducting, managing and reporting the clinical trial, and CQA must also be separate from QC functions. In general, QA audits are conducted on a sampling basis, for example only a limited number of investigator sites are selected for audit.

The independence of CQA should also be visible in that the reporting paths of CQA personnel are separate from operations: CQA usually reports directly to management. A properly composed CQA unit should therefore be able to conduct balanced, unbiased and independent audits of study processes and trial documents. The fact that CQA personnel are not involved in the day-to-day activities in clinical research helps develop a detached view of the processes. The predominant purpose of CQA is to evaluate whether the QC procedures were adequate to generate a quality product. In our example of the trial protocol, it would mean that the internal review process for the protocol is appropriate to capture all deficiencies in the development stage before the protocol is finalised.

Audits must not substitute for QC checks conducted by operations, but QC reviews and CQA audits are considered essential components of QM systems.

Typical Responsibilities of CQA Personnel

The range of responsibilities of CQA personnel is diverse. Although members of the CQA unit are usually called 'auditors', this term should not detract from the fact that there is more to QA than auditing.

Typical areas of responsibility for CQA auditors are described below.

Managing SOPs

In many companies and organisations, CQA is responsible for maintaining the SOPs, for initiating and managing the SOP review cycles and for verifying that the SOPs comply with GCP regulations and applicable guidelines, and that the SOPs remain current. SOP management encompasses many activities, e.g. preparing draft SOPs, reviewing and commenting on SOPs, and soliciting and incorporating comments from reviewers. CQA is also involved in revising and approving SOPs and in maintaining SOPs (as paper copies or in electronic format). Outdated SOP versions must be retrieved and new versions distributed. Further, CQA is often responsible for ensuring that all functional groups are properly trained on the SOPs (Hamrell and Wagman, 2001; Hattemer-Apostel, 2001b).

Conducting audits

Audits are usually divided into trial-specific audits and systems audits. Trial-specific audits are focused on one individual clinical study, whereas systems audits evaluate the adequacy of a subsystem in clinical research, e.g. the adverse event (AE) reporting process, and usually focus on several studies.

Trial-specific audits require review of key trial documents to assess the processes undertaken at the investigator site. Key trial documents include the investigator's brochure, the trial protocol and protocol amendments, the subject information sheet and informed consent form, the Case Report Form (CRF) and the final study report. These documents are audited to determine the compliance with GCP guidelines and regulations.

Audits at investigator sites are focused on the availability, completeness and accuracy of the trial documentation at the site and the transparency of the processes followed at the site. For example, the documentation relating to ethics committee approval and the notification of regulatory authorities is assessed. Auditors also check the signed informed consent forms for all subjects participating in the trial. Usually, data verification and validation of CRF entries is the time-consuming part during the investigator site audit. The reporting of AEs and serious AEs is also an important component of the site audit, as is the interview with the investigator and key site personnel to further assess the procedures followed for conducting the trial at the site. Handling, dispensing and return of trial medication are evaluated by checking the drug accountability forms and shipment/transfer documentation.

The audit of the clinical database compares the information in the clinical database with the entries in the CRFs and related query forms. Key objectives are to assess whether the clinical database is accurate (i.e. entries in the database and in the CRF must match) and complete (i.e. all CRF entries are included in the database and no entries are entered into the database which cannot be substantiated by the CRFs). Database audits are usually very time-critical, because they are conducted between database closure and unblinding of the trial (in case of blinded trials), before the trial data can be analysed.

Typical examples for systems audits are:

- Protocol/CRF/report generation;
- Clinical monitoring;
- Safety reporting;
- Data management and biostatistics;
- Training;
- Document management and archiving;
- SOPs;
- Computer validation;
- CRO/clinical laboratory/vendor (Hattemer-Apostel, 2000b).

Training and consulting

Many CQA auditors are involved in providing training on GCP regulations, regulatory requirements, SOPs and other related areas. Often, as a direct consequence of audits, feedback is provided to functional groups and departments of deficiencies and weaknesses observed during audits. The information on errors and non-compliance should prevent the recurrence of the observed weaknesses.

Education and Qualifications of CQA Auditors

There is no standard educational profile for CQA auditors, but typically, prospective CQA auditors should have completed secondary education, e.g. in nursing, natural sciences or medicine. They should be able to clearly express their ideas and concepts orally and in writing.

ISO 10011, part 2 suggests that auditors should have a minimum of four years' full-time relevant workplace experience and at least two years should have been in QA. Experience in the conduct of audits is also required, including at least the participation in a minimum of four audits with a total of 20 audit days (ISO, 1992; Hattemer-Apostel, 2000a).

Previous experience in the conduct, management or supervision of clinical trials, e.g. as a Clinical Research Associate (CRA), project manager or data manager, should be an entry qualification for CQA auditor candidates. Drug development is a specialist environment, and CQA is a small niche in clinical research. CQA staff are expected to be fully conversant with GCP regulations, applicable regulatory requirements and SOPs. Profound understanding of drug development in general and the conduct of clinical trials in particular is the basis for thorough and meaningful audits, and for arriving at valid conclusions.

Knowledge Base, Skills and Competencies of CQA Auditors

Willingness to travel is a prerequisite for auditors, as audits (particularly those at clinical investigator sites) must often be conducted in remote locations and foreign countries. The ability to speak and understand different languages paired with sensitivity to different cultures and operational constraints are typical requirements for auditors.

Proficiency in English, orally and in writing, is imperative, as this is the most common language used in audit reports and essential documents in clinical research. CQA auditors must also be computer literate and know 'standard' software packages used for word processing and calculation.

Interactions—Team, Professional, Inside and Outside the Organisation

CQA activities are not conducted in isolation; and the requirement for independence does not preclude communication and interaction.

Communication with other CQA members is vital, especially when a team of auditors conducts audits. Communication within CQA is essential to discuss audit observations, to share knowledge and to agree on the grading of findings and the suggested corrective actions.

Interaction with auditees requires seasoned communication skills, as not many auditees like the idea of being audited: they consider audits as a burden and as an interruption of the usual workflow. CQA auditors must, therefore, be sensitive to the different auditing situations and demonstrate diplomacy in handling stressful situations.

In all stages of an audit, from planning the audit to assessing the responses to the audit report, project teams and functional groups are important communication partners to CQA. Further, audit findings must be communicated to the organisation's management, either via audit reports or condensed summaries of the level of compliance observed. Objectivity, integrity and reliability are key requirements for CQA auditors.

Interfaces also exist with vendors (e.g. during pre-qualification audits) or contractors/CROs during the course of a trial. If an organisation is audited by an external audit group or inspected by representatives of regulatory authorities, CQA is usually serving as liaison during these events.

Further, networking with external QA colleagues is always helpful, especially when CQA auditors are working on their own. Attendance at conferences and seminars and active membership in QA and GCP associations provide good opportunities to meet colleagues.

Personal Attributes for the Auditing Role

Auditing requires good analytical skills to understand complex audit situations and documentation which is sometimes contradictory or misleading. Auditors should be open-minded, realistic, pragmatic and have a mature personality. Objectivity and integrity are essential attributes for auditors, otherwise the audit observations might be biased and the validity of the conclusions could be questioned.

CQA staff members must be able to handle multiple priorities and must be flexible and eager to learn so that they will remain up-to-date (Hattemer-Apostel, 2000a).

Training for and on the Job

While the scope, duration and focus of initial training will depend on the previous education and experience of the prospective CQA auditor, the following components provide an overview of the typical training modules for auditors. Depending on the specific work environment of the CQA auditor, additional training topics might be added.

1. Prior to starting work as an auditor, the regulatory framework for the design, conduct, analysis and reporting of clinical trials should be reviewed. On an international level, the Declaration of Helsinki (2000) and key ICH guidelines (ICH, 1995, 1996, 1997, 1998a,b) are important reading material. Knowledge must also be acquired on country-specific legal and regulatory requirements, e.g. FDA CFR.
2. Subsequently, training in the conduct of audits should follow, including the review of relevant CQA SOPs and additional auditing policies. The auditor should also be trained how to interact with the auditee(s), how to use checklists and how to complete templates of audit reports and audit certificates. Clear understanding of the use of these tools enhances the consistency of the auditing process.
3. The diversity of audits necessitates an introduction to each of the audit types and familiarisation with the relevant guidelines and regulations (e.g. for computer validation audits, a review of 21 CFR part 11 is essential). Review of previous audit reports is a suitable training method as is the conduct of co-audits with a more senior CQA auditor. Over time, the prospective auditor increasingly assumes responsibilities for all aspects of audit planning, preparation, conduct and reporting. The auditor's individual pace will determine the number of supervised audits (Hattemer-Apostel, 2000b).

Continuing Education and Training

The advances in drug development, the emergence of new and revised regulations and guidelines and the structural changes in the pharmaceutical industry force CQA members to keep abreast with current knowledge. Vast opportunities exist for continuous education and life-long learning (Hattemer-Apostel, 2001a).

Broadening of the knowledge base in QA could encompass familiarisation with additional audit types, which were not included in the initial training, e.g. systems audits. CQA auditors typically conduct the majority of audits at investigator sites. Auditing data management and biostatistics activities would extend the knowledge base significantly. Equally, computer systems validation and audits of computerised systems used in clinical research and development are useful skills for CQA auditors. The increasing importance of technology in drug development is undeniable.

Interesting opportunities to broaden the GCP auditing experience exist in the neighbouring disciplines of GMP and GLP. GMP regulations apply to the production and handling of investigational products; and knowledge of GLP guidelines is useful when assessing clinical laboratories. Familiarisation with fundamental quality management principles, independent of clinical research and even the pharmaceutical industry, can be achieved through training in ISO 9000 ff quality management.

Familiarisation with CQA responsibilities and on-the-job training as an auditor will take between six and 12 months, depending on previous experience and the pace of learning. The variety of audit types and the focus of the audits are largely dependent on the organisation's scope of services and, hence, need for audits. Typically, CQA auditors are first trained on a core set of audit types, which are most typical for the company or organisation they work with. Over time, and concurrent with the organisation's needs, the scope of audits may broaden.

Starting with being responsible for individual audits, CQA auditors will have the opportunity for assuming responsibility for a series of audits for a clinical study, managing the CQA resources for these audits and ensuring that the tight timelines for completing audits are met. Much more complex and demanding is the management of audit programmes for entire drug development programmes, spanning preclinical development to NDA submission.

Professional postgraduate qualifications, ranging from Certificates of Credit, MSc and even PhD, in research quality assurance or clinical research may be a valuable qualification for CQA auditors (ACRPI, 2002; BARQA, 2002; ICR, 2002).

Expanding the Scope of the CQA Role

Focus on auditing

Depending on the interest and the skills of the individual, specialisation of auditing skills may be an option, for example, the CQA auditor may undergo training as an expert in computer systems validation or as a specialist in auditing of biostatistics procedures. Given the increasing number of regulations and guidelines and the growing use of computers and electronic devices in clinical research, seasoned auditing skills in these areas are adding value to an auditor's knowledge base.

The CQA auditor may also decide to broaden her or his auditing knowledge and to learn how to conduct GLP and GMP audits. Although these areas are different to GCP, some interfaces exist, e.g. the production and handling of investigational products in clinical trials. Knowing the GLP and GMP requirements will provide the GCP auditor with additional expertise beyond the key areas in clinical research.

ISO 9000 ff is another route for CQA auditors to acquire knowledge in universal quality management techniques and approaches, which are independent of GCP and not typically related to the pharmaceutical industry. Certification in ISO 9000 ff opens opportunities outside clinical research and even outside the pharmaceutical industry.

Focus on training

Excellent teachers are rare. Some CQA auditors are specifically talented in providing training on GCP and related areas. They have the knack for making effective and innovative presentations which have a long-lasting effect on the participants. Experienced auditors can also specialise in training and coaching novice auditors within the CQA department.

Career Pathways

Many novice auditors have acquired previous work experience as a CRA, project manager or data manager when they decide to move into QA. However, prospective CQA auditors may come from other areas related to clinical research, and professional backgrounds in fields such as pharmacovigilance, regulatory affairs, document management and information technology are valid starting points for clinical auditors.

The globalisation of clinical drug development programmes and the involvement of investigator sites across many countries open up interesting opportunities for CQA auditors. Knowledge of regulatory requirements for foreign countries must be acquired for the conduct of site audits abroad. Auditing in (sometimes remote) locations challenges the flexibility of auditors and refines their ability to communicate with clinical researchers of various nationalities and with different cultural backgrounds.

Depending on the size and structure of the CQA department and the geographical spread of the CQA members, opportunities may arise to conduct audits in different company locations or even to relocate and work there for several months. Working abroad is a unique opportunity to obtain first-hand experience with foreign regulatory requirements and country-specific guidelines.

Following the classical career development, CQA auditors can also move into QA management positions, leading a team of auditors and managing complete audit programmes for research projects. Excellent time management, communication and coordination skills are the prerequisite for such promotions, and knowledge of budgetary and human resources considerations is an asset, too. QA manager or director positions usually encompass responsibilities such as the development of QA strategies and quality measurement tools in order to produce trend analyses.

Another option might be to pursue a career in the training and development function. The management of the training department and the development of a training curriculum is an interesting growth opportunity for those who are particularly interested in this area.

CQA auditors could also return to operational departments, either the same as before they entered CQA or another functional area, and start in a senior or a manager position. Their QA experience is a valuable asset in these positions as they are well aware of deficiencies and areas of possible improvement.

The Future

Quality assurance will continue to be a challenging area in drug development and clinical research. The growing complexity and increasing pace of drug development make it difficult for those performing clinical trials to be fully conversant with all applicable regulatory requirements and GCP guidelines. CQA auditors play an important role in securing compliance with these regulations. Their critical assessment of deficiencies and weaknesses across all areas and phases of drug development ensures that the subjects participating in research projects are adequately protected and that the data collected, analysed and reported are valid and credible.

Surely, the perception of auditing as a 'back end' service conducted by auditors with a 'check-box mentality' will turn into the vision of auditing as a tool of proactive quality management. Preventing errors from happening and problems from occurring is certainly the smartest way of securing compliance. It is the CQA auditor's role to make this happen through suitable CQA activities such as auditing, training and consulting.

Acknowledgements

The author gratefully acknowledges the assistance of Wendy Bohaychuk (Editor-in-Chief of the *Quality Assurance Journal* and Director, GCRP Consultants, Lakehurst General Delivery, Ontario, Canada) who kindly read the manuscript and provided critical review.

References

ACRPI (2002) Welsh School of Pharmacy, Cardiff University, in cooperation with Association for Clinical Research in the Pharmaceutical Industry (ACRPI). Information available at http://www.cf.ac.uk/phrmy/clinres/main.html or http://www.acrpi.com

Aschenbrenner, M. (2000) Qualitätssicherung in der klinischen Forschung. *Dtsch. Med. Wochenschr.*, **125**(7), A17–20.

BARQA (2002) Anglia Polytechnic University, in cooperation with British Association of Research Quality Assurance (BARQA). Information available at http://www.barqa.com

Declaration of Helsinki (2000) Available at http://www.wma.net

Hamrell, M.R. and Wagman, B. (2001) Standard operating procedures in clinical research: a beginner's guide. *Qual. Ass. J.*, 5(2), 93–97.

Hattemer-Apostel, R. (2000a) GCP auditors: hard to find—hard to develop—hard to keep. Part I. Criteria and methods for candidate selection. *Qual. Ass. J.*, 4(1), 3–8.

Hattemer-Apostel, R. (2000b) GCP auditors: hard to find—hard to develop—hard to keep. Part II. Initial training requirements for auditors. *Qual. Ass. J.*, 4(3), 123–135.

Hattemer-Apostel, R. (2001a) GCP auditors: hard to find—hard to develop—hard to keep. Part III. Continuous education and further development. *Qual. Ass. J.*, 5(4), 3–11.

Hattemer-Apostel, R. (2001b) Standard operating procedures—a novel perspective. *Qual. Ass. J.*, 5(4), 207–219.

ICH (1995) Note for Guidance on Definitions and Standards for Expedited Reporting (CPMP/ICH/377/95), June. Available at http://www.ifpma.org/ich1.html

ICH (1996) Note for Guidance on Structure and Content of Clinical Study Reports (CPMP/ICH/137/95), July. Available at http://www.ifpma.org/ich1.html

ICH (1997) Note for Guidance on Good Clinical Practice (CPMP/ICH/135/95), January. Available at http://www.ifpma.org/ich1.html

ICH (1998a) Note for Guidance on General Considerations for Clinical Trials (CPMP/ICH/291/96), March. Available at http://www.ifpma.org/ich1.html

ICH (1998b) Note for Guidance on Statistical Principles for Clinical Trials (CPMP/ICH/363/96), September. Available at http://www.ifpma.org/ich1.html

ICR (2002) John Moore's University, Liverpool, in cooperation with the Institute of Clinical Research. Information available at http://www.livjm.ac.uk/learning/postgrad/pac/4516.asp or http://www.instituteofclinicalresearch.com

ISO (1992) ISO 10011, Guidelines for Auditing Quality Systems. Part 2: Qualification Criteria for Quality Systems Auditors, June. Available at http://www.iso.ch

ISO (2000) ISO 9000:2000, Quality Management Systems—Fundamentals and Vocabulary, December. Available at http://www.iso.ch

Useful Websites

http://www.drugdev123.com
http://www.fda.gov
http://www.fda.gov/oc/gcp
http://www.emea.eu.int
http://www.ifpma.org/ich1.html
http://www.barqa.com
http://www.diahome.org
http://www.interscience.wiley.com
http://www.reg123.com
http://www.regsource.com
http://www.sqa.org

17

A Career in Product Registration and Regulatory Affairs

Pat Turmer

London, UK

Introduction

In almost all countries there is some form of governmental control before medicines for human and veterinary use can be sold or supplied. In its modern form this was probably encouraged in Europe by the thalidomide problem in the early 1960s. However, even before this event controls like the Therapeutic Substances Act in the Poisons Laws in the UK gave a legal structure to the sale of medicines and in the USA the Food and Drugs Acts of 1906 and 1912. Now with ever-increasing new chemical, biological and bioengineered drugs, formalistic controls exist almost everywhere.

The pharmaceutical industry, which produces these new drugs, is a high-risk industry in which long development times are usual. The process of 'drug registration' is the last step in the long process of introducing a new drug. This is the formal submission of documents to a regulatory agency in order to get approval to market. The regulatory process starts much earlier and should be seen right the way through the development process and must continue once the drug is marketed.

The aim of this chapter is a brief overview of product registration and regulatory affairs.

Careers with the Pharmaceutical Industry, Second edition. Edited by P. D. Stonier.
© 2003 John Wiley & Sons Ltd. ISBN 0 470 84328 4

Job Description

The task for product registration in its simplest aspect may be described as obtaining and maintaining authorisations to market medicinal products in as many countries worldwide as necessary. Within this all-encompassing statement lies a wide variety of actual jobs dependent on the geographical area, size and structure of company, type of product, head office or subsidiary location, size of department and structure of department. The headquarters of most major pharmaceutical companies are located in Europe, the USA or Japan, and these areas are where most regulatory positions are to be found. Other significant countries are Canada, South Africa, Australia and New Zealand.

To understand the job description it is necessary to know something about the general system of obtaining licences to market medicines. A certain amount of product development is described in other chapters of this book so a brief summary is all that will be given here relating to the various stages of development to the regulatory process.

Drug development starts with the synthesis of a chemical compound which is tested pharmacologically to determine its activity. It is also tested toxicologically to determine its possible unwanted effects and to estimate a therapeutic index or a ratio of activity to toxicity. At some point in this development a decision has to be made whether or not to progress to tests in humans. This is when the first formal regulatory activity becomes necessary, although it is hoped that there has been regulatory input in the preceding development phases.

In most countries there is some approval or registration procedure needed before potential drugs can be tested in humans. The degree of regulation varies considerably but in all cases a minimum level of toxicology is required, together with varying amounts of pharmacology, chemistry and pharmacy. A clinical protocol describing the study to be carried out is also required. This information has to be assembled and presented in the appropriate form to the concerned regulatory body. Any necessary updates, amendments and renewals have to be carried out.

During or following clinical trials a decision has to be made concerning the suitability of the trial drug for marketing. Many factors will influence this decision. If marketing is appropriate an application to obtain approval must be made in those countries in which it is planned to sell the product. This requires a Marketing Authorisation (MA) application (New Drug Application, NDA, in the USA). This varies in format and detail from country to country but the core data content is similar for most countries worldwide. There are three main parts to this application describing (a) chemistry and pharmacy (or technical aspects), (b) experimental, biological and toxicological aspects, and (c) clinical details. These three parts are accompanied by administrative details which will vary from country to country.

This registration application is presented to the regulatory authorities of the appropriate countries, whose professional staff will review the content. If it is acceptable, permission to market the product will be given. This may take several years in some countries and involve much dialogue with the regulators and often amendments to the data. Once on the market a product now enters another phase in its life cycle. It is now necessary to keep the various authorities updated with new findings or developments, obtain approval for any changes in manufacture, apply for new indications or additional pharmaceutical formulations, and keep the product information up-to-date.

At predefined intervals, which may vary according to country but which are usually every five years, the authorisation has to be renewed. The procedure to be followed varies according to country.

Regulatory Personnel: Numbers and Distribution

It is difficult to assess with any accuracy the total number and distribution of regulatory personnel. There is no formal register or exclusive qualification. Some estimate may be obtained from membership of institutions or societies of direct relevance to regulatory affairs professionals. European examples include the European Society of Regulatory Affairs (ESRA), the British Institute of Regulatory Affairs (BIRA), the French (AFAR), Italian (BRAS), German (MEGRA) and Belgian regulatory affairs societies. PEFRAS, the Pan-European Federation of Regulatory Affairs Societies, is a forum for all the 'national' regulatory affairs societies. In the USA there is the Regulatory Affairs Professional Society (RAPS).

As one example, in 2000–2001 BIRA had a total membership of 2135 drawn from over 30 countries (BIRA Annual Report 2000–2001).

Job Content

The job content is as varied as the industry itself. Regulatory input is required at all levels of the pharmaceutical industry, from the smallest company marketing and selling one medicinal product to the largest multinational. The involvement may vary from a purely organisational role, with the main work being done by contract research organisations (CROs), to an entire department of regulatory affairs with a staff of 100 or more reporting at board level.

The variety in the job may come from several sources, as indicated in the job description. The organisational set-up of companies varies and the regulatory aspects may be stratified by therapeutic groups with responsibility for 'cardiovascular' or 'respiratory' or 'dermatological' products, for example, depending on company interests. This is most likely in companies with a wide range of interests. The responsibilities may be geographical, with regional groupings such as Europe, the USA, Japan, South America, Africa, the Middle East and the Far East.

A division may be made between research compounds and marketed products, with separate sections responsible for clinical trial approvals, marketing authorisation applications and the maintenance of marketed products. Another option is to divide responsibility according to discipline, with separate groups responsible for the technical, experimental/ toxicological and clinical aspects of a registration file. Often a combination of the above groupings occurs in practice. The job location in 'head office' or in a subsidiary will play a major role in defining job content.

In multinational companies the head office is usually where most of the information will be assembled and collated and a 'basic documentation set' compiled. The work to generate these data may have been done in a variety of locations worldwide. This 'basic documentation' must then be adapted according to the authority to which it will be submitted. This may be done at 'head office' or it may be done locally. It may be a major undertaking, with significant additional items to be written or parts to be translated, or it may only require the addition of a local application form. This will vary according to the nature and structure of the 'basic documentation set', which may be very basic, consisting of reports and technical details and hence requiring considerable additional work or, as is more usual, a complete file based on either the European or American preferred format, in which a certain level of structure is imposed and detailed summary documents are included. The transposition of an American format file or NDA to a European file (EC file) or vice versa can involve a considerable amount of restructuring, although the basic information content is very similar. The process of international harmonisation is now well under way with regard to the actual data but the format aspects are still very varied. It is hoped that the Common Technical Document (CTD) will provide the means for further harmonisation.

Regulatory involvement may include considerable writing, particularly summarising of experimental, toxicological or clinical tests and detailed indexing and cross-referencing of files. It will certainly require the ability to handle large volumes of paperwork (in hard copy or electronic format) and to be able to extract quickly and accurately the key information from a document.

The ability to communicate, either with other regulatory specialists or with pharmaceutical, pharmacological, toxicological and clinical experts in the company, is also an essential requirement.

Depending on company structure, regulatory personnel may communicate entirely within the company, liaising with research and development staff and with other regulatory personnel, or they may communicate with professional experts from the national regulatory bodies. In all cases an ability to express oneself clearly and concisely is essential.

In some countries the pricing of a drug is part of, and closely allied to, the registration process; in others there is an environmental assessment needed and increasingly now a pharmacoeconomic consideration. These aspects may come into the regulatory portfolio.

Qualifications and Personal Attributes

As can be seen from the job content a good basic life sciences background is an almost essential prerequisite for a job in regulatory affairs. It is possible to enter regulatory affairs from many directions as there is no primary qualification directly relating to the area. For a direct entry into regulatory affairs as a first job after graduation a pharmacy degree is a good qualification, as it will have covered, albeit only briefly in some cases, most of the aspects of drug registration. However, qualifications in toxicology, pharmacology, microbiology or biochemistry are also relevant. There can be advantages in gaining industrial experience in a more specialised area before moving into regulatory affairs. Thus formulation or production pharmacists, analysts, pharmacologists, toxicologists, microbiologists, clinical research scientists or information specialists may all find their previous experience helpful and their specialist knowledge of value to the regulatory affairs department.

In positions where there is extensive writing or summarising involved, medical writing experience could be advantageous.

In a large multinational company with widespread interests, opportunities will exist for personnel with a wide range of qualifications, but many companies are small and specialised and here specific qualifications may be more important. Examples of these are companies specialising in ophthalmic products or in vaccines, blood or immunological products or biotechnology products. Here the regulatory requirements are of a more specialised nature although the same general procedures apply.

There is no ideal or typical regulatory affairs character. There are, however, certain characteristics which are helpful. A capacity to work under pressure is advantageous, if not essential, because the submission of a marketing authorisation application comes at the end of a long development process and often the time needed for this process is underestimated. When the clinical work is finished it is a commonly held view that marketing should follow soon after. Another useful skill is the ability to handle large amounts of data in hard copy or electronic format. Regulatory work is long-term: it can take six to 12 months to complete and file an application and then anything from six months to four years or more to complete the assessment procedure, thus the ability for long-range planning, good work scheduling and a retentive memory are advantages.

Communication skills have been mentioned earlier and cannot be over-emphasised.

Education and Training

As stated previously, there is no specific first qualification for regulatory affairs. However, it is now a complex and wide-ranging area of work. The main training is on-the-job. In a large department, this may involve rotation around several job areas or in a small unit, gaining general experience by the necessity of attending to all aspects of the job. In both cases it is very much a learning-by-experience situation.

Coming from another branch of industry may bring with it a knowledge of some aspects of regulatory affairs; for example, a clinical research scientist could have an awareness of the regulations applying to clinical trials, or a medical information officer might have useful product knowledge for handling post-licensing activities such as product information updates and labelling information, as well as information-handling skills which could be useful in preparing a variety of regulatory documents.

As well as on-the-job training there are a variety of commercially run training courses, meetings and seminars. Courses specific to regulatory affairs are run by BIRA, ESRA and RAPS among others, while many other organisations include meetings on regulatory affairs in their programmes. Specifically educational are the BIRA and ESRA Introductory Courses and the Diploma in Regulatory Affairs run by BIRA in association with the University of Wales at Cardiff. The regulatory authorities also run information meetings or seminars on topics of current importance.

Many national authorities issue newsletters or information sheets which contain detailed changes in legislation, new regulations or updates on items of regulatory importance. Some journals include material, the *Regulatory Affairs Journal* being one which contains entirely matters of regulatory interest. The Internet is a convenient source of information with most regulatory authorities having webpages. Current regulatory legislation and guidelines are to be found on these websites.

Career Course

Entry into regulatory affairs may be as a junior member of the team, with upward progress by specialisation in one area of regulatory affairs in management. A large multinational company may appear to offer more in terms of career development than a smaller or more specialised company. However, the latter can often offer more scope for development in specific areas of expertise.

It is important at an early stage in a career to acquire as wide a range of experience as possible before either specialising in a specific area or moving to a more managerial role or specialising in regulatory affairs in terms of general regulatory strategy, input into research and development (R&D) and legal aspects. It is very rarely as clear-cut as this and often senior regulatory positions involve all these aspects of the regulatory process.

Roles and Responsibilities in Medicines Research and Development

Roles and responsibilities are largely determined by what the company structure will allow and what the individual will or can respond to. Regulatory affairs ideally should be involved from the start to the end of the drug development, but whether this is active or passive involvement depends on the personalities involved. Does participation at a meeting mean sitting and listening, only responding when directly asked, or does it mean actively contributing to the discussion?

It is my belief that a well-informed, competent regulatory executive can contribute significantly to the drug development programme. There is a need for the contribution to be positive. Too often it seems that regulatory input is seen in a negative light, always putting difficulties in the way of progress. This should not be the case since appropriate input may enable time to be saved.

So what is the role of regulatory affairs in medicines R&D? To be taken seriously and given the opportunity to participate in drug development, the regulatory contribution must be able to provide accurate information on current guidelines, guidelines in development, current regulatory thinking, international requirements and local/national differences. Using this knowledge a regulatory strategy applicable to the product in question can be determined.

Much will depend on what responsibilities are given to the regulatory area. Speed in development is essential and often, once the experimental and clinical work is complete, it is expected that dossier submission will follow very rapidly. What opportunities are there for the regulatory department to facilitate preparation of reports? Delegation of work, organisation of resources, use of external consultants and contract houses should all be part of the strategic plan.

In order to fulfil this full and demanding role it is necessary to have the background and confidence to interact with scientists and clinicians at all levels of development. It is not, however, necessary to have in-depth expertise in all areas; the essential is a sound scientific background and the overall concept of the registration file which is often not available to the specialists. This overall view can sometimes be the most important contribution of the regulatory area to development, ensuring that there are no major inconsistencies between the various sections of the registration file.

In some cases, the regulatory department is only brought into the picture at the end of the development. At this stage the contribution is smaller but nonetheless important; the file still has to be put together and submitted. It needs to be checked for completeness and inconstancies overall. It must, however, be said that if a development is to be successful there has to have been someone taking the overall view as described earlier even if it has not been the regulatory department.

Career Development

Within regulatory affairs

The obvious career development is from a junior position in the department to a more senior post and then to a managerial role. Along the path there will be many diversions, possibly to section head or responsibility for a geographical area or therapeutic area or for chemical/pharmaceutical, toxicological or clinical aspects. Specialisation at this level often means continuing to play an active part in the day-to-day regulatory process, whereas at managerial level in a large department the emphasis will probably swing to strategic and personnel aspects rather than routine regulatory activities.

Here again company structure will play a part. Does the regulatory department play a role in strategic planning or is the role limited to dossier submission with strategy determined elsewhere? This might determine whether the upward route is also possibly the outward route, although regulatory strategy in this instance should be considered as the final goal in the regulatory career.

A problem with progressing upward in this manner is that the decision-making process could become divorced from the regulatory process. Good communications and information networks are necessary to keep optimum efficiency.

What can be an interesting career development is responsibility for a local development such as a line extension in one geographical region which may, if successful, be utilised more widely. Here experience can be gained in strategy and planning without the pressures inevitable with a large international project. Thus, career moves within the industry could progress from a position in a subsidiary with major activities on a national level to a major European responsibility through to an international role.

Once again the scope and responsibilities of the role will depend largely on the type of company and its internal structure. There are, however, sufficient companies and structures to offer considerable scope to the variety of ambitions that are found.

It must not be forgotten that there are other regulatory opportunities besides direct employment in the pharmaceutical industry. Many senior regulatory personnel are now to be found as consultants to the industry and it is in areas like this that experience gained from a career in regulatory affairs can be put to good use. It also offers the opportunity to continue to utilise such skills directly rather than take on greater managerial responsibility. There are also opportunities with contract research organisations either specialising in regulatory work or having a regulatory department within their structure.

Finally, and not to be forgotten, are careers within the regulatory agencies.

Outside regulatory affairs

Career development outward from regulatory affairs is more difficult to summarise. In theory there are many opportunities. In practice it may not be so easy. The obvious routes outward are into the legal area, particularly that concerned with labelling, product information and advertising approval. In some organisations these items may be covered by the regulatory affairs department. The commercial licensing department which handles the licensing of products from or to other companies is another possibility.

Patents, particularly with the introduction of the Supplementary Protection Certificate Scheme in Europe, could be an appropriate move. With the increasing legislation, health and safety or quality assurance are other areas worth considering.

At a higher level a move into corporate or strategic planning or project management could be considered but company structures vary considerably, so it is difficult to be precise about opportunities. Being in the right place at the right time is often the most important factor.

If a complete change of direction is sought a training period may be required. For example, moving into marketing often requires a period to be spent 'in the field' as a representative. Advertising, where a knowledge of both products and the legal requirements is required, is a thought worth pursuing; however, the caution and understatement of the regulatory affairs world might not be an ideal background for this area.

With the increasing dependency on electronic means of data handling and the increasing use of electronic submission of regulatory data there could be opportunities for regulatory personnel in information technology or information systems departments.

If all these ideas fail to satisfy it is always worth considering going back to the laboratory and finding out first hand why all the things that seem so obvious to the regulatory people just don't happen in practice!

Expanding the Scope of the Job

If this suggestion was put to most regulatory affairs managers they would look at you with amazement and say they had quite enough to cope with as it is, and this is probably true. However, for those who do find the horizons limited the answer probably lies in a closer involvement in the drug development programme, either overall or in a particular area, for example clinical trials or toxicology, such that the provision of regulatory advice could be related more closely to the R&D need. Alternatively a move to specialise in, for example, biotechnology products could be the answer.

Does expanding the scope of a job mean encompassing more aspects or does it mean becoming more specialised? Both approaches could be appropriate. Where a new requirement comes into being and there is an option of forming a new organisation to take it on or including it in the existing structure, opportunities for job expansion or enrichment may occur. Thus in recent years growth areas have been patient information, health and safety at work, particularly safety (COSHH) data sheets, electronic submission of regulatory data, Good Laboratory/ Manufacturing/Clinical Practice, and quality assurance/auditing.

All these impact to a greater or lesser extent on the activities of the regulatory department and could offer possibilities for job enrichment or, relating back to the previous subject, a change of direction.

The Future for this Job Role

The last few years have seen some significant changes. This particularly applies in the European region, where the European Medicines Evaluation Agency (EMEA) came into operation on 1 January 1995. This has had a major impact on procedure in Europe and by offering a unified system has reduced the duplication of effort that used to occur. However, this does not seem to have resulted in a reduction of personnel—as was once predicted. There may be a trend to relocation from small national units into large pan-European units or at least a different distribution of the work with major submissions being handled by the central unit and local work being retained by the national office. Depending on the working practice of the organisation, the various European procedures provide opportunities for local involvement.

When and if everything that can be regulated has been regulated, and closer regulatory relations, possibly facilitated by the CTD, have been established between Europe, the USA and Japan then job opportunities may decrease. At present, however, there are no signs of this happening. Increasing use of electronic data management, new legislation, including the new CTD in Europe, all seem to indicate that there will be a continuing need for the regulatory professional.

18
Careers in Drug Safety and Pharmacovigilance

Peter Barnes

Aventis Pharma Pty Ltd, New South Wales, Australia

Introduction

The safety of medicines is of prime concern to all who develop, prescribe or use them. No effective medicine is 100% safe, and the risks to a patient of developing side-effects (adverse drug reactions, ADRs) to their medicine must always be weighed against the expected benefits in treating a particular condition. The detection, confirmation, investigation and monitoring of suspected adverse reactions is a joint responsibility of prescribers, manufacturers and regulators. In this context the manufacturer has responsibilities for detecting and monitoring side-effects from the very earliest pre-clinical work in product development, through the clinical trial testing phase and into the post-marketing phase.

The term pharmacovigilance, used throughout this chapter, refers to the activities of prescribers, manufacturers and others when a medicine is marketed to detect drug safety signals and to confirm, count, investigate, monitor, report and communicate suspected and confirmed ADRs. The necessary actions can be taken based on the information and subsequent evaluation to ensure a positive risk/benefit ratio of the medicine and the optimum safety of patients and public with respect to their medicines.

The principles applied to pharmacovigilance, however, apply throughout the life cycle of medicine development from a newly discovered molecule to licensed and marketed medicine, and are not described in detail in this chapter.

Pharmacovigilance represents a good career choice for those wanting intellectual challenges together with exposure to a broad spectrum of drug development activities and the opportunity to apply their knowledge of the biomedical sciences. Recent widely published drug withdrawals from the market have highlighted the important role pharmacovigilance groups play in the modern pharmaceutical

Careers with the Pharmaceutical Industry, Second edition. Edited by P. D. Stonier.
© 2003 John Wiley & Sons Ltd. ISBN 0 470 84328 4

environment, both in commercial and public organisations. This chapter describes the roles within pharmacovigilance for both medical and non-medical personnel, as well as related subjects such as training, career progression and opportunities. As pharmacovigilance systems differ from one pharmaceutical company to another, from one regulatory agency to another and even one country to another, it is not possible to include all permutations of all possible jobs available. Rather, a general overview from a personal perspective is provided and suggestions made as to sources of more detailed information.

Pharmacovigilance is an essential aspect of the modern pharmaceutical environment, with ever-increasing demands for accurate information on the safety of medicines to be made available to governments, pharmaceutical companies, healthcare professionals and consumers. As such, there is a steady demand for professionals to manage what is a complex and demanding area, but one which allows the practitioner a broad view of pharmaceutical development, as well as the chance to contribute to the ethical and scientific debate that surrounds new products and technologies.

As pharmacovigilance is at the heart of product development, both pre- and post-marketing, it allows those who work within it the opportunity to make it their career or use it as a springboard to other opportunities within the pharmaceutical workplace. As it relies heavily on information technology, it is a good choice for those who enjoy the challenge of using modern computer tools to help solve complex problems. On the other hand it also requires the human skills of sound judgement, attention to detail and a broad medical knowledge. By its very nature, pharmacovigilance is sometimes unpredictable and stressful but, when performed well, can bring enormous satisfaction to those professionals involved as well as great benefit to organisations and public health in general.

Role and Responsibility

It is a truism that by protecting the patient, the product is protected and thus the company is protected. Therefore, to state it simply, the role of the pharmacovigilance professional is to contribute to public health by monitoring and reacting appropriately to changes in the risk/benefit ratio of a pharmaceutical product or medical device.

Job description

There are a number of different job functions within the scope of pharmacovigilance but this chapter will concentrate on those within the pharmaceutical industry. Government agencies and academic institutions also undertake pharmacovigilance activities and many of the tasks are the same as those employed by pharmaceutical companies.

Perhaps the most common is that of the receipt, coding, collating and reporting onwards of suspected ADRs. (Note: In a clinical trial setting, the term 'adverse event' is used, as this does not imply a causal relationship between the study drug and the unwanted event whereas, when the medicine is marketed, the terminology is 'adverse drug reaction' or 'suspected adverse drug reaction', as it is assumed that in order for a health professional or consumer to report an unwanted effect, a causal relationship is at least suspected.) Within the pharmaceutical industry, this role is often performed by a graduate of pharmacy, science or nursing.

This job is usually called Pharmacovigilance Associate or Drug Safety Executive. The medical interpretation of the individual and collated reports is usually performed, in large pharmaceutical companies and regulatory authorities at least, by a medical graduate. This job may have the title Drug Safety Physician, Pharmaco-vigilance Physician or Medical Assessor.

Pharmacovigilance associate

This job is responsible for receiving the reports of adverse events, from both within the pharmaceutical company (for example, from sales representatives, medical information, clinical research) and without (for example, consumers, pharmacists, doctors and the medical literature). This information will usually be immediately entered on to a computer database and initially processed. This will involve coding events, drugs and other details using special dictionaries established for this purpose. This coding may be performed entirely, or in part, by the computer programme.

The pharmacovigilance associate then assesses the quality of information provided and may, at that point, request additional information from the reporter. This will usually be requested by letter or telephone call. If additional information is received, the case will be updated on the database.

Depending on the nature of the case, at this point it may undergo assessment by the drug safety physician. If it fulfils certain predefined criteria, it will be printed out in a special form and sent to the relevant regulatory agency, or in some coun-tries, sent electronically. The associate is responsible for the processing and reporting of adverse event reports within specific internal company and external regulatory timeframes.

If the associate is working in an affiliate (i.e. a non-headquarters site), questions may be received from the corporate pharmacovigilance department, which normally maintains a worldwide adverse event database for the company's products. In addition to the processing of individual adverse event reports, the associate interrogates the database in order to answer specific questions about adverse events that arise, as well as produce regular summaries of collected reports, which are essential elements of Periodic Safety Update Reviews (PSURs). These documents are written reviews of a product's risk/benefit profile, submitted to regulatory authorities at predetermined intervals after a product's registration.

Drug safety physician

A major task of the drug safety physician is to provide a clinical interpretation of the safety data received by the employing company or agency. This interpretation can be made of individual case reports or of summaries of collected reports over time. It is important that the data collected be continuously monitored for 'signals' of a potential drug safety issue. This could take the form of an increased incidence of a particular adverse reaction or the emergence of a hitherto unknown adverse reaction to a product. Such monitoring is not simple and good clinical knowledge as well as experience of interpreting pharmacovigilance data are required. There is generally a lot of 'noise' in the background of adverse reaction reporting. This can take the form of poorly documented reports, erroneous reports, over- and under-reporting of reactions and confounding factors such as publicity in the media. The skill is to identify a 'real' signal from the mass of often confusing information that is routinely received on pharmaceutical products.

If a signal is identified, it may be further investigated using the techniques of pharmacoepidemiology, which uses the tools of epidemiology as applied to the use and effects of drugs on a population. This is a specialised area for which specific postgraduate training is usually required for those who practise it at a high level. If a new issue is identified that affects the risk/benefit ratio of a product, it is the responsibility of the drug safety physician to ensure that the most appropriate response is made. This could range from the relatively simple, e.g. notification to regulatory authorities, changes to the official product information (i.e. labelling) to the ultimate action of product withdrawal from the market. The drug safety physician also has an important role in contributing the medical interpretation of the accumulated adverse reaction experience of a product, as documented in the regular PSUR. This interpretation requires an appreciation of the pharmacology of the product, a thorough understanding of the disease it treats and other factors that might influence the number and nature of received adverse reaction reports.

Education and Qualifications

To be able to interpret effectively and act upon reports of adverse events, it is necessary to have a good understanding of normal and pathological physiological function. At a simpler level, the routine processing of adverse event reports by pharmacovigilance staff is facilitated if they have at least a basic understanding of human health and disease. Therefore, such staff often have qualifications in a biomedical science such as medicine, pharmacy, nursing or human biology. For pharmaceutical physicians employed to undertake pharmacovigilance activities, general training in the speciality is highly desirable and all recognised training courses in pharmaceutical medicine cover the basic principles and techniques of pharmacovigilance.

Specific courses are also available for non-medical pharmacovigilance personnel, ranging from those resulting in a university qualification to one-day workshops provided by commercial training organisations. In addition to specific training in the basics, it is essential that knowledge of the various company and external guidelines and regulatory requirements that apply be kept up-to-date. This can be achieved through assiduous reading of appropriate journals and websites but can often be most easily achieved by attendance at a specific workshop held under the auspices of a relevant professional organisation. If the size of a pharmacovigilance department is such that individuals specialise in a therapeutic area, it is useful for them to attend conferences and congresses in that subject in order to keep up-to-date with diagnostic and therapeutic advances, and thus be in a better position to provide expert analysis and opinion.

Knowledge base, skills, competencies

Knowledge of physiology in health and disease is essential within a pharmacovigilance department. In addition, familiarity with the effects, both wanted and unwanted, of commonly prescribed pharmacological and non-pharmacological treatments for disease is necessary. Therefore, depending on the level of sophistication required by a particular pharmacovigilance function (e.g. global centre versus small affiliate) the required knowledge base will vary. Likewise, the degrees of skill and competencies will also depend on the nature of the pharmacovigilance activity undertaken at a particular site. Information technology is playing an increasing role in the modern practice of pharmacovigilance, and so a good working knowledge and familiarity with computers is a prerequisite for most positions. In larger departments, specialised functions such as pharmacoepidemiology will be performed. This requires specific training in the discipline and experience in acquiring and utilising epidemiological data.

Interactions Within and Outside the Company

To provide an effective pharmacovigilance service, it is necessary to interact with all other sections of the company. In all but the smallest pharmacovigilance departments, a high degree of team working will be essential to cope with both the routine work and the unexpected issues that invariably arise with pharmaceutical products.

Production of PSURs requires that data are gathered from several areas of the company and this requires the ability to obtain information quickly and accurately from colleagues, as well as production of summary tables of information and medical interpretation of the significance of this information. On occasions there will be 'grey areas' where the course of action with regards to such things as labelling changes or protocol amendments is not clear. This can lead to differing interpretation as to the most appropriate course of action (or inaction) by the many internal and external stakeholders. A good pharmacovigilance professional will gather and assess all possible data on the topic, decide on the most appropriate action and then persuade others that this is indeed the 'way to go'. It is also the role of the pharmacovigilance department to train the staff of other departments, such as sales, on the processes surrounding the efficient collection of adverse event information from all sources. This commonly involves lectures to new staff members on the rationale of pharmacovigilance and the responsibilities all staff have to forward all suspected reports of adverse reactions, without delay, to the appropriate individuals within the company.

Demonstration of professionalism, openness and a high ethical standard will facilitate interactions with external health professionals and the regulatory agencies. Indeed, representatives of a company's pharmacovigilance department should be able to readily take a step back from their roles as company employees and act as agents of public health. Nothing is gained in the long run by attempting to ignore or trivialise potential drug hazards and a pharmacovigilance professional should be encouraged to make the tough decisions and give unpopular advice to management when required. To avoid this responsibility could have serious and far-reaching consequences for all concerned, not least patients.

Personal Attributes

Various roles within the pharmacovigilance department will attract different personality types. Those responsible for the collection, processing and collation of adverse event reports will need a disciplined and organised approach, as accuracy and adherence to systems and procedures is essential in this area. Attention to detail, persistence and finding satisfaction in accuracy and completeness are very valuable traits, as the quality of decision-making is influenced by the quality and amount of meaningful data collected on a particular pharmacovigilance issue. It has to be said that those involved with pharmacovigilance are often frustrated by the paucity of good-quality adverse events data and the apparent 'non-cooperation' of some clinicians, pharmacists and other individuals involved in the reporting of potential adverse reactions. Thus patience and diplomacy are also required. Those involved in decision-making need to have an ability to quickly assimilate data, problem solve and be able to influence and persuade their colleagues of the wisdom of their recommended approach. As drug safety issues are sometimes dealt with in circumstances of urgency and even alarm, such people need to be able to keep a cool head, focus on the important business at hand and not be diverted by extraneous influences. At times, this requires courage and a good deal of resolve. Such resolve comes most easily when the pharmacovigilance professional involved knows that he/she has collated all the available relevant information, consulted widely, considered all options and is confident that the approach recommended is the best available.

Training

As previously mentioned, pharmacovigilance professionals should bring to their jobs knowledge and experience relevant to medicine and pharmacology. The type of additional training required will depend, of course, on the role to be undertaken. Various courses are available on the basic principles of the practice of pharmacovigilance within the context of a pharmaceutical company. These courses are available from professional organisations as well as commercial training companies. All new associates of a pharmaceutical company should have a formal training programme which will result in them being fully equipped to undertake their role. This programme may include training in company Standard Operating Procedures, computer systems and in-house or external training in the relevant therapeutic area and specific products. Those employed in pharmacoepidemiology roles will need to have undertaken specific professional training in the discipline as well as be familiar with the various databases available to conduct relevant studies.

Continuing education and professional development

It is a requirement of Good Clinical Practice (GCP) that those undertaking specific activities with regard to pharmacovigilance have appropriate training and therefore a training record should be maintained for all staff members. Such a log will almost certainly be requested in any audit of a pharmacovigilance department. As a result of the pace of change within the area, it is mandatory that all pharmacovigilance professionals undergo Continuing Professional Development (CPD) training throughout their career in order to remain effective. This could include attending formal sessions of training in changes to regulatory requirements and GCP standards, new computer hardware and software, and in-house procedures such as application of causality assessments or adverse event coding. In addition to training related to pharmacovigilance, it may be appropriate that continued training be undertaken to fulfil professional registration requirements. For example, pharmaceutical physicians will be required to undertake specified amounts of Continuing Medical Education (CME) or CPD as a requirement of maintaining their medical registration.

Career pathways

Career progression within pharmacovigilance will depend largely on the interests of the employee as well as the size of the department in which they work. Typically, pharmaceutical companies will have a number of grades within a specific job function. For example, there may be positions with titles like Pharmacovigilance

Associate, Senior Pharmacovigilance Associate and Pharmacovigilance Manager, reflecting increasing seniority within the same department. The most junior title will usually be given to those new to the pharmaceutical industry or to the pharmacovigilance function and promotion to the next level will depend on increasing experience and good performance. Such promotion may be accompanied by managerial responsibility, for example, the running of a team within the larger pharmacovigilance department, which may include administrative staff as well as other pharmacovigilance professionals.

Depending on the structure of the organisation involved, a drug safety physician may be appointed to manage the pharmacovigilance department in addition to providing the medical interpretation. Alternatively, having gained initial experience within the pharmacovigilance area, the drug safety physician may broaden their experience by taking on responsibility for medical input to other areas of the medical department such as regulatory affairs and medical information.

Career development and advancement opportunities

Pharmacovigilance is increasingly an international undertaking, with pharmaceutical companies maintaining worldwide surveillance of their products and regulatory agencies sharing information across national boundaries. Therefore, opportunities commonly arise to work abroad, especially if employed by multinational organisations. This allows a valuable 'broadening of horizons' and can add to the attractiveness of a pharmacovigilance professional's CV. With a good grounding in pharmacovigilance, pharmaceutical physicians commonly branch out into other areas of a pharmaceutical company's activities. For example, clinical research, regulatory affairs and medical marketing roles are often undertaken by those who have started their careers within the pharmacovigilance department.

Expanding the scope of the job

As the practice of pharmacovigilance becomes ever more complex, there are often opportunities to broaden the scope of a particular job within the area by learning new skills. For example, as computer technology evolves, it is possible for those skilled in its use to develop powerful new tools to assist in the efficient monitoring and reporting of adverse reaction reports. Such individuals, with a good grasp of both computer technology and pharmacovigilance, are highly prized by organisations which are increasingly under pressure to install 'failsafe' systems and procedures, to ensure their legal and ethical commitments are met. Computer technology has also led to rapid maturation of pharmacoepidemiology as an important new discipline in public health. This has led to a subsequent demand for pharmacoepidemiologists by both pharmaceutical companies and government agencies.

Often these individuals began their careers in the pharmacovigilance department and undertook additional training in the techniques of pharmacoepidemiology.

Other ways the scope of a position within a pharmacovigilance department may be expanded include taking the leadership roles in issues/crisis management teams, undertaking post-marketing surveillance studies, managing external advisory panels of experts in a certain area of concern and acting as the media spokesperson for the company on safety issues.

Changing career course

As pharmacovigilance involves consideration of virtually all aspects of drug development (including toxicology, pharmacology, clinical research, marketing practices, corporate affairs, legal, etc.) it is an excellent area in which to obtain a 'grounding' in the pharmaceutical industry. A representative from the pharmacovigilance function should sit on virtually all project or cross-function teams established to develop and successfully commercialise a pharmaceutical product, thus providing exposure to many other areas of the business. Pharmacovigilance is also represented on the management committee of large companies and thus promotion to senior levels within the discipline is possible. Alternatively, careers within other areas of a pharmaceutical company are possible, using pharmacovigilance as the springboard. A pharmaceutical physician who begins his/her career in pharmacovigilance is well placed to move into a clinical research or medical marketing role. Pharmacovigilance associates can move easily into medical information and regulatory affairs departments.

Apart from intercompany moves, there has always been healthy two-way traffic of pharmacovigilance professionals between regulatory agencies and pharmaceutical companies. Staff members in both industry and government agencies are particularly well equipped to appreciate the problems encountered in providing a high-quality pharmacovigilance service in both sectors and bring valuable insights with them. Academic institutions also undertake some aspects of pharmacovigilance and jobs, sometimes as fixed-term research associates, are available in this field.

The Future

Expectations of patients, government regulators and company management with regard to early and accurate assessments of the risks of medicines means that pharmacovigilance is a 'growth' area within the pharmaceutical industry and those choosing to make it their career will find that many opportunities become available to them. Advances in information technology will impact upon virtually all areas of pharmacovigilance, and bring new possibilities as well as new problems to be addressed. The widespread use of 'smart cards' to be carried in patients' purses and wallets, and perhaps containing personal genetic information, will open up a whole new area of drug safety surveillance opportunities, as well as hopefully reducing the incidence of inappropriate prescribing decisions. The electronic linkage of various patient records, above and beyond that achieved by the handful of existing systems, will make possible more efficient post-marketing safety assessments. It is clear that the discipline of pharmacoepidemiology will grow in importance, and professionals trained in this area will be in demand by both pharmaceutical companies and government agencies.

Useful Websites

www.fda.gov   The Food and Drug Administration, the regulatory agency of the USA.

www.diahome.org   The Drug Information Association.

www.open.gov.uk/mca   The Medicines Control Agency, the regulatory agency of the UK.

www.aiopi.org.uk/sigar   The Special Interest Group for Adverse Reactions of the Association of Information Officers in the Pharmaceutical Industry, UK-based.

www.emea.eu.int   The European Medicines Evaluation Agency, the regulatory agency of the European Union.

www.herts.ac.uk/extrel/PGP99/faculties/natpharmacov.html   Information on the Diploma of Pharmacovigilance course run by the University of Hertfordshire in the UK.

www.lshtm.ac.uk/prospectus/study/other/short.html   Information on the Certificate in Pharmacoepidemiology & Pharmacovigilance course run by the London School of Hygiene & Tropical Medicine in the UK.

19
Careers in Medical Information

Janet Taylor

Janet Taylor Consultancy Services, London, UK

Introduction

The importance of the company medical information department to both its internal and external customers has gained increasing recognition over the last few years. Changes within the NHS, for example the increasing importance of bodies such as NICE, the National Institute of Clinical Excellence, have promoted the need within companies for a centre of expertise able to provide advice and information about the company's products.

For many doctors, pharmacists and other healthcare professionals, the company medical information department is their first point of contact when they need help with information about a company's products. Often, the industry is the only source of this information. Sometimes, the information required may be complex and is frequently required quickly in order for important decisions to be made about patient management. The customer therefore expects the medical information officer to be knowledgeable, even expert, on the use of the company's products. In addition he/she must have the interpersonal skills to deal professionally and helpfully with the enquirers.

Within the company, the medical information department is often the department called upon to provide detailed information, position statements and briefing documents to marketing colleagues. Similarly, on a daily basis, the company's own field-based representatives will contact the medical information department for help in satisfying a health professional's request for more information.

Therefore, because of its pivotal position servicing both internal and external customers, a company's medical information department has an important professional relations role. Its staff must be appropriately educated, well trained and fully equipped to fulfil this vital role on behalf of the company.

Careers with the Pharmaceutical Industry, Second edition. Edited by P. D. Stonier.
© 2003 John Wiley & Sons Ltd. ISBN 0 470 84328 4

The Role of a Medical Information Officer

The role of the medical information officer (the job title may vary, e.g. medical information executive, information pharmacist, product specialist, scientific adviser or product adviser) can vary greatly between companies, depending on the size of the company, the nature of its products and whether it is a head office or subsidiary site. For example, some companies may have predominantly external customers (healthcare professionals), others may have both internal and external customers and some may serve their medical information colleagues elsewhere in the world.

Over recent years, the effect of mergers within the industry has prompted companies to review all of their activities. When departments have merged, this has resulted in the need for staff to learn about new products, new colleagues and team structures and a review of working practices with the aim of adopting the best. Hopefully, despite being an unsettling period, this has been an opportunity for working practices to move forward faster than they might have. It has also been an opportunity to maximise the value of newer technology with the information departments often being some of the first to seize these opportunities within a company.

Within the UK it is a requirement for companies to have a scientific service that is responsible for information about the medicines which they market. With the increasingly fast pace of work, constraints on the NHS and improved access to information, customer expectations of the industry have increased. In addition, the increasing awareness in the industry of the needs of their customers has been heightened by the publication by the Association of Information Officers in the Pharmaceutical Industry (AIOPI) of *Guidelines for Standards in Medical Information*, which have been endorsed by the Association of the British Pharmaceutical Industry (ABPI). These standards were established through a consultative process with one of the key customer groups of industry medical information departments, the hospital medicines information pharmacists. The standards are reviewed on a continuing basis and regular customer surveys conducted in order to feed back information to companies so that they can improve their services.

In the UK, the main role of most medical information officers is connected with providing this scientific/medical information service. This could be summarised as 'to provide information and advice about the use of the company's medicines in response to enquiries from members of the medical, pharmaceutical and other healthcare professionals in support of the safe and effective use of the company's medicines'.

Besides offering a technical/medical information service to the medical and other healthcare professionals, most information officers will be heavily involved in providing information support to all areas of their own company including clinical research and commercial departments. In particular, the medical information department is now recognised as the company product centre of expertise. This means that the medical information product expert is the first choice when a position paper, briefing document or statement is required on the use of the company's product. Further details of these roles are discussed below under 'Job content'.

Numbers and Distribution

In the UK, all companies should have at least one person responsible for this function. In large companies or headquarters sites, there may be up to 20 medical information officers. However, in small companies, the provision of medical information may be combined with another role such as regulatory affairs or pharmacovigilance or may even be contracted out to an external organisation. In smaller companies or subsidiaries, it may be necessary to combine this role with another function such as regulatory affairs, drug safety or clinical research.

In total, there are probably approximately 400 graduates involved in the provision of medical information within pharmaceutical companies in the UK. In addition there are a further number of individuals and companies providing locum or contract medical information services. In fact, the locum route is often a common entry point to the industry, particularly for pharmacists.

In mainland Europe, the role, although generally less developed than in the UK, has been expanding in recent years, mainly in response to customer need. In the USA, companies usually have large medical information departments (sometimes called professional service/medical affairs) with similar roles to those found in the UK. As US-based companies and European-based companies have merged, this has created a blending of cultures and a number of major reorganisations in terms of how medical information has been provided on a global basis. Recent mergers have also created senior positions within the industry with a global or European perspective.

The role of medical information officer may have different emphases in different companies. For example, contacts may be internal, such as overseas subsidiaries, rather than external. With mergers taking place on a regular basis, department sizes are forever changing but generally getting larger. Also this increase in department size has resulted in specialist teams within the overall departments. It is therefore difficult to quote a size for an 'average' department.

Job Content

This will depend on the exact role of the site, be it headquarters or subsidiary, and how the different aspects of the overall function are split within the department. However, it can generally be expected to include at least the following roles.

The medical information service

This involves answering technical/medical enquiries from the healthcare professions mostly by telephone but also in writing. Customers generally include hospital pharmacists, doctors, retail pharmacists, nurses, other healthcare professionals, research scientists, students and members of the public. The exact nature of enquiries will depend on the product range, for example prescription-only products or over-the-counter (OTC) products, their maturity, that is, how long they have been in use, and the complexity of use. Companies may organise the provision of this service in different ways depending on their product range and the volume and nature of enquiries. For example, some companies will operate technical call centres staffed by medical information officers on a rota basis where members of staff answer enquiries on all products. Others may route calls directly to a product specialist. Some companies operate a combination of these methods.

Internal expert advisory service

This is increasingly becoming the role of experienced medical information staff within the industry who have a considerable level of knowledge of company products. The roles may include evaluation of new competitors, product position papers, for example, following the publication of a report by NICE, reviews of important new clinical studies, preparation of dossiers for NICE or drug and therapeutic committees.

Information requests from company staff

(a)   Company sales representatives;
(b)   Marketing;
(c)   Clinical research;
(d)   Regulatory affairs;
(e)   Other company staff.

Current awareness services

Keeping commercial and medical staff up-to-date with information relating to the company's products, competitors and advances in therapeutic areas within which the company operates.

Knowledge-base maintenance

This may include published and unpublished literature databases, common questions and answers, standard letters and information sheets on the company's products.

Review of promotional material

This important role ensures that the company's promotional material is technically accurate and conforms to the necessary codes of practice and legislation.

Other medical information officer roles

- Sales force training;
- Creation of SmPCs/patient leaflets;
- Writing, e.g. product monographs, training manuals;
- Management of a company's library;
- Management of a company's archives or records.

Role Content in Medical Information

Answering technical/medical enquiries

This will generally involve talking to a healthcare professional on the telephone, or receiving a written request, assessing their needs, and determining the most appropriate source of answer, for example a product question and answer database, company product database, or an in-depth literature search. Evaluating and summarising the information, and presenting the facts in a clear and balanced spoken or written reply within the timeframe the customer needs, which may often be minutes, not days, is one of the key professional contributions of the medical information officer's role for the company.

Provision of information to company staff

This is particularly an area where product expertise is required and therefore will require an experienced medical information professional with in-depth knowledge of how the company's products are used and the relevant literature, the therapy area as a whole plus a full appreciation of the marketing and sales position. It might involve an in-depth review or a critical evaluation of a competitor's promotional material.

In addition, the medical information department will provide technical support to the company's representatives on a daily basis. Customers inside the company may cover all levels up to the chief executive.

Proactive current awareness

In a competitive market, it is essential for relevant staff to be kept up-to-date with new information from the literature, trade and lay press. This is usually the role of the medical information department. A combination of both electronic and traditional journal scanning techniques might be used to review the data, extensively evaluate them, select relevant information and deliver it to customers in a timely and concise way.

Information needs to be tailored to each individual person's needs and therefore medical information staff will work closely with colleagues, who may be in marketing, sales, clinical research or pharmacovigilance roles, in order to establish their requirements.

Product safety

Most medium- to large-sized companies will have a separate group for this function although it is often located within the same department. However, medical information staff will frequently answer product enquiries relating to adverse effects and may well identify that an adverse reaction has taken place.

Promotional material approval

It is essential that all promotional material complies with the Pharmaceutical Industry Code of Practice, the UK Medicines Act and European legislation. The medical information department is commonly the group responsible for ensuring that information used in such materials and the material itself is up-to-date, accurate, represents current medical opinion and complies with the Code of Practice in all respects. This will involve a lot of contact with the company's own marketing department, advertising agency and medical staff. It also requires highly developed interpersonal skills!

Qualifications and Personal Attributes

Qualifications

Generally, entry qualifications are usually either a good life science degree (preferably pharmacology, physiology or biochemistry) or the candidate should be a registered pharmacist. The exact life science degree preferred will vary from company to company depending on their product range. Some medical information officers in the industry may also have a PhD. However, depending on the company's product range, staff with other appropriate backgrounds, for example nurses or nutritionists, may be employed. In addition, non-graduate-level staff may be employed within medical information departments, involved in answering some of the more routine enquiries.

In addition to an appropriate level of education, individuals must have the appropriate background and skills to enable them to understand and assimilate detailed scientific and medical knowledge.

Although some companies may take new graduates in a training role, with the high investment in time to train medical information staff and the need for them to be 'up and running' as quickly as possible, companies are now tending to prefer to recruit experienced medical information officers or pharmacists with medicines information experience.

When a company is looking at a group of otherwise similar candidates, they will consider any further relevant qualifications such as the Diploma/MSc in Pharmaceutical Information Management (discussed further under 'Training and education') or an MSc in information science. Individuals considering such a course as a way into medical information would be best advised to talk to companies first to assess current views.

Personal attributes

As the medical information department interacts with a wide range of people, external healthcare professionals through to internal colleagues in sales, marketing and clinical research, the skills required are many and it is often difficult to find all of these skills highly developed in one individual.

With the increasing demands on time and high level of mergers and partnership activities some of the most important personal skills for a future medical information officer are:

- Adaptability and flexibility;
- Assertiveness;
- Good time management;
- A good team worker;
- Plus, a good sense of humour is always extremely useful.

Some of the other personal skills required are:

- Quick-thinking, able to evaluate a situation and act appropriately;
- Good technical knowledge, able to use and remember knowledge gained during formal studies and from work experience;
- Willing and able to learn quickly, ability to assimilate knowledge. This is a daily task and will require self-motivation;
- High energy level, able to cope with high volumes of work and associated pressures;
- Customer-focused/personable/friendly;
- Good communicator;
- Even-tempered;

- Thorough with attention to detail;
- Confident and persuasive;
- Lateral thinking/creative;
- A good ambassador;
- Able to keep calm under pressure.

Besides well-developed personal skills, the medical information officer will either already have (depending on experience) or will need to develop a high level of competence in information management including:

- Sources of information;
- Information retrieval/searching including searching specialist databases;
- Information management;
- Information evaluation;
- Writing and presentation skills.

Because of the ever-increasing volume of information becoming available every day, keeping skills and knowledge up-to-date will be a continual process through a career in medical information.

Training and Education

Training is primarily on the job and will include such areas as:

- Product knowledge;
- Therapeutic area knowledge;
- Information skills

  o use of resources
  o enquiry handling
  o customer care
  o literature evaluation
  o use of external databases
  o writing
  o industry appreciation
  o advertising material review
  o current awareness
  o legal aspects of information use.

Training is generally provided within the company by more experienced senior medical information staff. However, internal and external courses may be used for therapeutic area knowledge and use of specialist external databases, depending on available company resources.

In addition, staff may require training in personal skill areas such as presentations, communication skills, interpersonal skills, time management and problem solving.

Initial training may be provided by internal or external courses, depending on the resources available inside the company. However, it may also be achieved through individual experiences, for example from projects within the company. Follow-up training and development will usually be by means of personal coaching and counselling by the manager or another experienced member of staff.

In addition to the training provided to an individual, it is important to remember that it is a personal responsibility for individuals to develop their own skills and competence on an ongoing basis.

In order to meet the specialist needs of those working in pharmaceutical information within the industry, City University, London in conjunction with AIOPI now runs a part-time postgraduate Diploma/MSc in Pharmaceutical Information Management. It is designed mainly for those working within pharmaceutical information in industry, the NHS or academia, and is taught by experienced industry staff, hospital pharmacists and specialist academics.

The course covers a wide range of subjects important to a career in pharmaceutical information, including management skills. Following the success of the course and for use by those unable to attend, a reference book has been written entitled *Pharmaceutical and Medicines Information Management. Principles and Practice* (Robson *et al.*, 2001).

The majority of medical information officers will join AIOPI, the professional association for medical information, and gain considerably from attendance at meetings, professional development seminars, the annual conference, and by receiving their regular newsletter.

For those also involved in drug safety, AIOPI also runs a Specialist Interest Group for Adverse Reactions (SIGAR). SIGAR also runs its own specialist meetings. Also, the University of Hertfordshire, in conjunction with AIOPI, runs a postgraduate Diploma/MSc in Pharmacovigilance.

As medical information officers continually need to update their skills and knowledge, reading of journals, attending meetings/exhibitions and meeting with colleagues play a vital part in their development.

Career Course

Depending on the level of entry of the individual into an organisation, a number of grades of medical information officers tend to exist. Even small companies will have developed career paths to encourage individual development and retention within the company.

This will vary from company to company depending on their product range and maturity and department staff numbers. However, areas of career development may include working on more high-profile or complex products, becoming products experts, team leaders, specialists and department managers. Titles will vary according to company culture.

Progress and development will depend on the size of the department, the size of the company, the opportunities available and the aptitude of the individual. Because of the wide variety within the job, there are always continual opportunities for personal development in terms of gaining new skills and broadening experience rather than traditional hierarchical promotion.

It is important to bear in mind that the exact job title may not always be an appropriate reflection of the individual's role and status in the company. A single person providing a medical information service in a company may still have the range of responsibilities of a manager in a larger department, with the exception of staff management responsibilities.

In some companies, medical information managers may progress to be in charge of international teams and may also be responsible for areas such as regulatory affairs, the library, drug safety, business information or public relations.

Although there is plenty of scope for an individual to expand his or her horizons within medical information, a number may wish to explore opportunities elsewhere, especially in the commercial areas of the business. Medical information officers liaise with so many other departments within the company that they gain a good appreciation of many other roles in the company. This does put them in a strong position to gain an appreciation of the role and build relationships with possible future colleagues and managers before considering a job move. Most medical information officers adapt well to their new roles, which may include:

- Sales;
- Product management;
- Market research;
- Clinical research;
- Drug safety;
- Regulatory affairs;
- Training;
- Public relations.

In fact, a number of senior business managers in the industry have had valuable early experience in medical information.

Outside the industry, medical information officers have developed successful careers with:

- External information providers;
- Public relations;
- Publishing;
- Training;
- Medical writing;
- Freelance/consultancy.

Expanding the Role

There is always plenty of opportunity for the proactive individual to expand their role for the benefit of company and him or herself. The position of the medical information officer at the hub of so many vital activities offers plenty of opportunity routes for those motivated to become involved in a number of other areas, as can be seen from the section on 'Job content'.

The Future

Information is becoming more and more important to all organisations, but it is particularly crucial in the pharmaceutical industry. The timely provision of appropriate information to the right individual at the right time is essential to help keep the company at the forefront of development in research and may help provide the competitive edge over its competitors.

The role of the medical information officer might be expected to develop in a number of areas particularly those of 'product expert' and information systems management.

Customer demands for information are likely to continue to increase and therefore an understanding of their needs will be crucial. It is likely that more and more companies may take the opportunity to allow healthcare professionals direct access to the company's information, which will be a new area of opportunity and challenge to the information professional. The company's own knowledge-base will become increasingly important as will individuals who have the skill to access this important resource.

Although the traditional medical information role would not be expected to disappear, an additional expanding role might be that of facilitator, guiding both healthcare professionals and company colleagues to the information they require.

Information overload is an increasing problem for everybody in the business world today. In the area of medicine, this is a particular problem as the number of articles published increases day by day. The specialist skills of the medical information professional both in identifying a customer's needs and in having the knowledge to find and retrieve relevant information could be expected to become highly valued.

There will always be a promising future for the adaptable and proactive medical information professional. In an industry where few individuals are as ideally placed to gain such an overview of the business and of the pharmaceutical industry as a whole, the opportunities are almost endless.

In addition, the individual who has a proactive approach to work is most likely to recognise such opportunities and where he or she as an individual can most be of benefit to the company.

References and Further Reading

Roberts, G. (2000) Medical information in the UK pharmaceutical industry. *Int. J. Pharma. Med.*, **14**, 159–162.

Robson, A.S., Bawden, D. and Judd, A. (eds) (2001) *Pharmaceutical and Medicines Information Management. Principles and Practice*, Churchill Livingstone, Edinburgh.

The AIOPI Standards Working Party (2001) A survey by medicines information pharmacists of the medical information services provided by drug companies. *Pharma. J.*, **266**, 66–67.

Useful Websites

Association of Information Officers in the Pharmaceutical Industry (AIOPI): www.aiopi. org.uk

Association of the British Pharmaceutical Industry (ABPI): www.abpi.org.uk

Diploma/MSc in Pharmaceutical Information Management: www.city.ac.uk/pgrad/ informatics/pharmaceutical

20

Medical Writing as a Career

Brenda M. Mullinger

Wordpower Projects, Shipbourne, UK

Introduction

The role of a medical writer is to produce high-quality materials within specified timelines. These materials will relate to the use of pharmaceutical and healthcare-related products in man, and may appear as written, visual or verbal output through conventional or electronic media. Medical writers fall into two broad categories—those providing regulatory documents and those supporting sales and marketing activities. In either category they provide a service to others. The career opportunities for medical writers have increased considerably within the past decade and openings are now available within the pharmaceutical and allied industries, contract research organisations and communications agencies. Although no formalised career pathway exists, the medical writer may progress through two or three levels of seniority and assume additional editorial, project or man-management roles. There is ample opportunity to interface with complementary roles and those with aptitude may transfer into either research-orientated or commercially focused positions. The ability to write well is an eminently transferable skill and one that, coupled with relevant experience, can lead to a rewarding long-term career.

Good communication skills are regarded as a prerequisite for many of the careers outlined in this book. Nowhere is this more relevant than in the capacity of medical writer, a broad title that encompasses many job descriptions. Common to all is the need to use words effectively, so that the end result fulfils its function—whether that be within a technical or more commercial environment.

Medical writers provide a service to others, such as those responsible for international clinical research, product registration (regulatory affairs), or sales and marketing activities. The discipline of medical writing within pharmaceutical and allied industries has expanded enormously over the past decade and is now receiving increasing attention. As a consequence, there is a growing need for specialist writers who not only relish the challenge of communicating medical

Careers with the Pharmaceutical Industry, Second edition. Edited by P. D. Stonier.
© 2003 John Wiley & Sons Ltd. ISBN 0 470 84328 4

findings in an accurate and responsible manner but who also enjoy using language effectively.

Role and Responsibilities

Medical writers can make a significant contribution within today's highly competitive pharmaceutical business where rapid regulatory approval for a new product as well as effective marketing are paramount to success. The role of the medical writer is therefore to provide high-quality materials within specified, and often tight, timelines. Individual responsibilities can best be understood by considering the many types of output that fall under the general heading of medical writing. These can be divided into two broad categories—regulatory or marketing (Table 20.1).

Regulatory documents, required at various stages of the drug development process, are often of considerable volume and in exacting detail. By contrast, a much broader range of communication modes is used to support sales and marketing activities.

All pharmaceutical and biotechnology companies are faced with producing a similar range of documents and materials but responsibility for writing them can fall within several departments and to many and various personnel. Consequently the work of a medical writer will vary from one company to the next and from one communications agency to the next. In my experience, most company and CRO writers fall under the regulatory category; they generally concentrate on a limited range of documents in support of one main function or therapeutic area within their organisation. By contrast freelance and, in particular, agency writers have to

Table 20.1 Materials prepared by medical writers

Regulatory	Marketing/other
End-of-study reports (clinical study reports)	Papers for publication
Efficacy and safety summaries/updates	Literature reviews
Expert reports	Conference presentations (with slides),
Study protocols (may include case record	abstracts and posters
forms, patient information, patient	Post-conference highlights or full proceedings
consent forms)	Product monographs
Investigator brochures	Exhibition/conference support materials
Patient information leaflets/package inserts	(e.g. commercial stands, graphic displays,
Summary of product characteristics (SPC)	on-line quizzes, handouts, web-casts)
Standard Operating Procedures	Sales support materials (e.g. detail aids, slide
	kits, questions and answers, videos)
	Marketing support (e.g. competitor analysis,
	training materials, press releases, websites)

be 'jacks of all trades' in the medical communications field, responding to their client's current needs.

A brief description of the purpose and contents of some of the key materials follows.

End-of-study reports (clinical study reports)

At the end of each clinical trial a full report must be prepared which details every aspect of the investigation, such as who did it, where, when, in what disease and patient population, using which medications and methods, what was found and what the results mean. These substantial reports are needed for internal record keeping, as part of quality assurance activities and Good Clinical Practice (GCP), to meet statutory requirements of the regulatory authorities and often as part of a submission for marketing authorisation.

Writing a study report is a demanding and time-consuming activity which, owing to the day-to-day demands of running clinical trials, is increasingly relinquished by clinical research personnel. Such reports are the *raison d'être* for the majority of medical writers within pharmaceutical R&D and for many freelancers. They are generally written using a standardised and often highly circumscribed format, specified by a company's Standard Operating Procedures (SOPs); this is facilitated by use of a common template based on the company's house-style but also accommodating guidelines from the International Conference on Harmonisation (ICH). Introduced in 1996, these guidelines call for an 'integrated' clinical study report that incorporates clinical and statistical information, with extensive supporting appendices. The challenge here for the medical writer is not one of structuring the document but rather of providing unambiguous, relevant text that supports the tables, graphs and flow-charts.

Expert reports and integrated summaries

These important components of the dossiers are needed for product licence applications and may well be drafted by a medical writer for use by the national or international regulatory department. Expert reports are key documents that not only provide an unbiased distillation of the important clinical research findings detailed in the individual study reports but also a critique of the methodologies, studies and, indeed, the whole development plan. Their preparation requires skill and experience. The final copy must appear above the signature of an appropriately qualified expert. Similarly, integrated summaries provide an overall analysis of, for example, all safety issues relevant to a regulatory application, including pre-clinical data as well as those from controlled or uncontrolled clinical trials. Once again they call for an experienced writer.

Investigator's brochure

This comprehensive document is written at the beginning of a clinical research programme on a new medicine and it is updated as additional information becomes available. It informs staff at an investigational centre about the new medicine, its pharmacological and toxicological profile in animals, its pharmacological and pharmacokinetic properties in healthy volunteers, and presents any preliminary data from studies in patients. Investigator's brochures are often prepared by members of a project team, with a medical writer working alongside pharmaceutical physicians or clinical research scientists.

Protocols

Every clinical trial requires a protocol detailing the objectives and methodology of the trial. When a new clinical research programme becomes established the medical writer may be involved in producing a core protocol, containing many standard sections, that can be amplified as needed for individual trials. Some of these sections may subsequently be used in the end-of-study report.

Papers for publication

The pressure to publish the results of clinical trials in one of the thousands of biomedical journals around the world stems from a commercial desire to publicise the new medicine, coupled with the investigator's wish for recognition. Once the treasured responsibility of investigators or company research personnel, manuscript drafting is now very much within the medical writer's domain. The principal reason for this is one of speed. Writing a good paper is neither a simple nor a straightforward task; it requires ordered thinking, succinct writing and a feel for the language. A medical writer who has honed these skills is in a strong position to facilitate the process. This not only saves time but also increases the chances of a paper reporting a good scientific study being accepted by a prestigious journal; paying attention to that journal's requirements on structure, length, style of references and so forth is second nature to an experienced writer.

The role of the medical writer in the production of papers for publication can vary. As an 'author's editor' they can help the original authors prune and improve a draft manuscript, a particularly valuable service to busy authors or those wishing to publish in a 'foreign' language. Alternatively they may act as a 'ghost-writer' producing a draft for discussion and modification by the acknowledged authors. This is a legitimate activity since it ensures an accurate and well-written paper that, if the science is good, should not be returned by the journal for lack of information, muddled presentation, ambiguity or inconsistent arguments (all common criticisms by journal editors!).

Finally, reviews of all published and/or unpublished data on a particular medicine can provide valuable marketing support. Whereas some companies employ their own marketing-based medical writer, such projects are often commissioned outside the company. Indeed, some independent communication agencies specialise in producing their own reviews of pharmaceutical products.

International conference communications

Conferences provide an opportunity for the rapid dissemination of important new research data, a chance to access an international audience with specialist interests and a forum for promoting the company's image and products. These conferences can, therefore, generate a lot of work for the marketing-orientated medical writer both within and outside the pharmaceutical industry.

Research findings may be presented as a talk or through a poster session; either way, the first step is the submission of an abstract to the conference organisers. Preparing the abstract is an art in itself since a lot of data must be condensed into a small space. The actual presentation is a similar challenge in view of the limited time available and the accompanying visual aids (whether slides or a PowerPoint presentation) will make or mar the event. Finally, the production of posters has become big business, as each vies with the next to catch the eye and communicate a message. In all these activities the medical writer with a flair for design and appearance can make a significant contribution.

The commercial opportunities offered by international conferences go far beyond these activities, however. Post-conference reports or highlights may be posted on a website or published either in a newsletter format or as detailed proceedings; as such they provide a service to healthcare professionals and increase company awareness. The drawback for the writer is the necessary speed of turnaround after the conference—there is little value in 'old' news.

The exhibitions that accompany most big meetings also generate medical writing activities. Often undertaken by communications agencies, these can include the design and building of the stand itself. Innovation is key, as each stand must attract as many delegates as possible and clearly communicate the company's messages. This may be achieved through visual effects, competitions or interactive displays, all of which require input from a medical writer with strong commercial awareness.

Product monographs

Written to inform doctors and pharmacists, the product monograph provides a comprehensive picture of a new medicine, including the rationale for its prescription and an outline of prescribing information. This is a key marketing support document that provides a factual overview of the product, without the fine detail invariably found in research reports.

Educational, training and marketing support materials

Medical writers, particularly in communication agencies, help to provide a large variety of educational or training materials on, for instance, a specific disease or health problem, or product-orientated therapeutics. These may be used in-house or to support sales and marketing activities. There are now very many ways in which such information can be disseminated. From detail aids used by representatives, through slide kits or videos for local affiliate companies, to company intranets, CD-ROMs and websites providing a service to healthcare professionals, all require some component of medical writing. Versatility and creativity are essential in this highly competitive field.

Other specialist areas/tasks

Medical information is a speciality in itself that is the subject of another chapter (Chapter 19). Suffice it to say, some medical information officers spend much of their time writing: answering queries on products from the public or professions and providing reviews or abstracts of current literature in specified fields.

Writing advertising copy is another specialised field, this time calling more for flair in advertising than a sound technical background. Most pharmaceutical companies retain one or more independent agencies—this encourages originality through access to a number of copy-writers.

None of the documents mentioned so far is the exclusive province of a medical writer. Some may form part of the wider job of colleagues; nearly all will attract appraisal and input from others. Equally, writing may not be the sole task of a medical writer. For instance, critiquing and editing the contributions of others is a common responsibility—one that requires a somewhat different set of skills. Project management responsibilities may also arise, either through interaction with agencies or freelances when in-house resources are limited, or when seeing a project from inception to completion, by interacting with designers, studio or sometimes the printers.

Job Description

A medical writer is someone whose primary function is to produce written, verbal or visual communications about the use of pharmaceutical and healthcare-related products in man, either through original writing or substantive editing. Tasks may also include taking in editorial changes made by others, reference searches, selecting appropriate artwork, marking up copy, reviewing page proofs from printers and checking colour proofs. According to seniority, the position may involve either project-management or man-management roles. Job titles vary; the terms 'medical writer' or 'medical editor' are often used by CROs, independent communication agencies and freelance writers. Within the British pharmaceutical industry titles such as 'clinical documentation scientist', 'reports production unit', 'medical affairs scientist' and 'editorial executive/assistant' may also be encountered.

Education and Qualifications

There are no obligatory requirements for qualifications and experience. Most medical writers are graduate scientists—many have a second degree. Degrees in one of the biomedical sciences provide the most useful background, particularly for an R&D-related writing job, although any science degree may be acceptable. Despite what seems to be implied by the job title, medical writers in the UK, USA and Australia do not generally need a medical degree; in some other European countries the opposite may be true.

Relevant experience is as important as formal qualifications. Previous industrial experience in laboratory or clinical research is particularly useful for technical writers although some come from academic or hospital medicine. The most important qualification is the hardest to define—an affinity with writing! Any prospective medical writer must provide evidence of their writing ability: research papers, a degree thesis, even an article for the local newspaper will help. In addition, all must expect some sort of writing test as part of the interview process. This may vary from preparing a précis of a technical report or editing a paper, to proof-reading an article or preparing a newsletter. Needless to say, the CV and accompanying letter will be scrutinised too.

Knowledge base, skills, competencies

Strong language skills are very important; it is a misconception, however, that a good writer is also a grammarian. The key ingredients are a genuine interest in writing coupled with an intuitive feel for the use of language. While some understanding of the healthcare industry is a great asset to anyone wishing to become a medical writer, it is not essential. Likewise, in a role that relies on modern technology, good keyboarding skills coupled with a sound understanding of standard computer programs (Word, PowerPoint, Excel and the like) are also valuable.

Technical writers working with R&D findings need to be logical thinkers with an eye for detail and a tidy mind. An interest in data is necessary, coupled with the ability to evaluate and communicate numerical findings. Being able to identify the key points and present them in a clear and concise manner is the challenge here. By contrast, on the commercial side, writers must be able to 'add value' by creating strong marketing messages while maintaining an understanding of the technical background.

Time is of the essence in medical writing. Time management skills must therefore be developed; it takes experience to be able to evaluate just how long is needed to write, re-write, edit and polish a piece of work. As there is rarely enough time to do a lot of background reading a medical writer must be able to move into a new area with ease and quickly assimilate the salient points.

Interactions

The process of writing is essentially a solitary occupation; however, the job of a medical writer can involve varying degrees of interaction. At the most basic level all writers receive a brief for each project; this may be arrived at through discussion with an external client or through participation in a team meeting. Progress reports on larger projects generate further interaction; however, it is the draft stage(s) that is most likely to involve interaction with colleagues, within and often also outside the organisation.

Personal Attributes

Self-motivation is a necessity for all writers but particularly those working free-lance. In-house, there is also a need for flexibility, stamina, good humour and a thick skin! The very nature of the work means that writers must be able to take criticism. Burnout is recognised by many as a real problem for writers, for some due to the volume and repetitive nature of the reports, for others due to constant pressure and tight deadlines. Successful writers develop resilience and their own ways of coping.

To be a successful writer requires a finisher/completer temperament that ensures the project reaches its rightful conclusion. Text is often the tip of the iceberg; much more work lies beneath the surface, whether it be checking references, discussing successive drafts with the client or ensuring copy coming back from the printers meets the brief in every way. A person who cannot be bothered with such details is unlikely to enjoy the role of medical writer.

Tact, diplomacy and negotiating skills are not the most obvious attributes of a writer, and yet all come in useful. The writer often interacts with others when agreeing strategies or content, resolving differing views or negotiating contracts. Those with leadership skills become team leaders working towards a consensus and a goal, while others in their capacity as editors may assume the role of teacher to aspiring authors, or mentor to key researchers.

Finally, all potential writers should seek to set and maintain high standards and derive satisfaction from seeing a job completed within given time limits.

Available Training

Training for medical writers either externally or on the job has been sadly lacking for many years. The situation is slowly improving as the number of writers increases and the importance of the role is recognised. The European Medical Writers Association (EMWA) and the American Medical Writers Association (AMWA), now independent organisations, each provide conferences and programmes of workshops that are led by experienced medical writers. Their focus is meeting the needs of the regulatory-based writer. However, some topics such as punctuation and grammar obviously have a wider appeal. These programmes can lead to recognised professional credits (in Europe) or qualifications (in North America).

There are now a number of commercial organisations that, from time to time, provide introductory training days for medical or technical writers. In addition, the principles of copy-editing and proof-reading can be learnt either through day or evening classes, or by distance learning.

Pharmaceutical companies and CROs vary enormously in the provision of in-house training for the job of a medical writer; most seek candidates with established writing skills, then provide necessary training on specific products or therapeutic areas. Even less training support has been apparent in the agency world. However, the situation is changing all round. As the number of experienced writers no longer meets demand, employers are now considering the needs of new graduates by providing some training—the way this is delivered will vary between establishments. The provision of training is definitely a worthwhile topic for discussion at interview.

Continuous education/training

No formalised facilities for continuous education are available in the field of medical writing; no doubt they will evolve as the discipline expands.

Career Pathways, Development and Opportunities

There are no clear career pathways for medical writers as the speciality is still evolving. That said, opportunities for advancement are growing apace. Within the larger pharmaceutical companies, contract houses and communications agencies there are generally two or three levels of seniority for writers, which may involve increasing editorial, administrative and/or management responsibilities. Perceptions of opportunity after that vary enormously.

In the industry, medical writing is increasingly viewed as a good point from which to enter planning, regulatory affairs, quality assurance, international medical affairs or even clinical research, since the medical writer becomes well aware of what is going on elsewhere in the company. On the marketing side, the role of communications manager is an obvious choice and one that provides key support to product managers. A good medical writer, with broad experience, is generally welcomed by the communications agencies, where career progression can be rapid. Agencies provide the opportunity to work on a wide variety of projects, both in terms of the product area and type of communication. Within the agency world, writers who develop good commercial awareness can progress to become project managers or account directors, taking responsibility for winning and executing the business.

It is not possible to assess the number of job opportunities for medical writers; with their varying titles and areas of responsibility they do not form a homogenous or easily identifiable group of employees. In-house writing groups and CROs providing medical writing services have expanded considerably in recent years; so too have the size of communications agencies and the number of freelance writers. Since medical writers provide a service, groups are generally located within the pharmaceutical company's head office or regional centre. The differing priorities and occasional language barriers often mean that subsidiaries choose to use local freelance writers or communication agencies, to be found almost anywhere!

Within the UK, advertisements generally appear in the national newspapers, journals such as *Nature* and *New Scientist* and pharmaceutical industry communications. Recruitment agencies may also be involved in finding candidates.

Freelance writers

Many people consider becoming a freelance medical writer, often for the wrong reasons. It is not an ideal career solution for everyone. Not only is an enjoyment of writing essential but so, also, is the right personality. Self-motivation and self-discipline are obvious attributes; so too are an ability to work alone, generate business, negotiate realistic deadlines and establish a reputation. These are not easy tasks when starting from scratch; networking is essential and a contract from former colleagues is generally the way most freelances get started.

Confidentiality, integrity and reliability play an important part; clients must be able to rely on all three. Anyone who works independently is only as good as their next contract, so repeat business and good recommendations from a client are essential for survival. But however good, the freelance will always have to handle the irregular ebb and flow of the work load and income, while being psychologically prepared to refuse work when time constraints are impractical.

The uncertainty of work, together with the isolation, lack of training opportunities and the limited sense of involvement and feedback mean that working on a freelance basis does not suit everyone. Additionally, there is the knowledge that only rarely does an outsider get projects on the latest pharmaceutical breakthrough. More often, communications concern lower-priority products for which the company medical writer may lack motivation or rush jobs from an agency short of resources.

All this should be of little concern to the freelance writer who welcomes the opportunity to work in as diverse fields as possible. The variety, flexibility, opportunity to exercise choice and above all, the independence, make freelance writing an ideal outlet for those with the necessary experience.

Challenges, Opportunities and Changing Course

Each individual medical writer must identify their own opportunities and tackle the associated challenges. Although the more enlightened organisations may provide access to a senior writer or mentor to guide the fledgling writer, in most cases individual initiative is key to career advancement. Likewise, expanding the scope of the job very much falls to the writers themselves. Particularly within the more commercially orientated writing environment, there are many opportunities to observe complementary functions, from the work of graphic designers and IT specialists to the role of product manager or conference organiser. The medical writer with aptitude can consider a transition to many related careers.

The Future

In the field of medical writing each individual has a chance to develop their own position and carve their own career path. They are not bound by long-established traditions or expectations. For anyone with an interest and ability in medical writing, the range of opportunities is expanding all the time. Since the ability to write well is an eminently transferable skill, and the need for written communications is unlikely to diminish, the long-term future for medical writers is encouraging.

Further Reading

Albert, T. (2000) *Winning the Publications Game*, Radcliffe Medical Press, Abingdon, 2nd edn.

Glenny, H. and Mullinger, B. (2001) Communicating effectively, in *Principles of Clinical Research* (eds I. Di Giovanna and G. Hayes), Wrightson Biomedical Publishing Ltd, Petersfield, chap. 18, pp. 379–403.

Hall, G.M. (ed.) (1998) *How to Write a Paper*, BMJ Publishing Group, London, 2nd edn.

Kingdom, W. (2001) So you want to be a medical writer? *Clin. Res. focus*, **12**(2), 39–41.

The CONSORT statement (2001) Revised recommendations for improving the quality of reports of parallel-group randomised trials. *Lancet*, **357**, 1191–1194.

Useful Addresses/Websites

European Medical Writers Association (EMWA), 10 Batchworth Lane, Northwood, Middlesex HA6 3AT, UK: http://www.emwa.org

Society of Freelance Editors and Proofreaders: http://www.sfep.org.uk

European Association of Science Editors: http://www.ease.org.uk

Book House Publishing Training Centre: http://www.train4publishing.co.uk/ bookhouse

Institute of Clinical Research, PO Box 1208, Maidenhead, Berks SL6 3DG, UK: http://www.instituteofclinicalresearch.org

Tim Albert Training: http://www.timalbert.co.uk, Tel.: 01306 877993

The John Kirkman Communication Consultancy, Witcha Cottage, Ramsbury, Marlborough, Wilts SN8 2HQ, UK: Tel.: 01672 520429

21

Career Opportunities in Medicines Regulation— The Medical Assessor

Nigel Baber*

Medicines Control Agency, London, UK

Introduction

It may be considered that a chapter on medicines regulation fits uncomfortably in a book on careers with the pharmaceutical industry. At first sight it may be thought that the aims of pharmaceutical companies, which ultimately are to realise maximum profits for shareholders, are the antithesis of those of the regulator.

However, the primary responsibilities of the Medicines Control Agency (MCA), as captured in its Mission Statement, puts this in perspective: 'To promote and safeguard public health through ensuring appropriate standards of safety, quality and efficacy for all medicines on the UK market. Also, to apply other relevant controls and provide information which will contribute to the safe and effective use of medicines'.

Moreover, marketing authorisation holders and regulators do have a mutual interdependence; without the need for new medicines, agencies would not exist and without regulatory authorities, pharmaceutical companies may have even more stringent barriers placed on their activities.

The Medicines Control Agency seeks to foster an environment in which the pharmaceutical industry in the UK is successful in serving the requirements of patients, and the wider interests of the UK economy. The Agency is also required to advise ministers on policies relating to pharmaceutical and regulatory issues and to assist

---

* The views expressed in this chapter are those of the author, and do not seek to represent any official position of the Medicines Control Agency.

Careers with the Pharmaceutical Industry, Second edition. Edited by P. D. Stonier.
© 2003 John Wiley & Sons Ltd. ISBN 0 470 84328 4

ministers in achieving their high level objectives on health. Finally, it is a fact to the mutual benefit of both, that physicians and other scientific staff move from one type of organisation to the other and not infrequently, back again.

This chapter gives a view from the perspective of a national competent authority in the UK. It does not comment on career structure or opportunities in the European Medicines Evaluation Agency (EMEA) which is responsible for centralised procedures of medicines regulation throughout Europe. Nor does it comment on careers in other national agencies in Europe, the FDA or other major agencies such as those in Japan and Australia.

Roles and Responsibilities of Clinical and Scientific Staff Within the MCA

Physicians and other professionals—scientists, toxicologists, pharmacists, statisticians and administrative staff—are civil servants in the Department of Health. They are, broadly, organised in multidisciplinary teams, the size and composition of which depend on the function and workload within the Agency. The primary roles physicians may fulfil are: Assessor (associate, accredited, senior, expert), Manager and Inspector of good clinical practice. Currently there are some 50 medical staff at the Agency and the great majority of these are assessors. All professional staff listed above hold assessor ranking.

The assessment of data supporting applications for Marketing Authorisation Holders (MAHs) or assessment of issues raised as a result of safety signals in pharmacovigilance is the core work of the physicians. The organisation of the Agency reflects this. There are three operational divisions. Licensing is responsible for new (including biologicals) and abridged applications and for clinical trial applications. Post-Licensing is responsible for variations, renewals, reclassification of medicines and for pharmacovigilance. Inspection and Enforcement deals with good clinical practice, among a number of its responsibilities. The Clinical Trials Unit within the Licensing Division is responsible for assessment, granting and modifying applications for the start up and continuation of clinical trials.

In broad terms, assessment of an application or a safety issue consists of weighing the benefits and risks of a medicinal product in the context of use for the individual patient and the protection of public health. This is a challenging undertaking and requires mastery of medical and scientific facts as presented by the applicant, searching for supportive information, summarising the findings and forming a judgement on efficacy and safety. Statistical, pharmaceutical and toxicological assessment is frequently required, depending on the type of application, and this expertise is available within the Agency. Assessment reports are frequently submitted to the Agency's main advisory committee, the Committee on Safety of Medicines (CSM) for its advice. Assessors need to be able to present their work succinctly to the Committee and to answer questions on the data and on regulatory implications.

As far as the medical assessor is concerned, one of the main deliverables from an assessment procedure is an approvable Summary of Product Characteristics and the patient information that accompanies it. Pharmacovigilance, i.e. the discipline that detects and assesses signals, requires a knowledge of the origin and reliability of the signal (e.g. by the Yellow Card reporting system, or from specifically designed studies or from the Periodic Safety Update Reports), the research for supporting evidence, hypothesis generation and the seeking of advice from advisory committees. Monitoring of the safety of medicines is intensive in the first two years, or more in some instances, after marketing approval.

Regulatory medicine is a global specialty and in particular a European one. Although many national licences still exist, the formal European basis for medicines regulation has been in place since 1995 with a previous period of transition. The significance of the international perspective in regulation cannot be overstated. It takes two paths. First, efficacy, safety and quality information has to be shared with other agencies and with the EMEA. Second, European procedures for new applications, variations, renewal of licences basically follow two routes; mutual recognition (or decentralised procedure) and centralised procedures. Both are subject to strict timetables and, in the case of centralised procedures, directed by the Committee on Proprietary Medicinal Products (CPMP).

These processing aspects of regulation have to be integrated with a technical assessment in order to make a fulfilling job for the medical regulator. It can, at times, seem that the need to follow timetables, and ensure that correct hierarchical procedures are followed, outweigh the fundamental aim of the assessment, i.e. to obtain the optimal European opinion for the benefit of patients.

The Medicines Control Agency, as a national competent authority, has the overriding responsibility of serving health ministers in the UK. This responsibility takes a variety of forms. For example, the drafting of responses to official enquiries from ministers' offices, which may be raised by the general public or by Members of Parliament, or informing ministers of drug-related public health issues and the anticipation of public concern, are frequent duties for assessors. The drafting and circulation of memoranda is a skilled discipline often performed against tight deadlines. Medical staff responsible will need to fully understand the technical and public health issues and be able to express themselves with clarity and brevity. On occasions, medical assessors and senior medical managers may need to brief ministers directly.

Medical assessors and managers receive letters from members of the general public and from healthcare professionals concerning the regulation of medicines. It is their responsibility to respond to these in an informed and helpful manner, giving professional advice, but avoiding commenting directly on individual patient care.

Another important duty of assessors is to interact with pharmaceutical companies. Formal written correspondence is still the commonest medium used, but use of e-mail is becoming more frequent. Agency medical staff and company representatives meet face to face for a number of reasons. MAHs often need advice on the suitability of a clinical development plan, the content of an application, or to bring specific issues to the table such as reasons for negative advice from an advisory committee. Meetings between regulators and MAHs are always formal but this does not inhibit constructive and interactive discussion. It is incumbent upon medical assessors chairing or attending such meetings to be fully briefed.

Centralised and mutual recognition procedures require interactions with staff at the EMEA and with colleagues in other member states. This is nearly always conducted by e-mail or fax, but occasionally medical assessors are required to attend the EMEA to give expert advice or, rarely, to be involved in arbitration procedures when consensus cannot be reached between member states.

Career Development and Opportunities

The assessment of scientific data supporting applications for new drugs and abridged applications, clinical trial start-up, variations, renewals, reclassifications and pharmacovigilance form the mainstay of medical assessor work. Assessors may be asked to take on special projects relating to individual drugs or a class of drugs. This is particularly so in pharmacovigilance where reviews of the safety aspects of a drug class may be triggered by a public health issue from one product in the class. Reviews may be much broader based such as drugs and driving or the use of medicines in children. These reviews can be challenging, but rewarding to carry out and always involve presentations to and advice from experts on advisory committees. There is always a European perspective to be brought to these issues and there may be opportunity for academic publications. Assessors may also be invited to work on a CPMP working party to produce a guideline, for example on drug development in a particular class.

Medical assessors are appointed to particular positions in the Licensing or Post-Licensing Divisions. They are expected to develop their regulatory knowledge and competencies across a number of therapeutic areas but they frequently come with experience in a particular medical specialty and their expertise is fully utilised. Perhaps one of the most prestigious roles is to be one of the two representatives to the CPMP.

Medical assessors may be expected to give advice to Agency units which do not have their own medical staff. Two such areas are in advertising and in borderline products. The inappropriate advertising of medicines is brought to the attention of the Agency in various ways, and certain physicians may be asked to give an opinion and will need to be familiar with advertising regulations. Borderline products are those which fall between medicines and food products and are heavily promoted for the enhancement of various bodily functions. Advice is most frequently required on whether the product has pharmacological effect, or whether the claims being made are those that should be applied only to medicinal products. This can be an interesting and challenging aspect of the assessor's work.

Management opportunities

The MCA has a linear hierarchical management structure. Each of the five divisions has a Director, and the current incumbents of the Licensing and Post-Licensing Divisions are medically qualified. The Directors, who report to the Chief Executive, have group managers reporting to them who in turn have unit managers responsible for medical assessors and other staff. Most managers at the Agency have 'come up through the ranks', which gives them a thorough knowledge of regulatory procedures. At an operational level, the Licensing and Post-Licensing Divisions are organised into multidisciplinary teams of medical, scientific and pharmaceutical assessors, with administrative and expert support, such as statisticians.

Until recently, management training has been largely experiential; skills and competencies have been acquired by use and practice, supported by occasional off-site or internal management training. The Agency is now committed to a major leadership and management training programme, for established and new managers.

Managers at all levels are expected to retain a high level of technical competence in their field. Most managers will have their own case work, as well as advising and approving the assessment reports of their staff. Among standard management responsibilities, Agency managers have in particular an active participation in the appointment, performance appraisal and personal development programme of their staff.

Education, Qualifications and Personal Qualities for Medical Assessor Positions

Medical assessors join the Agency from a variety of previous posts, including pharmaceutical industry, contract research organisations (CROs), general practice, National Health Service and academia. The Agency has a well-developed equal opportunities policy and provided the individual has a General Medical Council (GMC) registration and requisite qualifications and skills, he/she can apply. Most medics have a higher qualification, e.g. MRCP, PhD, FRCS, and it would be unusual for an assessor to be recruited in the first two to three years after registration. Practical experience of therapeutics and an appreciation of the risks and benefits of medicines at individual and preferably at public health level are definitely an advantage. Pharmacokinetics and statistics are competencies that are frequently needed in all forms of assessment. The Agency has a small number of its own statisticians and expert kinetics advice is available internally and from advisory committees.

However, these are two skills worth developing to a high degree. In Post-Licensing, pharmacoepidemiology is a valued skill to have, but training is offered in this specialty.

Medicinal products for assessment cover all therapeutic classes. Some assessors come with and are able to develop a new specialist skill, e.g. in infectious diseases, obstetrics and gynaecology, respiratory medicine, but this is to some extent opportunity driven. The stress in the Agency is on general regulatory assessment work. Most physicians who come into the Agency know little, if anything, about the regulation of medicines unless they have previously worked in the regulatory part of pharmaceutical industry. Some have a basic knowledge from the Diploma of Pharmaceutical Medicine. Knowledge of regulatory procedures takes time to acquire; all physicians will develop a working knowledge of European directives and regulations that inform the regulatory work, and a few will acquire in-depth competence in European regulatory affairs.

Some of the personal qualities required to be a good assessor include:

- An enquiring and critical mind;
- Ability to assimilate, and assess objectively, large quantities of data;
- Ability to balance the risks and benefits of a medicine and to assess the overall public health issues;
- A desire to work in a European environment;
- Ability to adopt varying leadership and team member styles, from the directive to the consensual;
- A genuine and rigorous concern for patient welfare that is not lost in the day-to-day routine;
- Resilience and a positive liking to work to tight deadlines.

Training, Continuing Education and Revalidation

Medical staff, like all Agency employees, have an annual appraisal which evaluates performance against objectives. The Agency recognises the need for CME and CPD and the importance this will have on career opportunities and in revalidation. There are regular professional forums and seminars with both internal and external speakers, and many physicians attend further education courses, usually in regulatory or therapeutic specialties. Agency staff are in great demand as speakers at symposia and workshops, and within limits, this is permissible. Many physicians are fellows or members of the Faculty of Pharmaceutical Medicine and there are always three or four assessors each year undertaking a postgraduate course in pharmaceutical medicine in order to sit for the Diploma in Pharmaceutical Medicine. In addition, there is the opportunity for those in pharmacovigilance to study for the Diploma in Pharmacoepidemiology at the London School of Hygiene and Tropical Medicine.

The Agency recognises a need for broader professional development and a number of medical staff write papers, referee journals, are lecturers, editors or examiners for the Diploma in Pharmaceutical Medicine and for postgraduate and undergraduate students. At present the Agency is actively pursuing a programme with the GMC for revalidation of its members and recognises the need to capture the unique experience and competencies that assessors have.

The Future

The environment in which the Agency, in common with other national regulatory agencies, is operating is changing. There are four main 'drivers' of change.

First, the globalisation of the pharmaceutical industry together with mergers of larger numbers of companies leads to challenges and opportunities for the pharmaceutical companies which are based in the UK. The Agency can respond to this by ensuring a swift and efficient provision of services such as the licensing of new medicines, the establishment of fruitful dialogue and having an effective post-marketing surveillance system. It has recently been announced that the Medical Devices Agency (MDA) will merge with the MCA. This is planned for the first to second quarter of 2003. There are some synergies between the two agencies and most European regulatory agencies have integrated functions.

Second, the scientific base on which drug discovery and development is founded has changed and will continue to do so through biotechnology, genomics and proteomics. The Agency will continue to seek to appoint high-calibre staff to assess these new kinds of applications.

Third, the regulatory environment is changing. The 2001 review of the new European licensing system will result in significant legislative change that may not be in place for some years but which nevertheless will have a profound effect on the Agency's business and how it operates to protect public health.

Finally, the public expectation of health care services, including easier access to medicines, is changing. Patients expect, and can get, more information about medicines and the government is responding to the public demand for provision of more medicines. The Agency will have a crucial role in contributing to the safe introduction of new medicines and making more older medicines available without prescriptions, yet at the same time striving to monitor the safety of these products and provide information to all interested groups.

The regulatory physician will continue to have a crucial role in this new environment. Assessment of efficacy and safety data will remain at the heart of their work, but availability of and access to wider sources of information will impact on the assessment process. The challenge of seeking to reach consensus in key issues in an ever-widening European Community which is increasingly centrally controlled, while meeting national health requirements, will become ever more demanding. National agencies also need to consider how to appoint and develop physicians in specialist roles to tackle the assessment of medicines developed on the basis of new biological techniques. The wider government policy to make more medicines available to the public will require assessors to be familiar with the use of meta-analysis and systematic reviews, and have an awareness of government and public health expectations. These will be exciting times but quite different from the traditional role physicians have been trained for in the past.

22

Pharmaceutical Law—A Growing Legal Specialty

Ian Dodds-Smith

Arnold & Porter, London, UK

It is perhaps surprising that, until recently, a student of law would have searched in vain for textbooks in the English language even remotely concerned with European pharmaceutical law as a special subject. The industry has naturally been a fertile field for the practice of intellectual property law for a long time but most lawyers in the patent and trademark field would have a practice where pharmaceutical matters were common rather than their exclusive diet. Legal texts on subjects such as medical negligence now often have a token chapter on specific issues relating to the supply of medicinal products but even this is a relatively recent development. However, there are no legal texts that deal with the relevant law in the type of detail so common in other areas of activity such as the aviation industry.

This is despite the fact that the pharmaceutical industry is one of the more discrete industrial sectors, European industry is at the top of the world league and has had specific European Community (EC) legislation, let alone national legislation, devoted to its activities since 1965. The picture is changing fast and it can confidently be stated that a new legal speciality has developed that springs largely from the unusual regulatory features of the industry, the special ethical and legal problems relating to clinical research and the complexities of personal injury litigation concerning its products.

Regulation in the Pharmaceutical Industry

The pharmaceutical industry is today undoubtedly the most regulated of all industrial sectors. At every stage in the marketing of products there is governmental intervention. The normal way in which such intervention is achieved is through

Careers with the Pharmaceutical Industry, Second edition. Edited by P. D. Stonier.
© 2003 John Wiley & Sons Ltd. ISBN 0 470 84328 4

detailed legislation backed by criminal sanctions. On some matters voluntary government schemes exist (e.g. pricing) but the control is no less formal for that.

In comparison to the USA, which has had extensive regulatory controls for more than 50 years, most controls within Europe have been imposed in the last 20 years, with the thalidomide tragedy adding a new urgency to the political pressure that already existed for control of dealings in medicinal products. In the UK, from the relatively small beginnings of product licensing under the Medicines Act of 1968 (in fact, not operational until 1971), virtually every aspect of supply has been controlled, partly in response to harmonising directives within the EC. Within the EC regulatory control of the industry was an early candidate for attention, with Directive 65/65/EEC laying down the framework for licensing based upon safety, efficacy and quality, but the pace of adoption of directives quickened in the last five years with attempts to complete the internal market by 1992. Twenty-five out of 29 of the directives relating to human medicines were adopted in the period 1983–1993.

Legal specialities develop out of the demands of commerce for advice, which in turn tend to be dictated by the increase in the complexity of relevant laws and uncertainties in their application. Whilst lawyers working within industry naturally develop knowledge and skills specific to their employer's business, legal knowledge in private practice will only develop if companies find the need to seek legal advice in a particular field on a regular basis. Until recently, that simply did not happen in the regulatory field.

One of the reasons is that regulatory control was not treated as a natural arena for lawyers. Initially such control focused upon obtained marketing approvals and despite the fact that the controls ultimately had their origin in legislation—often some of the most detailed and opaque texts on the statute book—regulation was treated essentially as an issue of administrative rote in most companies. Regulatory personnel tended to operate as adjuncts to either the medical or marketing function and legal input was minimal. Even in-house lawyers seldom became involved in the licensing process. The ethos of such groups was to get the product to market as soon as possible, and companies would operate the procedures imposed by the regula-tory authorities, frequently without any real understanding of the statutory basis for such procedures. If a regulatory authority wanted something done, it was done and with little or no thought being given to whether there was a sound legal basis for the request or restriction imposed. This is not to be critical of such an approach because in most cases the interests of a company may be better served commercially by complying with a request rather than questioning the powers of the regulator.

One feature of the regulatory framework in the UK is that the full expression of the controls is not to be found in statutes in any event but rather in 'administrative directions' issued under the Act through notices published in the Medicines Act Information Letters (MAIL). Perhaps the best example is in the field of adverse drug reactions, where the statutory controls are, in fact, described very simply as a requirement to maintain a record and provide details as and when the licensing authority direct. However, based on this simple statement, periodic and changing directions (often of a very detailed nature) were issued in MAIL. In short, the practical controls on companies were to be found as much in interpretive and 'how to do' guidelines and notices of the Department of Health as in the statute book. For many years industry was very comfortable with this.

What changed to cause the demand for regulatory advice to increase? First, national regulation has increased not only the complexity of controls (and particularly the relationship between them) but also the potential for conflict with the regulatory authorities. Controls developed progressively in the UK through the late 1970s to cover commercially critical areas such as advertising. The prosecution in 1986 of one company and a responsible officer in relation to the advertising of a product undoubtedly increased the concern of companies to ensure compliance. Legal as well as medical sign-off of advertising copy became much commoner. More generally, with increasing controls companies became more concerned that one could not always be confident that different companies were being treated fairly and consistently in relation to the same issues. Undoubtedly, the authorities were sometimes grappling with similar problems of interpretation and positions changed from time to time, sometimes depending upon the attitude of individual assessors or officials. As a result companies became more concerned to establish that their 'rights' were not being infringed in an increasingly competitive marketplace.

The second complicating factor has been the addition of a raft of European legislation, often with limited consultation and text that is frequently not a great advertisement for careful thought and precise drafting. In fact, of course, if directives are to harmonise practices and decision-making within the European agencies, drafting that is imprecise merely facilitates (and frequently enshrines) lack of consistency in approach. English lawyers are sometimes criticised for applying a too rigid interpretation based upon what the words alone mean and are told that in the European context one must apply a 'purposive approach' to interpretation based upon the recitals to the directive. If a purposive approach is adopted it is suggested that all will become clear and the need for lawyers will evaporate. This is, of course, fallacious because few directives have a single, clearly defined purpose; most seek to balance somewhat conflicting principles, namely the need to ensure safety and promote public health, but to do so without hindering the free movement of goods and the innovation and development of the European pharmaceutical industry. It is therefore not difficult to reach different interpretations of a directive's provisions according to the weight you attach on any given matter to one or other of these underlying principles. Moreover, sometimes provisions are so vague and conflicting that incorporation into national law is delayed. The difficulties experienced in the UK in implementing the Advertising Directive and Labelling Directive illustrate such problems very clearly.

Explanatory documents such as the Notice to Applicants and Guidelines from the Committee for Proprietary Medicinal Products (CPMP) seek to assist in interpreting directives, and these documents frequently go into considerable and useful detail not found in the directives themselves. Companies are guided in their planning by such documents but in fact the documents carefully eschew any claim to be legally authoritative and at the end of the day they reflect an opinion that the courts can, and do, frequently disregard when asked to adjudicate on the law. It is small wonder that companies, perplexed by the uncertainty that European legislation injects for a business that must take long-term decisions, and for which uncertainty is therefore particularly unwelcome, turn increasingly to their lawyers for assistance and hopefully a degree of certainty.

The problems are compounded by the need to translate directives into the domestic legal framework. Frequently, member states persuade themselves that their existing legal provisions will already comply but often, while the main thrust is consistent, the wording of key provisions is, in fact, different. Thus when Organon sought the assistance of the English courts in determining their rights in relation to the product Bolvidon (mianserin), the judges identified a significant number of ways in which even relatively basic provisions of European law were not accurately reflected in the Medicines Act legislation. This was of great significance because as a matter of European law a company is entitled to rely either upon the provisions of the domestic law (in which case the licensing authority cannot seek to apply a European provision that it has failed properly to implement) or, if they are more favourable to the company, the provisions of European law (and the licensing authority cannot rely upon domestic provisions that are at odds with the European law that the state was obliged to implement). Companies consider it novel to have an option in the law they may follow and the demand for legal advice will obviously rise in such circumstances!

An additional factor predisposing to uncertainty and, therefore, the need for legal advice is that directives may be implemented not by legislation but merely by administrative action. The latter converts into statements of practice which the Medicines Control Agency in the UK usually issue in MAIL. It is normally considered optimal that when the law changes on a given matter those affected by it should receive a clear statement of the new position at the time the change becomes effective. In the UK there have been several instances where statements of administrative practice have been issued many months after the operative date. Such was the case with the far-reaching changes in relation to abridged applications generated by Directive 87/21/EEC. It was not until the SmithKline French litigation concerning generic copies of Tagamet had raised one of the issues arising out of that directive that the Department of Health issued a statement in MAIL in August 1988 describing the administrative action that implemented the new law which had become effective long before in July 1987. Total absence of information creates the most uncertainty of all!

Finally, whilst the EC has not yet fully implemented the Future Systems, the European regulatory authorities are in certain cases (e.g. pharmacovigilance) already acting as though they were in place. Often this makes extremely good sense, particularly with a view to getting consistent and speedy decisions on safety issues. However, the existing legal function of the CPMP, outside the concertation procedures for multi-state and biotech/hi-tech applications for marketing authorisation, is to advise member state authorities rather than to issue directions to the holders of national marketing authorisations. Such *de facto* developments towards centralised decision-making add a new dimension to the problems of those in regulatory affairs, who in the pharmacovigilance field, for instance, increasingly have to understand the legal requirements in all member states because adverse drug reaction (ADR) reporting remains unharmonised as to both type and timing of reports and the controls remain firmly rooted in national law.

Not only are companies keener to establish their legal position, but also as the relationship between the regulatory authorities and industry has become more open it has perhaps also become more professional. There has developed a greater willingness on the part of companies to defend their interests, if necessary by resort to law. The traditional concern that to argue with the authorities over the licensing of one product would only provoke difficulties for the company with other product applications, is giving way to an appreciation on both sides that where uncertainty exists or companies are aggrieved by an issue it may be necessary to seek clarification of the law by judicial review. This naturally increases the demand for lawyers with expertise in regulatory affairs.

There are, of course, dangers in assuming that the courts are equipped to resolve all regulatory disputes, particularly those that genuinely arise from scientific assessment. However, as successfully prosecuted cases of judicial review show, there are cases where a company has little choice but to seek judicial review and it would be strange if, against the complexities of law described above, there is not an increase in cases of judicial review. Recent case law has clarified that European law gives standing to any person aggrieved by the wrongful application of European law by a regulatory authority to seek the assistance of the courts. In contrast, in the Medicines Act itself (S. 107) an attempt is made to restrict any challenge to the regulatory decision to the licence holder or prospective licence holder rather than a third party directly affected. This, together with the development of European law suggesting that in appropriate circumstances damages may be obtained from the regulatory authority for breach of European law obligations and the possibilities of obtaining interim relief pending the substantive hearing such as the suspension of the licence in issue, will increase the willingness of companies to litigate to protect their interests. On one view, regulatory law alone will provide sufficient material for specialisation, without necessarily encompassing expertise in the matters that are discussed below.

Clinical Research and Ethical Issues

Regulation of commercial activities—in the broadest sense of the word—takes many forms ranging from legislation to application of the general law principle requiring the exercise of reasonable care at all times. Despite the growth of European regulation described above, at the present time no directive has been adopted directly controlling clinical research. This reflects in part the difficulties of harmonising activities that touch upon different medical traditions and practices. A few countries such as France and Ireland have legislated in advance of European harmonisation. Phase I research in healthy volunteers is not directly regulated at all in some countries, including the UK. Nevertheless, the last 10 years have witnessed markedly increased interest in issues relating to the ethics of research and its organisation. Of particular concern have been issues of 'informed consent', the increased commercialisation of research notably with healthy volunteers at phase I, and compensation for injury suffered during the course of research. Lacunae or uncertainties in the law have been partially filled by a plethora of guidelines from various organisations, some European (e.g. the Guidelines for Good Clinical Practice (GCP) of the CPMP), some national/governmental (e.g. the Department of Health Ethics Committee Guidelines), some trade association (e.g. the GCP Guidelines and Compensation Guidelines of the Association of the British Pharmaceutical Industry) and some professional (e.g. the Royal College of Physicians of London Guidelines on Research).

To a large extent ethics committees, operating by reference to these guidelines, have filled the regulatory gap and during recent years both their constitution and procedures have been formalised. Ethics committee approval is now of considerable importance and more problematical. Delay in obtaining it can have significant commercial implications. The application of ethical guidelines (which by their nature tend to be flexible) to different factual situations creates significant problems of interpretation which are accentuated when, as is often the case, pharmaceutical companies conduct multi-centre (including foreign centre) trials. Legal training is seen as an advantage in considering the interrelationship between such guidelines and general law principles, and very many ethics committees now include a lawyer. Expertise in the law and ethical guidelines relevant to research is now very much a requirement for lawyers advising pharmaceutical companies and the contract research organisations that serve such companies.

Product Liability

The trend towards legal specialisation arising from regulatory developments has been given added impetus by the significant increase in litigation concerning the products of the pharmaceutical industry. The thalidomide tragedy led to the first major case, but in the event the litigation was fairly limited as media pressure brought about a settlement of claims that had become bogged down in legal and technical uncertainties. Many of the uncertainties remain and it is still the case that no litigation in England involving a pharmaceutical product has yet proceeded to trial and judgement on both negligence and causation—the two key components that traditionally a plaintiff has had to prove to establish a right to compensation. In the mid-1970s claims concerning the marketing of Eraldin (practolol) by ICI were settled by a compensation scheme established very quickly after withdrawal of the drug. The Primodos litigation (concerning a hormone pregnancy test) which began in the late 1970s was the first case to proceed any distance and involved several hundred claimants and allegations of teratogenicity. However, the proceedings were discontinued after four years by the plaintiffs (a matter of weeks from trial) on the basis that the expert evidence exchanged showed that there was no real possibility of the plaintiffs establishing that the product was capable of causing the alleged injuries at all.

However, the 1980s witnessed an explosion of major cases with claims in respect of particular drugs being numbered in the hundreds and sometimes in the thousands. Claims involving pertussis vaccine, steroids, oral contraceptives, blood products, non-steroidal anti-inflammatory agents, intrauterine devices, contrast media and benzodiazepines have been raised. One of the most significant was that involving pertussis vaccine, where the court ordered a preliminary issue on causation and the Wellcome Foundation was able to demonstrate that on balance of probabilities the vaccine was not capable of causing brain damage. This result was achieved in large measure by dissecting the principal epidemiological studies upon which the association was based and showing that the epidemiology was severely flawed, mirroring to a considerable degree a key factor in the discontinuation of the Primodos litigation where base data underlying central epidemiological studies had also been obtained and assessed for the first time with a critical eye. The relationship between legal principles of probability (each component of a cause of action including causation must be established on the balance of probability) and tests of statistical significance in epidemiology raises interesting issues.

Other cases were either discontinued, settled or, in a few instances, are still pending. The largest pending litigation concerns benzodiazepines and has involved directly or indirectly all of the manufacturers of benzodiazepines from the 1960s onwards. It is unusual in that physicians prescribing the drugs have been made defendants in a number of cases. It is also noteworthy that the Legal Aid Boards in Northern Ireland and Scotland have in this litigation contributed to the funding of the more advanced litigation in England on the basis that there should not be parallel proceedings in all jurisdictions within the UK based on public funds. The benzodiazepine litigation developed into the largest personal injury litigation that has ever been seen in the UK where the nature of the claims (the essential allegations concern dependence), the long period of usage of products and the similarity between the symptoms of the underlying conditions for which benzodiazepines were prescribed and the symptoms alleged as injuries, obviously contribute to its complexity.

The 1990s have seen new additions to the lists of products where material litigation is or has been threatened including human insulin and, for the first time, veterinary products in the shape of products used to dip sheep. Indeed, if today one opens the 'Help Please' column of the *Law Society Gazette* (where solicitors advertise to other solicitors their interest in particular types of claims and their desire for coordination) in some weeks well over half the entries relate to possible claims in respect of medicinal products. Of course, many of these claims do not develop and others develop very slowly. Frequently claimants are encouraged to 'forum-shop', and if the UK licence holder has an American parent one will often find that an attempt is made to have the claims heard against the parent in the USA, arguing that testing took place there or the product information was 'controlled' by the parent company. In recent years the American courts have become firmer in their resolve to dismiss such claims on the grounds that the American forum is not convenient, but lawyers advising pharmaceutical companies need to have a working knowledge of the jurisdictional and choice of law rules applicable in other countries.

Most major pharmaceutical companies are multinational and the possible international dimensions of litigation are increasingly important. Publicity surrounding claims in the UK are picked up by the foreign press and there is then a considerable potential for claims developing in other countries, particularly in Australia or New Zealand where the legal system and legal remedies are similar. Finally, an added difficulty for companies is that one can no longer assume that claimants in Scotland or Northern Ireland will join in, or await the outcome of, English litigation relating to the same product. The same factors at work in England are present in those jurisdictions and a company can quickly find itself fighting on a number of fronts. Careful coordination is at a premium both to safeguard the client's interest and control costs, with the result that the English lawyer advising the pharmaceutical industry today needs to have a good knowledge of the relevant procedural rules in those jurisdictions too and have developed contacts with lawyers there in whom he has confidence.

What are the factors that have led to the pharmaceutical sector being at the forefront of product liability litigation? Clearly we have a more litigious environment, where the public are quicker to sue if they believe (or more accurately have been led to believe) that use of a product might be to blame. The explosion in claims certainly does not reflect reduced standards in the industry (controls are greater than ever before) and increased litigation has affected the practice of medicine too. The fees for membership of the medical defence organisations in the UK continue to soar, reflecting the legal costs of defending and sometimes settling claims. The trend is not restricted to the UK; in the Republic of Ireland premiums have risen by 139% for surgeons and 143% for physicians over the past two years, reflecting both the increase in litigation and the higher personal injury awards (40% higher on average than in the UK). Procedural changes have in some respects made litigation easier in the UK and the Republic of Ireland than in many other European countries, but primarily it is the very nature of medical treatment and the use of medical products that makes it easy to commence (though usually difficult to prove) claims. Relevant factors are the inevitability of an association (though very often not causal) between the symptoms of illness and use of a drug or other medical intervention, the relative ease with which negligence can be alleged in fields with few absolute standards and the difficulties in proving the negative in relation to medical causation.

Media interest and changes in the approach of the legal profession to advertising have also contributed. The media (and public) love health issues and this, combined with the 'David and Goliath' scenario to which claims against multinational corporations automatically give rise, is an irresistible combination. Invariably unbalanced publicity about one claimant's 'battle' with a 'drug giant' can quickly create a snowball effect, with anyone who has taken the drug in question and contemporaneously experienced ill-effects quickly discounting the possible relevance of the underlying condition for which the drug was taken in the first place and believing that he or she may have a valid claim for compensation. Moreover, media interest is now fuelled by solicitors seeking to develop their own reputation in this specialist field who, since changes in the rules of professional conduct in 1990, may now more freely advertise their involvement in particular cases. This is accepted as a legitimate way of promoting the client's case and bringing further pressure to bear on the manufacturer to settle claims. Media comment often invites other patients who believe they may have a claim to contact particular lawyers already involved on behalf of claimants. While all of this is perfectly legitimate, in the pharmaceutical field there are certain risks attached because many patients are naturally suggestible; if such patients are eligible for legal aid they can participate in litigation at no cost to themselves, and the question arises: what have they got to lose by putting forward their case for consideration? In recent years some firms of solicitors have advertised in the press by reference to named drugs that have been withdrawn or had their licences suspended. Such advertisements note that patients might be entitled to compensation if they have used the particular drug and offer free first consultations. Whilst defendant corporations are much less comfortable about their own lawyers participating in the media debate, lawyers advising pharmaceutical companies need to have experience in dealing in the media with what are frequently highly emotive issues.

A further factor in the growth of litigation is ironically the development of court procedures for 'controlling' multi-claimant (and sometimes defendant) cases in the management sense. The concept of a 'group action' is not unknown in other fields but most experience has been gained in the pharmaceutical field. Part of the aim of these procedures is to ensure that claims are coordinated and proceed roughly in parallel, usually under the supervision of a single judge. Such procedures can only operate efficiently according to a strict timetable with the imposition of 'cut-off' dates by which all claims must be notified. In fairness, however, such dates have to be given some publicity and the courts have encouraged plaintiff lawyers to advertise the dates freely. The effect, of course, may be to encourage the submission of claims of varying merits and viability solely to ensure that the opportunity to proceed is not lost. In the benzodiazepine litigation, the increase in claims following advertisement of the names of the various benzodiazepine drugs marketed over the years was phenomenal, with almost 20 000 claims notified by the cut-off date. Whilst some of these factors ought also to encourage litigation in other sectors (and environmental claims are certainly increasing), the fact remains that the pharmaceutical sector is particularly vulnerable to product liability litigation and this is reflected in the fact that nearly all the group actions raised have been in the pharmaceutical field.

As regards the future, there is little reason to imagine that pressure from claims will abate. First, substantive law has moved in favour of claimants. Strict liability was introduced in 1988 under the Consumer Protection Act 1987 and adds an additional cause of action that is meant to facilitate the pursuit of compensation for injury due to defective products. If a product fails to offer the safety persons are entitled to expect, it is deemed 'defective', and if causation is demonstrated the manufacturer is left with the burden of proving one of the statutory defences, the most important of which is the 'development risks defence'. This bars liability if the manufacturer can show that at the date he put the product into circulation it was not possible, in the state of scientific and technical knowledge, to discover the defect in the product. Strict liability only applies to a product that was put into circulation after 1 March 1988 and so virtually all the litigation to date has required proof of negligence. Although there is little experience with strict liability (in either the pharmaceutical or any other commercial sector) the effect is not likely to be to reduce litigation, and the general principle of 'a consumer's expectation of safety' and the 'development risk defence' raise special problems of interpretation in pharmaceutical cases.

Secondly, plaintiffs are increasingly better advised than they used to be. Lawyers in private practice instructed by companies have developed expertise in the field, although in practice defendants tend to go to a few firms with a 'track record'—a sure sign that the need for specialist advice is recognised. In parallel and perhaps to an even greater extent, as instructions have been more widely spread, considerable expertise and knowledge of the sector have been developed within firms traditionally acting for plaintiffs in the personal injury field. The English Law Society's proposals for panels of specialists in personal injury and medical negligence work and the Legal Aid Board's move towards franchising of firms to conduct major litigation for claimants based on proof of expertise are expected to lead to greater specialisation. Whilst the number of firms handling the work for plaintiffs will diminish, identifying where specialist legal advice can be obtained should become easier. The Law Society's plans for a specialist panel for personal injury is well advanced and curiously pharmaceutical product liability has been assigned to the personal injury panel rather than to the medical negligence panel, despite the overlap with the latter. As an adjunct to these developments, specialist support services have blossomed in recent years. The Association for Victims of Medical Accidents (AVMA) has become increasingly important in advising people who may have claims. The recently formed Association of Personal Injury Lawyers (APIL) and even more recent formation of the Forum of Insurance Lawyers (FOIL) is further evidence of increasing specialisation. There is also an international dimension, with lawyers acting for plaintiffs in different countries getting together and exchanging know-how and thoughts on strategy, and information and documents relating to particular products and the way they have been marketed in different countries. With the help of such technical advisers and with greater coordination of effort, lawyers are in general more willing to take on, and more adept at conducting, claims against pharmaceutical companies.

Finally, there is the issue of contingency fees. The financial limits for eligibility of legal aid have not kept pace with inflation and very recently, amidst much criticism, the government has restricted eligibility still further in the UK. In response, the government has bowed to pressure to revoke the prohibition on contingency fees and allow them, albeit not in the form of the American model. The new rules will allow conditional fee arrangements to be made between solicitors and their clients, thereby facilitating litigation and shifting some of the risk and financial burden onto the legal profession and away from the individual litigant and the public purse. In the USA the lawyer is able to agree with his client that a charge will be made only if the litigation is successful. In those circumstances the lawyer becomes entitled to a percentage of the damages, normally about 40%. The UK proposal is not to give the solicitor a direct interest in the damages but rather to allow him to increase his fees above the norm in the event of success. It was, at first, proposed that a limit of 20% uplift would apply but this was clearly too low to make the option attractive and the government very recently agreed that the uplift may be 100%. Whilst conditional fee arrangements are unlikely to cause an increase in personal injury claims generally which is outweighed by the reduction in eligibility for full legal aid, there is real concern that the identity of the defendant rather than the merits of the claim will more frequently be a factor in determining the decision of the lawyer to take on the case or avoid it. The 'deep pocket' principle of which American lawyers speak not only reflects the natural consideration that litigation should not be commenced against someone without resources to meet a judgement, but also tends to encompass the principle that some litigation may be 'viable' because the defendant is likely to be more willing to settle a case for (quite high) nuisance value to avoid cost, management disruption and adverse publicity. It is too early to say how precisely these new arrangements will affect litigation in the pharmaceutical sector but there are reasonable grounds for suggesting that they will increase litigation, and as they incorporate a performance incentive they will, in their own way, encourage specialisation still further by plaintiffs' lawyers.

Litigation in the pharmaceutical field is characterised by wide allegations, normally including failure to research and failure to warn. This translates into the need to collate and disclose massive quantities of documentations, invariably covering the whole life of the product. Such litigation combines the special nature of personal injury law and practice with the law relating to product liability, as applied in an industry with distinct characteristics. The procedural problems are accentuated by its propensity to be multi-plaintiff. For its optimal conduct it requires a thorough appreciation of the nature of the pharmaceutical industry and the regulatory system within which the industry operates (the regulatory authorities may also be co-defendants), together with an appreciation of the legal issues to which the interposition of the prescribing physician between the supplier of the product and the patient gives rise. The concept of the learned intermediary (as US lawyers call such physicians) in its purest form is peculiar to the pharmaceutical field and creates special problems related to the application of general law principles, particularly in 'failure to warn' cases.

Also required is an understanding of the scientific disciplines raised by the issues in the action, which invariably include pharmacology, toxicology, epidemiology and pathology. Dependent upon the nature of the claims and disease the drug was marketed to treat, lawyers must also become conversant in other disciplines as diverse as teratology and psychiatry. The instruction of experts and the assessment of the cogency of their opinions depend upon an understanding of the scientific fields within which they are practising. In the author's own firm this has led to the recruitment of a number of physicians, some but not all of whom have gained a further professional qualification in law. This reflects the fact that as many cases turn on science as upon a substantive or procedural law issue. The major multi-plaintiff pharmaceutical cases are administratively onerous and extremely costly to conduct. Optimal conduct requires the legal advisers to both plaintiffs and defendants to possess special skills and knowledge. Neither the Legal Aid Board nor the industry is prepared any longer to pay to take the lawyers they appoint 'up the learning curve'.

Conclusion

Although as yet aviation law finds a special place in legal directories but pharmaceutical law does not, this reflects only a lack of appreciation by the authors of these texts of the complexities of the regulatory environment and the fact that most pharmaceutical cases have been settled or discontinued with limited publicity. Behind the scenes a specialisation has recently developed in response to an explosion of regulation and litigation, and while it is not as widely developed as in the USA it is likely to become so in the next decade and be European in focus.

23
Industry Careers for Pharmacoeconomists

Nick Bosanquet

Imperial College, London, UK

Introduction

The last five years have seen a shift in pharmacoeconomics to the centre of corporate concerns. Pharmacoeconomics used to be seen as part of the world of strategic planning and drug development. Now drug acceptance and sales may often depend on the results of economic studies. The next generation of chief executives will want to show this experience on their curricula vitae. Pharmacoeconomists have come out of the backroom into the arena where company reputations are won or lost.

Pharmacoeconomics used to be seen in the industry as a negative force, which would be used by regulators to block the introduction of new therapies. However, companies have shown how they can adapt and use the new discipline to a more positive end. Pharmacoeconomics has generally provided evidence which has favoured new therapies. The coming of pharmacoeconomics has been associated with a period of rapid growth in spending on pharmaceuticals first in the USA and then in the UK. While clinical trials of effectiveness have become more difficult and expensive and have shown a higher failure rate, economic studies have tended to show more positive results.

The greater use of economics has been associated with a new healthcare paradigm. Healthcare is not just about doctors treating individual patients. It is about reducing risks across local populations. Health funders have to reach out to ensure that high-risk individuals get access to treatment. For agencies such as health maintenance organisations (HMOs) there is an element of interest as well as a professional duty in this. Preventive treatment now may reduce hospital admissions and treatment costs in the future.

Within the UK the new paradigm has been expressed in the graduated treatment plans of the National Service Frameworks (NSFs) which have encouraged rapid

Careers with the Pharmaceutical Industry, Second edition. Edited by P. D. Stonier.
© 2003 John Wiley & Sons Ltd. ISBN 0 470 84328 4

diffusion of statin use for coronary heart disease (CHD) and set standards for reducing risk of progressive disability in diabetes.

The use of economics has also coincided with the rise in influence of informed groups of patients. Such groups have been able to use economics to get much more focus on rarer diseases with smaller patient groups. Economic studies have brought into focus the longer-term costs and benefits involved in treatment of these groups. This has reinforced the supply side change by which smaller pharmaceutical companies have sought to develop new niche markets. Ten years ago the industry was organised around a rather small number of blockbuster drugs. Now there is a more diverse range of effective new therapies. Health economics has been a powerful support for smaller groups of patients whose interests might have been lost in the broad social calculations of governments and giant pharmaceutical firms.

The increased influence of health economics has also been assisted by the rise of a new range of lifestyle drugs. These depended more than drugs for specific diseases on modelling future risk factors since the newness of these drugs meant that there was no actual experience of use with large patient populations. These drugs also required links to be made between healthcare and changes in the social and economic environment. Calculations of indirect costs and benefits (those to patients and to carers rather than to the health agencies) were particularly important for these therapies. There were also close links between pharmacoeconomics and marketing.

Educational Background

Health economists and pharmacoeconomists have expanded in numbers. They have also become more diverse in terms of background. The traditional route into the new roles has been through a Master's degree, usually at the University of York. However the majority of these health economists have gone to work in the academic world. The outcomes groups, which employ most pharmacoeconomists, have usually recruited from within the industry, mainly from managers/researchers with a background in the natural sciences. This has worked well in outcomes analysis which was in any case disputed territory between economics and psychology and where the actual content of specialist economics may have been quite low: however, such transfers may well be more difficult as the role of economists expands into such areas as pricing where a more formal background in economics is essential.

The Work of Pharmacoeconomists

The range of jobs open to economists in this field is now much wider. They can work directly within companies in carrying out studies and developing submissions to regulatory authorities. They can work with marketing specialists within companies. They can also work for the regulators, or for academic units to which the regulators have outsourced work. The general effect has been to create a severe shortage of pharmacoeconomists, and as a result some people within companies have moved across into outcome divisions from other backgrounds and activities. Pharmacoeconomics has been a function which people learnt on the job or through distance learning.

There is a new group of new or temporary economists as well as those who have taken more formal courses, usually at the University of York. This influx has helped to revitalise the field and contributed to new perspectives. It has also created a new range of job opportunities for people who have developed an interest in the area since finishing their university degree or postgraduate course.

Pharmacoeconomics has also become a route for people who want to move from the natural sciences towards management.

The subject has also become much more international. With increasing numbers of governments now requiring cost-effectiveness studies for reimbursement, health/pharmacoeconomists are no longer concentrated in the USA and the UK: they are found around the globe. An international labour market is likely to develop and expand, and future careers are likely to involve an increasing amount of international experience and travel.

Clinical trials

The original role of economists was in contributing an additional dimension to clinical trials. Data would be collected during the course of the trial and then towards the end of the trial additional economic analysis would be carried out. This would cover:

- Detailed costing of alternative therapies;
- Estimates of resource savings from more effective therapies;
- Estimates of costs to patients from treatment.

Many companies adopted this model of involvement in clinical trials in the early 1990s. For example Schering Plough's Annual Report for 1992 stated that 'The Company's new pharmacoeconomic and Quality of Life (QOL) research unit is integrating economic and QOL evaluations into world-wide clinical trials and new product development, providing support to therapeutic and marketing teams' (Schering Plough, 1992).

This role of economics in adding to clinical trials has indeed expanded so that a large clinical trial will have an economics component, which will be reported separately. Clinical trial results may also be used for modelling economic costs and benefits in the future.

Cost-effectiveness

To the old hurdles of safety, efficacy and quality has now been added the fourth hurdle of cost-effectiveness. This means in effect a second period of time before the general adoption of new therapies after the initial period while agencies make decisions on the first three issues. The coming of the fourth hurdle of economic efficiency has been the single most important event affecting health economics over the past decade (Maynard and Cookson, 2001). The new role of economists is in using trial evidence for external presentation for regulators, and the central place here of cost-effectiveness has transformed their role and workload, bringing them and the frontline company success or failure.

A new range of agencies has begun to emerge. The first country to introduce this fourth hurdle was Australia. The Australian Pharmaceutical Benefits Scheme will not reimburse the use of new pharmaceuticals unless appropriate economic evidence is provided.

Since 1997 Denmark, England and Wales, Finland and the Netherlands have all introduced systems for collecting economic evidence to justify reimbursement. The National Institute for Clinical Excellence (NICE) in England and Wales is emerging as a key international leader.

With respect to pharmaceutical products, the stated aim of NICE is to speed the take-up of effective therapies and to ensure equity by ending postcode rationing by which there were discrepancies in funding the new therapies between different areas of the country. Companies present cases based on clinical and cost-effectiveness data. NICE also carries out an independent appraisal which is usually outsourced to an academic unit. The NICE Appraisal Committee gives an appraisal determination of clinical and cost-effectiveness, which when finalised is issued with guidance for use of the product within the National Health Service.

The NICE appraisal generates a great deal of work for economists. In the first stage they are helping to prepare the companies' submissions—where £50–100m of sales may typically hang on the decision or they are working with the agencies to appraise the evidence. The main work in the first waves of appraisals by NICE has been to try to make the best use of such evidence as is available, but NICE will soon begin to have an impact on the way clinical trials are conducted and on the supplementary activities in collecting additional data on cost-effectiveness.

NICE adds an extra element of intense scrutiny drawing on experience from a wide range of reports, reviewing 40–50 new and existing technologies a year. The NICE approach will also increase and sharpen comparisons between drug therapy and other types of therapy in surgery or health promotion. For the first time an agency will be reviewing all kinds of therapy on a consistent basis. NICE sees its role as moving up the quality care in healthcare and it has gained credibility with health professionals although not with the wider public. In practice most new technologies and therapies submitted to NICE have generally been accepted. The failure rate has been far lower than with the US Food and Drug Administration (FDA), which is now the main source of scrutiny of the two-thirds of new drugs which are first launched in the US market.

Within the USA the new challenge of cost-effectiveness has come not from the Federal government but from HMOs and insurers. The FDA's initial assessment and approval of new products is made purely on the basis of safety, quality and efficacy, although the FDA does have a later role in approving any promotional material which mentions economic assessment or economic evidence.

The main health economics challenge comes from funders such as HMOs and insurers. They are facing severe tests in managing within budgets and have set up annual capitation amounts for enrolees. As a result they have moved towards care which is based on protocols and formularies. Companies have to submit cases for inclusion in formularies: and in the USA there is intense negotiation about prices as well as about actual market entry. The free pricing situation in the early 1990s is giving way to one in which local funders are seeking to discount.

Change in the public sector is adding to this pressure. US government programmes for Medicare and Medicaid used to be centrally funded with one set of rules. Now there is more state autonomy in Medicaid and in Medicare, where there has never been one pharmaceutical benefit in Medicare, but there is state pressure to extend. In effect the market expansion of the 1990s—with increasing sales of 10–15% a year for prescription medicines—has raised some very difficult questions about access and ability to pay. The use of economic evaluation is now spreading to most of Europe.

Commercial

In all countries except Germany economic evaluations are used for reimbursement decisions and in others economic evidence is used for a wide range of functions including price negotiations, local decisions on formularies, developing clinical practice guidelines and communication to prescribers. As the use of economic evaluation spreads so will career opportunities for economists. These used to be confined to a few organisations: now a much wider range of agencies at insurance fund or regional level are likely to be using the services of health economists.

Marketing

Pharmacoeconomists also contribute to marketing once a drug therapy is accepted for funding. There are many new challenges in relating to patient groups. One particular kind of study provides a vital link between marketing and the concerns of the regulators. These are the studies of the burden of disease. These provide estimates of current and prospective treatment costs together with estimates of the economic and personal losses arising from morbidity. They bring together data from the health service on admission rates and treatment patterns with data from the wider society about the impact of illness on income and on withdrawal from the workforce. The burden of disease studies has provided new evidence both on costs to patients and on longer-term treatment costs. They have powerfully reinforced the case for early intervention. These studies have given positive results for regulators: they have also assisted in communication with patients.

Supply

So far we have mainly been reviewing the impact of change on the side of funders or the demand for pharmaceuticals but there have also been important changes on the supply side in the range of companies. In the mid-1990s the industry was dominated by a small number of mainly American firms. The US market has become even more the focus for the buying, funding and launch of pharmaceuticals, moving from 31% of world sales in 1990 to 46% in 2001, while the share of sales in Europe fell from 32% to 22%. The supply side of the industry has become more diverse even though the demand has much more concentration on the USA.

International

Since the mid-1990s the most significant change was the increased market role of companies which had been little involved internationally. European companies such as Sanofi-Synthelabo, Schering AG, Pharmacia and Lundbeck scored significant success in developing niche markets for new products (Bosanquet and Atun, 2001). The European presence was particularly strong in cancer treatment which American majors had seen as an unpromising area for development. These firms recruited economists who tended to work in smaller groups closer to development and marketing managers. The economists also have to carry out a greater range of work, as there was less internal specialisation. The changes opened up employment at many more points. Pharmacoeconomists used to be employed by a few large firms, now they had the chance to work for many more medium-sized firms.

Pharmacoeconomists used also to be concentrated in the USA and the UK: they are now an international group with numbers in every European country and also a growing number in Latin America, Asia and working for international institutions. The main research centres however remain in the USA and the UK, although there is a notable increase in high-quality research from Scandinavia.

The Future

For the future the outlook for increased numbers and range of employment for pharmacoeconomists seems good. There seems little prospect of any reduction in regulation or lowering of the fourth hurdle. Indeed it is likely that more countries will make cost-effectiveness data a formal requirement and where this is already the case there will be more intensive use of it. There is also likely to be more use of pharmacoeconomics from new groups of patients/consumers and such use will become much more international.

Within companies the effective use of pharmacoeconomics is likely to become even more critical to survival. This will be especially so for larger companies struggling with the loss of patent protection. It will also be important for newer companies seeking to expand their role in world markets. In 10 years pharmacoeconomics has moved a long way from a backroom research activity to a critical area of company growth and even survival. The next five years seem likely to strengthen employment prospects and add to the diversity of roles for economists in pharmaceuticals.

References

Bosanquet, N. and Atun, R. (2001) 1998–2001 in the pharma industry: from deep river to white water rapids. *Eur. Business J.*, **13**(2), 74–82.

Maynard, A. and Cookson, R. (2001) Money or your life? The health–wealth trade-off in pharmaceutical regulation. *J. Health Service Res. Policy*, **6**(3), 186–189.

Schering Plough (1992) Annual Report, Schering Plough Corporation, Maddison, NJ.

24

Consultant in Pharmaceutical Medicine

Brian Gennery

Gennery Associates, Bracknell, UK

Introduction

The idea of being a totally independent person who both earns a living and obtains job satisfaction by using intellectual and personal resources is an attractive one for many people. Some such people leave the environs of a pharmaceutical company or contract research organisation and set themselves up as a consultant in pharmaceutical medicine. It is difficult to quantify how many individuals have taken this step but the number is growing on both sides of the Atlantic. Some estimates put it at over 300 in the UK alone. The reasons for this growth are partly because of the numbers of separations or lay-offs of even quite senior medical staff from corporations who are struggling to cut back costs in view of the squeeze in healthcare budgets in all developed countries.

In this chapter an attempt will be made to analyse the reasons for people going into consultancy, the planning required and the steps that need to be taken, the characteristics and qualities needed to succeed, the type of work which is available and finally the problems and risks of making this particular choice of career. This chapter will not cover consultancy work carried out by contract research organisations or by full-time academic and hospital physicians who offer part-time consultancy services to various companies.

Reasons for Going into Consultancy

Anyone entering consultancy or contemplating a career in this direction should always look upon it as part of a career plan. It is a step which should only be taken after a careful analysis of the various career opportunities open to an individual and

Careers with the Pharmaceutical Industry, Second edition. Edited by P. D. Stonier.
© 2003 John Wiley & Sons Ltd. ISBN 0 470 84328 4

a thought-out decision that this is absolutely the right step for that person. It is no use going into consultancy just to have a 'try at it'. Unless one is committed to this career option it is not likely that anyone would be successful at it.

Having said this it is not at all uncommon, and this is a quite different scenario, for people who have reached retirement age and are in receipt of a full company pension to do some occasional or part-time consultancy as a way of maintaining an intellectual challenge. This is, of course, open to anyone who so desires to take up such a challenge, and the risks from it are obviously considerably less than if consultancy is considered to be a deliberate career move at an earlier stage, from which one wishes to earn sufficient money to replace a salary or a pension. The problem for such people is how to regulate the amount of work that they do. Often there is more available than is wanted, but to turn away work too often results in acquiring a reputation for not being willing to take on tasks.

Assuming that one is moving into consultancy as part of a planned career move, it is important as part of the analysis to look at the risks and benefits of the opportunity and to ensure that at least in the medium to long-term the benefits are likely to outweigh the risks.

Risks

The biggest risk of moving into consultancy from a company position is the immediate cessation of all the benefits package associated with working for a large company. One no longer has the comfort of a regular and predictable monthly income which would normally be expected to take care of all the necessities of life with perhaps a little bit over. Equally there will be no further bonuses which in the past may have been an important source of income and form the basis of such important events as family holidays and Christmas presents. The car will almost certainly have gone, as will the pension, contributory or non-contributory, free life assurance, chronic sickness benefit packages and private healthcare insurance. Suddenly you are on your own and you have to provide for all of this list of things. Clearly some priorities will be decided as to which are the most important and this will vary as to an individual's personal circumstances.

One of the most important is whether to transfer the company pension into a personal policy. This will depend on a number of factors and professional financial advice should be taken as early as possible.

Benefits

The potential benefit of being a consultant is the idea of being able to plan one's own life pattern; associated with this is being one's own boss! In practice of course one no longer has a single boss but hopefully a multitude of bosses who are all pulling for their project to be done at the fastest possible pace and for the least possible cost. A consultant would hope to do only those jobs which are really of interest and have a variety of different projects moving forward at the same time which provide intellectual challenge and a large amount of interesting work.

There is also the hope and possibility of working with a variety of different companies and benefiting from seeing their various corporate cultures in operation. Finally, if one is successful, there is the hope of considerable personal reward both financially and in terms of job satisfaction.

Consultancy by Default

It is becoming increasingly common to come across individuals who are setting themselves up in a consultancy operation not out of choice or desire but because they have been the victim of a major corporate reorganisation or merger and are unable to find employment in any other company. This is not the way to move into consultancy because it means that the individual is probably not committed to that type of career, has not planned for such a move and thought through the type of services that they are able or prepared to offer, and has not got the necessary resources behind them to enable them to establish their position within the scope of consultancy opportunities before they become successful.

Planning for Consultancy

As with any business a consultancy package offered by an individual should be viewed as a 'product' and as such should be marketed, preferably with some unique features about it which makes it attractive to potential clients, who will usually be pharmaceutical companies. As with any product launch the product needs to be thoroughly researched and worked out, and the time of the launch planned so as to maximise the opportunity available. This usually means reviewing the attributes of the individual providing the consultancy service and seeing what they can offer potential clients.

'Product' characteristics

The following is a list of experiences and skills that a pharmaceutical physician might have had and that might be appropriate for him or her to use as part of their consultancy product package which they are going to offer to clients.

The first of these is the amount of time spent in the industry. As in so many aspects of life, time means experience gained and types of events experienced, both of which may be unique to an individual and if in demand will put that individual into a good position to offer a consultancy service. All too often people who have spent three to five years in the industry set themselves up in a consultancy position, only to find they have almost nothing to offer beyond the experience of a few clinical trials, putting together one or two CTXs (Clinical Trial Certificate Exemptions) and attending a few symposia. Whilst there can be no hard and fast rules on timing, it is difficult to imagine that anyone who has less than 15–20 years' experience in the industry has had sufficient variety and depth of experience to make what they have of value to potential clients. Having said that there are a number of people who have made the move successfully at an earlier stage and only worked within the limit of their experience. The limitation of this is that their horizon may also be limited.

The types of experience that should have been acquired during a career in pharmaceutical medicine will inevitably include those in clinical research and associated activities such as product registration. It would have been important to list the number of products for which one has had responsibility in phases I, II, III and IV, whether there is any experience with post-marketing surveillance studies, activities with the Code of Practice Authority, putting together CTX applications and marketing authorisation applications, and finally what experience an individual has with the various European procedures. Wider international experience, particularly with the FDA, is a real bonus.

It will also be important to list the breadth of an individual's experience in the clinical research and registration arena, taking into account not only Europe but also the USA and Japan.

Other attributes that need to be examined and brought together are an analysis of training programmes that have been undertaken and the length and depth of an individual's management experience in a variety of different positions.

Other important aspects that will be helpful in demonstrating one's stature within the environment of pharmaceutical medicine is to have demonstrated wide experience in a number of organisations, such as serving on committees and helping with activities of various organisations such as the British Association of Pharmaceutical Physicians, the Society of Pharmaceutical Medicine, the Faculty of Pharmaceutical Medicine or the Association of the British Pharmaceutical Industry.

Also of importance will be a list of publications demonstrating an individual's knowledge and experience and whether or not a person serves on the editorial board of a journal.

These then are the elements that go to make the 'product'. It now needs to be put in the context of the market in which it is to operate and be merchandised and presented to potential clients so that they take advantage of the opportunity presented.

Resources

It is important to view a pharmaceutical consultancy as a business and the content of the type of consultancy being offered as a product. The elements which go to make up the product have already been discussed, but it needs to be presented in the same way as any other product.

The first thing to do is to write out a business plan in exactly the same way as one would for a large multinational corporation. This should include a mission statement, a set of objectives against which you can measure your own performance, and a financial plan including a cash flow analysis for at least the first three years.

The next thing to look at is to determine what finance is going to need to be invested into the business before it becomes a viable self-sustaining operation. This is where long-term planning for consultancy comes into play, as few people are likely to be able to sustain themselves by generating enough income over the first few months or a year and therefore need some personal financial resources to fall back on to carry them through this period. The only alternative of course is to solicit a bank loan, which may be perfectly possible but inevitably involves interest charges and arrangement fees. These come more expensive for a business than for a personal loan and this option should be avoided if at all possible. Venture capital is not an option for straightforward consultancy businesses.

The business plan should be shared widely with a variety of professional people such as legal advisers, financial advisers, accountants and the bank manager. The reason for doing this is twofold: one is to solicit their views as they will often have considerable experience in helping people start up small businesses, and second is to show that you have a grasp of what you are trying to do and that you are setting about it in a structured, organised way.

The next decision is to decide whether one is going to work from home or to find a small office. This will often be determined by availability of space at home, the price of office accommodation to be found in the locality and finally personal preference. Some people just cannot work at home and feel that they have to go to an office in order to be able to change their mind-set into a work mode. Others can happily get up and work at home just as though they were going out into an office environment. Wherever one is going to work from, it is important to get the necessary facilities to be able to operate effectively; as a minimum, these include a high-quality computer with a considerable range of software, a fax machine and in the absence of full-time secretarial help an answer-phone facility. A mobile phone is an absolute must these days.

The next thing is to register with the Customs and Excise for Value Added Tax. This is not a critical requirement in the first instance, but as soon as one is approaching the thresholds for VAT it is important to register so as not to fall foul of the law. A critical decision is whether or not to incorporate, that is form a limited company. The arguments around this are complex and involve taxation and insurance. The situation can also change from budget to budget. Again, professional tax and financial advice is crucial.

The next exercise is to market the product, and this should be approached in exactly the same way as with any other marketing operation. There should be efforts at direct selling by personal contact with colleagues either individually in their offices or at meetings; this network can be widened by writing personal letters to colleagues explaining the types of consultancy on offer and if appropriate asking for a personal meeting. It may be appropriate to produce a brochure describing the range of facilities being offered, and this can be mailed widely across the industry either to personal contacts and friends or just in a somewhat more blind fashion. Finally it may be appropriate to take out advertisements in journals to make sure that everybody knows exactly what programmes and facilities are being offered.

Characteristics and Qualities Required for Success

As with any marketing operation, it will only be as successful as the quality of the product on offer and the way it is presented to potential clients. There are a number of characteristics about the consultancy business which make it somewhat distinctive from many other areas of endeavour and there are qualities required of somebody going into consultancy which are probably a prerequisite to success.

What is on offer

In order to be successful in consultancy it is necessary to have a long history of achievements in the pharmaceutical industry. It is better if these are in more than one company, cover a wide range of functions within pharmaceutical medicine, include some experience in management at a senior level, and cover a wide geographical area and are not just confined to the UK. It is also helpful to have served on a wide variety of committees and organisations as this establishes a substantial network. This network is necessary not just for potential clients but also as a resource to be called upon for help when uncertainty about a particular issue or problem arises and it is important to get reassurance from a senior colleague or friend. This network should include other consultants in pharmaceutical medicine. Obviously to some extent one is in competition with such individuals but to exclude them from one's network of contacts is not in one's own interest and there is no harm in offering sound advice to a colleague who hopefully one day will return the favour.

Defining areas of expertise

It is crucial only to offer services in areas in which one has experience and know-how and something to offer. In the common jargon this means bringing 'added value'. Developing and maintaining credibility is critical and there is nothing better designed to destroy such credibility than to offer services ranging from discovery research, through clinical R&D, registration, post-marketing surveillance, sales, marketing, public relations, crisis management and treasury operations when one has worked in only one or two of these areas and has no knowledge of any of the others. This means going back to the simple basics of knowing one's own strengths and weaknesses and having the courage to turn away work that is simply outside one's experience. This is clearly difficult to do early on when the number of projects on offer may be somewhat limited, but it never does any good to take on a project that clearly cannot be tackled effectively and with the appropriate degree of skill and knowledge. One's credibility as a consultant can rapidly be destroyed by totally letting a client down with regard to a particular project.

Being resourceful

The first thing that one learns on leaving a corporate organisation is that suddenly you have none of the facilities available in the way of secretarial resources, computer back-up resources, library facilities, etc. Therefore one has to do everything from arranging hotels and travel plans through to carrying out literature searches and writing up reports.

Many of the resources that one would want are not immediately to hand. Examples are a lack of the wide range of journals normally found in most companies and access to critical documents such as those coming from the European Community Commission and from the Medicines Control Agency. Fortunately the Internet has made most of these available at one's fingertips and there is now no excuse for not being up-to-date in an area where one claims to have expertise. The problem is one of information overload and filtering out only that which is important.

Work ethic

Most consultants will say that their time in consultancy is the busiest of their life. With luck they are working harder than ever before but this in its own way brings a number of problems. There is sometimes great difficulty in managing one's time effectively. Work comes in peaks and troughs, at least early on in consultancy, and the tendency is to take anything and everything that comes along, thereby creating continuous peaks and fewer and fewer troughs. The ideal of being one's own boss, planning one's own lifestyle, and controlling one's own workload rapidly evaporates as one quickly realises that one no longer has a single boss but a hundred people pulling in different directions, all wanting their project done by the day before yesterday. This is an important point and needs to be continuously borne in mind, particularly as the temptation early on in the consultancy career is to take any project that becomes available.

Types of Work

Companies will only employ consultants when they have to fill some type of gap in their resources. These gaps occur in a variety of interesting and unusual areas and different consultants will feel that they are better able to fill one gap than another.

Gaps in head count

With the increasing uncertainty in the healthcare area and the various pressures being put on pharmaceutical companies, most managements these days are trying to man for the troughs and manage the peaks. However, the work that comes with the peaks has to be done and this is where consultants can usefully be employed. It is possible that a consultant will simply be asked to act as a 'locum' to fill the role of a medical adviser or senior medical adviser for a particular project over a defined period of time. This may be whilst the company is recruiting a new full-time member of staff or it may be on a longer contract, with the consultant spending one or two days a week in the company. Other projects which require this type of gap to be filled include protocol writing, report writing, monitoring studies and sites, and ghost-writing either expert opinions or articles for journal publication.

Gaps in experience

Whilst most of the very large companies find that within their staff they have people with experience in most areas of therapeutics, many medium to small companies do not have this luxury. Therefore they will seek outside help in order to find out about a new therapeutic area, and a pharmaceutical medicine consultant with wide experience can often fill this gap. These projects tend to be somewhat short-term and involve explaining the area, offering some kind of training for people within the company and leaving them able to cope with the new challenges ahead of them.

A second gap in experience is in the limitation of territory in which a company has operated, and a consultant with wide international experience may be able to help a company start new programmes in new territories.

The third gap in experience is with registration problems, often of a transnational nature, and a consultant with a great depth of experience will be able to help a company through some of these issues.

Finally a consultant with wide experience in different types of organisations may be able to help a company which is trying to reorganise its medical function to cope with the developing concept of globalisation.

Gaps in expertise

Whilst most large companies will have within their organisation the necessary resources to tackle all aspects of pharmaceutical medicines, there are still a number of areas which are rapidly developing and changing where a consultant may be of use to both large companies and smaller ones.

The first of these is training, and whilst many organisations run a variety of training programmes sometimes a consultant has a particular area of expertise and knowledge which is valuable to a company and is able to offer training in that particular area. Indeed sometimes companies may ask consultants to run significant training programmes for them covering many layers of staff and embracing many aspects of pharmaceutical medicine.

The second area is in quality assurance and the need to be able to satisfy registration authorities that clinical studies have been done to Good Clinical Practice standards and a certificate of quality assurance inspection can be proffered. Even some quite big companies do not yet have quality assurance units in place capable of carrying out this function, and even those companies that do have such units in place may find themselves short of resources on occasions. Therefore consultants with the appropriate know-how and expertise in this area will be invited in to fulfil this growingly important function.

Thirdly, some companies still do not have full sets of Standard Operating Procedures (SOPs) in place and even those who have sometimes feel unhappy with what they have available to them. They might therefore invite in a consultant to review their SOPs and to advise how these may be changed and developed so as to be more user friendly and therefore used more frequently.

Finally, in this age of medico-legal problems and a litigious society, companies are frequently finding themselves faced with not only the threat but also the reality of litigation and all the crisis management issues that surround that problem, and often will bring in a consultant who has had some experience in this area to help them through a variety of aspects of this difficulty.

Bridging a gap

An interesting and somewhat surprising function of a consultant is sometimes to act as a reconciling person within a company. There are situations where there are strong divisions of opinion as to how a particular project should be developed within a company, and a consultant is sometimes brought in to act as the 'referee'. The consultant has no face to lose either way and can quite often bring new light to bear on the problem, reconciling the different opinions within the company and hopefully helping the company to develop its product in a more effective way.

Pitfalls and Minefields

As with any business there are a number of pitfalls and minefields which need to be avoided if the business is to thrive and be successful.

Size of operation

If a consultant is successful there will be the temptation to expand the organisation and operation so as to cope with bigger and bigger projects, perhaps branching out into contract clinical research, and offering a variety of other services. This will be perhaps the most important decision the consultant ever has to make about the way he or she is going to manage the business and how they are going to let it develop and grow. Most companies when they call in a consultant expect the undivided and personal attention of that individual and not for the programme to be delegated down to a junior member of staff or associate of some sort.

Whilst other members of staff may be useful in terms of carrying out background research, in the end a consultant and his or her organisation only thrives on reputation and that can be destroyed very quickly. Therefore the decision to stay small as a one-person organisation or to expand into a small group is a critical one from a business point of view and it is also a risky one from a financial point of view. If one has been operating without an outside office previously this now becomes necessary and one also becomes responsible for other people's mortgages, pension plans, life assurance, etc., as well as one's own. This means that the revenue generated by the business has to expand very dramatically and whilst what has been coming in up to date has been perfectly adequate to support the consultant and his or her immediate family, whether it can take the quantum leap to support other members of staff is something that needs to be looked at very critically. An alternative may be to go and seek financial bridging to help the business to expand but again this requires critical review and analysis before making such a decision.

Buffers

Inevitably with consultancy, work tends to come in peaks and troughs and it is essential when there are a number of good peaks to put some of that income into a high-interest deposit account so as to cope with the troughs. As has been stated previously, one of the great difficulties is not having that regular salaried income coming in every month from a company and therefore one has to plan financially on a somewhat longer term than when working for a corporate organisation. Another part of having a buffer is to ensure that there is enough 'work' available to cover the troughs. This may mean storing up articles and other literature that needs to be read, having some pet project which one can never quite get round to but could cope with if there was no other work to be done for a few days or weeks, going to meetings and training courses if the opportunities avail themselves and doing something very lateral such as learning a new language.

Speaking

If one has expertise in one or more areas it is not uncommon to be invited to speak at a variety of seminars and meetings. This is a very good method of meeting potential clients and demonstrating one's skills and expertise in a particular area. However, invitations to speak should be reviewed critically and carefully as for every hour of presentation one needs something like one working day of preparation. As the fees for speaking at many such seminars tend to be somewhat mediocre, to say the least, one has to weigh up very carefully if the potential value of accepting an invitation to speak is justified in view of the potential lost income that it involves.

Conflict of interest

Clients of consultants assume that the work that they ask their consultants to do will be treated as confidential and some companies will ask for a confidentiality agreement to be signed. This is particularly true of biotechnology companies, where the guarding of intellectual property is seen as crucial to the survival of the business. Indeed it may be as well for the consultant to have their own confidentiality agreement prepared and offered to clients so as to demonstrate their commitment to confidentiality. However, there is another type of conflict of interest which must be borne in mind and that is not to accept assignments on products from two or more companies which clearly are in conflict with each other. This would be highly unethical and would rapidly destroy one's credibility. Equally important is for the consultant to protect their own long-term interest and ensure that the reports that they produce for clients are exclusive to the client only inasmuch as they are particular to that product under investigation and evaluation and not the consultant's generic skills.

Conclusion

If one goes into consultancy for the right reasons and it has been properly planned for it is very likely that the individual will succeed. He or she will probably have the right qualities and resourcefulness to find appropriate projects and will eventually find enough to provide an interesting, wide variety of work which is both enjoyable and rewarding.

PART V
CAREER PROGRESSION

Careers with the Pharmaceutical Industry, Second edition. Edited by P. D. Stonier.
© 2003 John Wiley & Sons Ltd. ISBN 0 470 84328 4

25

Landing that Job—Recruitment, CVs and Interviews

Sue Ransom

AXESS Ltd, Richmond, Surrey, UK

Introduction

Career planning should be the start of every new foray into the job market. Too many people find themselves vaguely dissatisfied at work, happen to see an advert that takes their eye and find themselves on a treadmill of interviews. Your career deserves a more considered and structured approach—after all, this next job could well define your career path for the next 20 years. Within this chapter, we will explore not only how to look for and secure a new position, but also how to tackle the process to ensure that you end up in a role which is the best one for your career aims. There is also useful information for the new entrant into the industry, giving insights into the types of selection procedures you may go through, and hints on where to start.

The pharmaceutical industry is a mature one; it has a fairly well-defined set of careers, a number of well-regarded organisations which can help in career planning, and a wide selection of opportunities. The UK industry employs around 70 000 people directly, with another 250 000 in support roles. It is regarded as a 'safe' industry, as there are rarely any significant numbers of redundancies, and the stocks and shares are generally a low-risk investment. This inevitably makes the industry a popular choice for new graduates, and once in, people often stay for their entire careers. Competition for jobs is therefore often fierce, so you must make the most of all the opportunities which come your way.

Recruitment in the Internet Age

With the advent of widespread use of the Internet and e-mail, recruiters and human resource (HR) departments are becoming overwhelmed with the volume of

---

Careers with the Pharmaceutical Industry, Second edition. Edited by P. D. Stonier.
© 2003 John Wiley & Sons Ltd. ISBN 0 470 84328 4

applicants. It takes very little effort for an individual to send off a standard curriculum vitae (CV) for 10 or more potential roles in a trade journal such as *CRFocus*. However, whilst increasing exposure, this approach rarely includes any element of tailoring of the CV, and in a huge number of cases, even a covering letter. People are increasingly using technology as a substitute for quality and focus, in the hope that if they throw the net wide, they will land the job they want.

With the growth of the Internet there has been a corresponding growth in the number of places where you can look for a new role. Pre-Internet it was fairly simple: trade journals, the *New Scientist* on a Thursday, the national papers if you were senior enough, plus the few agencies which specialised in your specific field. Now the choice is almost overwhelming. There are hundreds of Internet recruitment sites, some very general and others covering a niche market. All offer but few deliver, and there were some well-publicised collapses of job sites when the dotcom bubble burst.

This new technology can be used to your advantage in your search for a new, rewarding position, but it must be used with the full understanding of the consequences, and how your application will actually be processed. Throughout this chapter I hope to be able to give you some insight into the recruitment process from the recruiter's perspective, and how you can help yourself in your search for a new role by understanding the needs of your customer—your prospective employer.

Recruitment and the Law

Over the last few years the recruitment process has become much more constrained by both the Data Protection Act and the requirements of new legislation within the recruitment industry. The aim of both is to protect the interests of the applicant from discrimination and unfair practice. All reputable agencies and HR departments are in the throes of adapting the process to take into account the new requirements.

As an applicant you will have the right to review any information held about you by the interviewer, including interview notes. You may also find that in dealing with an agency you are required to give formal written consent to your CV being forwarded to prospective clients, or that you are asked to produce documents such as a passport early on in the process.

Whilst in some cases these new procedures will result in the process becoming slower, applicants should be aware that the end result is a higher level of protection afforded to them by the law.

Planning your Campaign

If you are a new entrant into the job market, having just left school or graduated, you need to consider what skills you have acquired and how they could best be used. Analyse these and see how they compare to the requirements outlined in the other chapters. For example, if you have a biological science degree, enjoy working with computers and have a good eye for detail, you may want to consider data management as a step into the industry.

If you are already in the industry and keen to move on, the first and most obvious question to ask yourself is—what are you looking for in a new role? Is it more responsibility, more money and more travel, or less travel, greater breadth of role and the opportunity to develop staff? To best answer these questions consider your current role: which aspects of your job do you enjoy the most, and which are you perceived as being best at? Do you want to manage people, or do you prefer projects? Do you want to stay in your specialisation long term (e.g. statistics), or are you happy to use that to leverage your career into general management?

You should also review your transferable skills—can you motivate staff or lead teams, are you the person who is asked to solve the tricky technical problems, or to take on the project running behind schedule? This area is particularly important if you are looking to move into a different job area. You will potentially be up against people with more relevant experience, so you need to make the best of the skills you already possess. You should also consider whether you would be prepared to take a salary drop if you are looking to move in a new career direction.

Location is another key issue. Are you prepared to relocate? The majority of office-based positions within the pharmaceutical industry are located in the south east of England, and management positions in the field are rare.

Answers to these sorts of questions will help to direct you towards your best next role. Once you have identified the role, start doing some research into the types of companies which offer this role. For example, if you are looking to move into a role which will allow you to spend some of your time on research, you are likely to need to move to a major pharmaceutical company with a significant R&D presence, rather than a local marketing affiliate or a contract research organisation.

Having identified your chosen role and the types of companies to approach, you need to consider your approach—direct or via an agency. Direct approaches or responses to adverts mean you are in direct control of the process, but can take up a significant amount of time. Agencies can be very helpful in distilling your career thoughts with you, providing advice and guidance, but are another hurdle to cross before you get in front of your potential employer. However, agencies also offer access to a wide range of jobs which never make it onto the open market, and can consider a large number of jobs on your behalf.

Where to look

When looking for a new position you should concentrate your efforts in looking where the agencies in your specialty advertise—they will have spent a lot of time researching where the majority of their target audience will search, and as a result, most adverts gravitate towards a few key places, of which the three main ones are:

- Trade press;
- National press;
- Websites—specialist or general.

The majority of professions within the industry have their own associations, and most of these have journals. Recruiters are always very keen to use these types of journals for advertising, as the targeting of the audience is so specific—you can be guaranteed that a high percentage of the readership will be the people who are potential candidates. If you are trying to get into the area, contact the appropriate association and see if you can become an affiliate member. This will usually give you access to the journals and a lot of useful career information.

The national press is still used a lot by the major blue-chip companies, so it is worth keeping under review. However, for a lot of the more specialised roles within the industry, or for some of the smaller companies, national advertising is a rarity.

The *New Scientist* carries some interesting opportunities, and can be particularly useful if you are investigating a range of different roles.

All major publications now duplicate their recruitment advertising on their websites, which allows you to keep up-to-date with vacancies even if you do not purchase the paper or journal regularly.

By far the most popular place for advertising at the present time is on the web. It is quick, there is no need to wait for weeks for publishing dates, it can be updated (often in real time), and in some cases it allows for interactive responses from potential applicants, greatly reducing the time the whole process can take. Each company will usually have an 'Opportunities' section on their own sites, and the recruitment agencies always have large numbers of positions listed.

Covering all these can take a considerable amount of time, so you may want to consider using some of the industry-specific sites. The pharmaceutical industry is supported by a small number of specialist job sites, such as *Pharmiweb*, which carry thousands of vacancies at any time. It is possible to register your interest and as jobs are posted by the companies and agencies, any which match your requirements will be automatically e-mailed to you. In addition, most specialist associations have their own jobs boards, which can be variable in quality and in the quantity of vacancies.

Finally, you should not overlook the importance of your network of contacts in finding a new role. Talk to your contacts about forthcoming change within their organisations, or if people are moving on. A well-timed speculative approach arriving on an employing manager's desk will put you well ahead of any other potential applicants, and can allow the company to bypass the whole process of advertising.

Your Curriculum Vitae

Your CV will be one of the most important documents you ever write. It has only one purpose—to get you an interview with the company of your choice. It is a sales document, selling you, and it has to be easy for your customer to use.

Ideally, you should review your CV on a regular basis even if you are not actively looking for a job. It is difficult to do well in a hurry, and occasionally opportunities present themselves which you don't want to miss. If you are already in the industry never be tempted to use the CV that your company uses for audit purposes—it won't give the information you need to sell yourself properly, and it tells the recruiter that you are not organised enough to do one of your own.

There are three areas to consider when reviewing your CV:

- Structure,
- Content,
- Presentation.

There are two usual CV structures; one based on a chronological breakdown of your career, the other based on the skills you have acquired. Within the pharmaceutical industry the chronological CV is the norm, and most recruiting managers will expect to see your details presented in this way.

The CV should be kept short, ideally no more than two pages, with a third page of supporting information, such as publications. The longest CV I have seen was 27 pages, which had the only relevant experience listed on the final page. The applicant didn't get an interview.

Most CVs should follow the same general format, and keeping to this will make your CV easier to use. If recruiters have to search hard for the information they want, you have less chance of getting through. Many CVs are screened through an HR department, and they are often looking to 'tick the boxes', so ensure that you present the information in a way that they can use it.

The following format is fairly standard:

- Name;
- Brief synopsis of experience and career aims;
- Personal details;
- Education;
- Employment;
- Specific skills;
- Additional information.

Name: Use the name that you are known by, rather than your given name, if different. One applicant I knew had always been known by her middle name, but didn't specify this on her CV or mention it during the process. She got the position and arrived to find that the company had printed business cards and included her in the internal telephone directory, all using the wrong name.

Brief synopsis of experience and career aims: This should be no more than about four lines, and should give the reader an immediate understanding of where you are now, your major personal characteristics, and what you are hoping to achieve longer-term. This is often written in the third person.

A well-qualified clinical research professional with over 4 years' experience working in the CRO sector. Therapeutic expertise includes CNS, oncology and urology. Excellent organisational and communication skills, now looking to move into a position of greater responsibility within a pharmaceutical company.

Personal details: This should include your home address, home and mobile telephone numbers, e-mail address, date of birth, nationality and marital status. Other information is not usually necessary, but could include professional registration and insurance numbers and details of driving licence.

Education: Education and qualifications should be presented in reverse chronological order, and should clearly state the name of each qualification, the establishment, and the relevant dates. If you have a good degree grade, add it in, otherwise leave the grade out. Only include A-level qualifications or lower if you are a new graduate.

Employment: This should be presented in reverse chronological order, with the greatest amount of information given for the most recent or current position. If you have been promoted a number of times within the same organisation, show each job separately but under the overall banner of the company—recruiters like to see stability. Identify your major achievements in each role, and any specific benefits you have given to the company. Do not give reasons for leaving, as you will have ample opportunity to discuss this at interview.

Endeavour to show job changes running in smooth chronological sequence with no overlapping dates, but if there are gaps in your employment add reference to them, e.g. 'Career break to go travelling'. If you have been in employment for some time, your earlier experience becomes rather less relevant, and should therefore be edited down to one or two lines per company.

Specific skills: The content and size of this area will depend on the specialisation in which you are working. You should identify any particular IT skills, therapeutic expertise, management experience or relevant training.

Additional information: This section allows you to add information on interests and non-work-related achievements. It is also a good place to cover language skills, or international experience if this is not covered in the education or employment sections. Interests should be concise: 'amateur dramatics' conveys as much useful information to the reader as a description of your last starring role. Humour is not always a good idea at this point. Some people find it irritating and you are not looking to be remembered for the wrong reasons.

If you have voluntary work or charitable achievements, add them here. For example, 'Raised £3000 for the charity Mencap by running in the London Marathon', or 'Successfully completed the Duke of Edinburgh Gold Award'. These can be excellent talking points at interview, and allow you the opportunity to present a broader picture of yourself.

Some interests can be used to demonstrate qualities which you wish to build on in your career. For example, being captain and manager of the local football team can be useful if you are looking to secure a first-line management role.

When people are reviewing CVs they tend not to notice if a CV is particularly well presented, but they definitely remember if it is presented badly. If you are sending a hard copy, use high-quality paper, and print the CV every time—do not photocopy. Use an A4 envelope so that it does not have to be folded, and use a paper-clip or one staple to secure the pages together. Never be tempted to bind a CV or to put it in a fancy folder. Folders get immediately discarded and binding makes copying and storage very difficult. If you are sending an electronic CV, attach it as a Word document. This will help to ensure that the formatting is not corrupted by the transfer.

Keep the document as plain as possible. Be consistent with your formatting, particularly if you are applying for a job which requires a good eye for detail like CRA or Data Manager. Use the spell and grammar checkers on your PC, or the services of a reliable friend. Do not put in lots of borders and avoid the temptation to add colour, fancy graphics or photographs. Keep to a simple typeface such as *Arial* or *Times New Roman*, and use a readable font size, e.g. 12pt. It is better to go to three readable pages than to squash too much information illegibly onto two.

Having built a generic CV, you should always tailor it for each specific job, as the most relevant aspects of your career need to be highlighted. This may seem like a lot of work, but if you can reflect back the skills that are listed in the advertisement, you are much more likely to get into the interview pile. Always make sure that you keep a copy of each tailored CV to take with you to any potential interview.

Covering letter

Many people seem to think that the informality of the Internet is an acceptable excuse for not bothering with a proper covering letter. This letter is the ideal place for you to present yourself and your credentials in the best light—your initial sales document.

Use the opportunity of the covering letter to highlight your key skills, and to show how well you match the brief for the role. This will make the recruiter's job easier and will increase your likelihood of success. Reflect back some of the wording in the advert and demonstrate understanding of the role and the company. However, avoid the temptation to repeat large sections of your CV as this wastes time and makes the letter over-long.

Agencies and HR groups are always recruiting for a large number of positions, so it is important to state clearly the role in which you are interested. An e-mail with

'Please find attached my CV' is not sufficient. They cannot help you if you don't tell them what they need to know. This is particularly important when you are making speculative approaches to a company, and an astonishing number of applicants are guilty of omitting this essential covering letter.

The letter needs to contain the following elements:

- Job reference number or job requirement (e.g. Enquiry for the Position of Statistician);
- Introductory paragraph—who you are, what experience you have;
- Why you are applying for the role, including examples of what you can bring to the job should you get it;
- Follow-up and timescale—always suggest that you will call to check the progress of your application, and then do it.

The letter should be on a single side of A4, and if sent hard copy, should be on the same type of paper as the CV. It should always be typed unless the advert specifically states otherwise. Use a standard letter format with the same typeface as the CV.

The Interview

Once you have secured an interview you should invest some time and effort in preparation. Research the company, its jobs and the likely interview structure. Check the website for the latest financial and scientific results, keep up-to-date with recent news items from publications such as *Scrip*, and see if you can find someone from your existing network of contacts who may know the company from inside. Use your recruitment agent—he/she may have been working with this client for years, and could have a great deal of useful information.

Revisit your CV and the job description, and try to see where the interviewer is likely to focus. What skills do you need to demonstrate to show that you will be good for the job? Identify past situations which show you have these skills. For example, if you are likely to be asked about management experience but have had no actual line responsibility, try and find some instances where you have had to direct and motivate teams of people. Experience outside the workplace is equally valid.

Find out who will be interviewing you and what format this is going to take. If the interview invitation does not specify job titles, ring the agent and ask. If it is a direct application, call the company and ask reception or the interviewer's secretary.

Ensure that you have adequate directions to the company and understand the route you are going to take. If you are driving, check that there will be parking on site.

Types of interview

There are many different types of interview, but within the pharmaceutical industry the usual types are:

- Initial telephone screening;
- Informal;
- Technical;
- Human resources.

There may be multiple interviews, with some sequentially during the same day. You should make the same preparations for informal or telephone interviews as you would for a more formal meeting—if you don't come across well you may not get another chance. For telephone interviews ensure that you are in a quiet place, sitting at a desk so that you can write, and that you will not be disturbed. If possible do not have telephone interviews on a mobile phone.

Some interviews include an element of testing. This can range from a fairly straightforward written test examining your understanding of a topic, to full assessment centres where you may be observed in group situations. Personality profiles are still relatively common, but seem to have become less prevalent in recent years. For all tests ask for feedback. You may want to counterbalance the outcome of the test with other examples of your performance.

Increased technology is in the process of making other things possible. For example, some agencies are now using video to capture candidate responses to a set of standard questions.

Personal presentation

The dress code for interviews has become much more difficult since companies started adopting a smart casual dress code. However, the pharmaceutical industry is relatively conservative compared with some other sectors, and it is usually safe to assume that business dress is most appropriate for interviews. Men should wear suits and ties, and women should wear suits or smart jackets. Trouser suits are fine, but skirts should not be too short. For both, shoes should be dark and polished, and men should wear dark socks. Jewellery should be kept to a minimum, and perfume and aftershave toned down. There is nothing more off-putting to an interviewer than to be sitting in a cloud of strong scent.

You should also consider how you will be getting there. If it is on public transport make sure you have a decent coat with you in case it rains. If you are driving don't assume that you will be able to park close to the building in the visitors' spaces. Many pharmaceutical companies have large car parks but limited visitor parking, so you could end up walking some distance. You should take with you your CV, covering letter, invitation to the interview and a copy of the advert. You may also want to take examples of work, if relevant. All this is best contained in a document wallet or briefcase, not just the interview letter envelope.

Arrival

You should aim to arrive with a reasonable amount of time to spare (generally at least 15 minutes). Use the time waiting in reception to browse through any company literature on display. Always be polite and friendly to the receptionist and any secretaries you meet, even if you are made to wait. Interviewers often ask their opinion about candidates.

If you are offered a drink it is usually best to refuse, unless you are already in the interview room. Trying to greet the interviewer, carry your case and the drink can prove difficult. One candidate I interviewed took a sip of his coffee as he was being shown through to the interview room, and spilt it all down his front. Again, not a good way to be remembered!

During the interview

When you meet the interviewer your handshake should be firm but not gripping. If there are others present whom you were not expecting, check out who they are and what they do. You may want to answer questions differently if they are a technical expert, for example.

Put your relevant papers on the table, with a pen, and then try not to touch them again until it is time to make some notes. Candidates who fidget come across as nervous, so try and avoid this by sitting with your hands neatly folded on the desk. Sit upright, as this will make you come across as more assertive.

It is vitally important to maintain correct eye contact during an interview. You would generally be expected to have direct eye contact for about 70% of the time. Any more and you can seem aggressive, much less and you appear evasive, particularly if you spend your time looking over your interviewer's shoulder.

Don't worry about the interviewer taking notes. Good note taking is vital to the eventual outcome of the interview, as most people's memories are not good enough to remember the details later. If you have answered a question and the interviewer is still writing, be wary of saying more to cover the silence. Let them finish writing and ask the next question.

Frequently asked questions

Most interview questions are designed to identify experience, competence and interpersonal abilities. Usually the interviewer will ask you a few simple questions about your CV to break the ice, and then move on to the more taxing questions. Good interviewers will also use your answers to generate supplementary questions to get what they need, rather than just reading down a list.

It is always best to be prepared for the nervous interviewer. Some people ask closed questions and don't follow up, which can leave you with a limited chance to get yourself across. In these circumstances always expand upon your answers and make sure that the information you wanted to impart about yourself has been aired.

You should prepare some responses to these common questions:

- What are your strengths and weaknesses?
- What has been your most challenging management situation?
- How would your staff/peers describe your management style?
- How do you manage your time effectively?
- What has been your greatest organisational challenge?
- How do you deal with difficult people?
- What is your greatest achievement?
- Why are you leaving your current role?
- Why should we employ you for this role?

Questions and checking for objections

At the end of most interviews you will be given the opportunity of asking some questions. Always have a list prepared to indicate that you are interested in the position. For example, at an interview for a commercial role you should ask informed questions about the business, for clinical positions you could ask about the clinical research programme. At the early stages avoid asking about terms and conditions or remuneration.

At this final stage you should ensure you give yourself the opportunity to identify and counter any outstanding objections from the interviewer. Ask if you have the skills that they are looking for. If they suggest that you are weak in a particular area, you then have the opportunity to offer additional information which could get you through to the next round.

Before you leave, get an understanding of the process, including where you are now, what will happen next and over what timeframe. Make sure that you thank the interviewer for their time, and say that you look forward to meeting them again. If you are shown out by a secretary be friendly and enthusiastic about the position. It will probably be fed back.

After the interview

If your interview has been arranged by an agency phone them as soon as possible to give feedback. Make sure that you sound enthusiastic and keen to proceed to the next stage—the agent will convey your enthusiasm to the client. If possible send a short e-mail to the interviewer thanking them for their time and saying that you are looking forward to meeting them again.

The agent should be able to give you feedback. If you are not successful get as much information as possible about why, so that you can tackle those issues at your next interview.

At the interview you will have determined the next steps. If that doesn't happen in the expected timeframe, chase the agent or the client. Do not be over-pushy at this stage, as it is easy to tip enthusiasm into being annoying.

The Offer and Beyond

If you are fortunate enough to be offered the position you need to negotiate an acceptable package. At this point it can be very useful to have an agent to act as a go-between. Decide on your minimum requirements and don't push too far. It's often easier to get additional benefits rather than additional salary, as salaries can be determined across a group and therefore difficult to vary. Accept the offer in writing as soon as you are satisfied.

At this point you should send letters withdrawing from all other outstanding applications, thanking people for their time where applicable. You never know when you might want to apply there again.

When you move on maintain your networking contacts in your old company and with others you have met during your search—the pharmaceutical industry is not large, and these people could be invaluable to you in the future.

Conclusion

Getting a new job is hard work, but you can make the whole process easier by using the information available to ensure that you are focused. You must always have the end in sight, and be clear that it is really where you want to go. Spend some time doing your research, because if you start out on the wrong professional track it can be extremely difficult to change it further down the line.

Always remember that the CV and the interview are sales tools. You are trying to persuade them to buy your services, so step back and evaluate, and see if you can present yourself in a more compelling way. Ideally you want to convince people to be disappointed if they have missed the opportunity of interviewing or employing you. Maintain a positive attitude, even if you have received setbacks. Use every rejection as an opportunity to learn why, that way you can improve your performance next time.

Finally, remember that the interviewer sat on your side of the table once, and agonised over their own CV. They made it, and so can you. Good Luck!

26

Career Development in Pharmaceuticals

Roger D. Stephens

RSA Consulting Ltd, Old Hatfield, UK

Introduction

If a high flier joins the pharmaceutical industry at 27 and retires at 62 having enjoyed an average package of c. £85 000 p.a. his or her career earnings will be about £3 million. Adjust these figures how you like for personal career progression and local market conditions, but your career decisions may still have multi-million pound implications.

It's amazing how people who cheerfully write pages of justification for a new photocopier or car take back-of-the-envelope decisions about their careers. Career development literature hardly helps. Mostly it's written from a management perspective and designed to help human resources people to plan training and organisational change. Very little has been written from the perspective of the people who actually own their careers. Few companies seem to have career development programmes that really work. None manages its programmes to recognise the primacy of individual employees as stakeholders in their own personal development: all are (quite rightly) based on organisational needs.

This chapter assumes that you—not your employer—have the primary responsibility to manage your own career. Because the decisions involved may be megabuck decisions, they deserve at least the attention you'd give to any meaningful project at work. It's based largely on a talk I gave at a career development symposium some years ago, when I acknowledged the debt I owed to Dave Francis, author of *Managing Your Own Career*. This is a book that defined the practical, person-centred approach to career development that I still recommend to people who want to take charge of their own lives. I am glad to acknowledge it again here. Since then, I've also learned a lot from Golzen and Garner's wise and subtle book *Smart Moves*, which is also well worth reading.

Careers with the Pharmaceutical Industry, Second edition. Edited by P. D. Stonier.
© 2003 John Wiley & Sons Ltd. ISBN 0 470 84328 4

A Working Process for Developing your Career

The general approach is marketing-driven and quality/customer-orientated. It starts by asking you to regard yourself as a product which exists to maximise the opportunities or solve the problems of organisations. It is like the process used in the pharmaceutical industry to develop drugs and market them. Thus, given that a compound is emerging from some university or discovery programme, the first questions, designed to define its potential, might include:

- What is its structure?
- How does it work?
- What benefits will it offer to its users?
- Are there contraindications?
- Who needs one of these?
- Do the customers know they need one?
- What differential advantages are they seeking?
- Does my product offer such advantages?
- If not, can I develop it to meet their needs?
- In short, how can I fit my product to meet real world needs?

Serious Introspection—Defining Yourself as a Product

Analyse yourself as if you were a product. You may already have done some work on a curriculum vitae (CV). This can be a valuable start, but it isn't the right basis for a strategic career development programme. Indeed, there is a school of thought that calls CVs 'fictions about the past to help us feel better about the future'. If your CV is like that, throw it away!

To understand and define where your career is going, you need to understand where you are now, and exactly how you really got there. Collect factual information about your past and your present, and put it into a big lever arch file or scan it into your PC. Make a kind of 'Book of Your Life'. Include:

- Family memorabilia, notes of the addresses where you have lived and periods you were there—things you liked and disliked about each place.
- Brief descriptions of the characters of parents, grandparents, uncles, aunts, cousins, teachers, bosses and very close friends you have had over the years.
- Copies of your school reports, matriculation, degree and other certificates of competence or qualifications.
- Letters of appointment, psychometric or other test results, performance appraisal forms, congratulatory letters which came with bonus awards.

- If you have a family of your own, copies of your marriage certificate and the children's birth certificates; brief descriptions of the characters and aspirations of your spouse and children.
- Any other documentation or image which tells other people who you are and anchors you in your own personal reality.
- A page about why you chose your career specialism in the first place—what influenced you; who influenced you; what personal values were involved.
- Another page or two about the rationale behind each separate step of your career to date, and the pluses and minuses of each move.

Write each chapter and file it in the relevant place in the Book of Your Life. Leave each piece of writing for a few days, then review it. Try hard to make it 100% accurate and honest. Be rigorous. When you have finished, ask your closest friend to read and review it. He or she will confirm whether you have developed the clearest, most reliable characterisation possible of the history and structure of the product which is you. If you have, go on to the next step.

Defining your Aims and Objectives

To help you define your future strategy, you'll need to think hard about your personal values, aims and objectives. You probably started out with some wonderful dreams—to win a Nobel Prize, to be a master surgeon, to be as rich as Croesus. Now you're probably more realistic, and your situation may be more constrained by the real world. So prepare statements of the short-, medium- and long-term objectives that you have set for yourself and each member of your family. If you haven't set any, then get some down on paper and agree them with the people concerned. You cannot begin to plan without them. Try defining them under headings like wealth, power over people, expertise, creativity, working with like-minded colleagues, independence, security and personal status in the community, at work, at home, etc.

If you really want to be rich, then you are probably wasting your time being an employee: taxes and social security contributions will see to that. Try the Lottery, or start your own business. If you seek power and influence, an obvious thing might be to go into politics, or if you're really talented, to make your way to the top of a big company, academic institution, trade association or regulatory body. If exercising expertise excites you, then perhaps you should be a consultant or work in the more intellectually demanding areas of industry. Employers seem to prefer steadiness to creativity in their staff, so if you want to be creative perhaps you should get into the media or learn to paint. Autonomy and independence are contraindicated in industrial organisations: even at the very top you will be constrained by governments, stock exchanges, banks, lawyers, the press and television.

Security, in the sense of lifetime jobs with guaranteed pensions at the end of them, has gone right out of fashion, even in the government service. But the consolation is that it's getting more straightforward for people with marketable competencies (leadership ability is the most bankable) to build themselves secure lives, either as independents or as employees.

When you have completed your analysis of these things—your personal drivers—you'll be ready to work out two or three alternative sets of possible career steps that might give you a fulfilling career. Then you can assess the likelihood or otherwise of taking these steps with your present organisation.

Development Moves Inside the Organisation

Matching people to the current and future needs of companies is a key management responsibility. It's absolutely in accordance with your own self-interest as a career manager to help your company management fulfil this responsibility. Alert them to your own career interests and objectives. Don't wait until the annual performance appraisal interview to do this. Initiate discussions—especially if you have changed your plans in ways that might help the company achieve its own objectives. Remember: advancement may depend on developing and using competences you don't need in your present job. So co-operate with your management to design personal development activities that meet new challenges and improve your ability to remove obstacles that currently worry or frighten them.

Get the widest possible experience. To do this, you can either 'sit still for long enough, and maybe the whole lot will come to you' or move from unit to unit, or country to country. Get the widest possible exposure to successful executives in your own and other organisations: watch and follow what they do; make sure they and other influencers are aware of your plans. Become a volunteer in your company, relevant specialist societies and clubs. Approach opinion formers and senior figures when you see them in conferences, symposia and meetings; seek their advice and counsel: you'll be getting somewhere when they know your name and seek your advice in return. If this happens, make sure your company knows about it. Note that people who are doing well in their careers almost always manage to look good. They may not be especially handsome or expensively dressed, but there is usually a certain harmony between their grooming, clothing, colouration, body language and presence. Study how they do this and learn to emulate, or hire an image consultant or personal shopper of your own (free at John Lewis or Marks & Spencer if you can't afford to 'go private'). Be strong and energetic.

In situations of uncertainty, give management the benefit of the doubt. Don't whinge or cringe. Help identify and remove the obstacles that are in the way of your seniors. Be known as the provider of solutions, not the describer of problems. In short, make yourself the logical choice for the right next job when it comes along. But don't rely on your company as the only source of training or new opportunities. It may not always be able to provide them at the right time for you, or in the right sequence. So your strategic plan should also include self-motivated training and development, and if necessary, career moves which take you away from the company.

Development Moves Outside the Organisation

The structure of your company is almost certainly pyramidal, setting natural geometric limits to your promotion prospects. However, upward opportunities are not the only kind of career development. You can move further into a function, or move sideways via a lateral job change or move out altogether. The important thing is that your career should continue to develop at reasonable (say three-year) intervals. It is not always right to focus on the external trappings and higher salary of a more senior assignment. But it's natural sometimes to feel that your company is taking too long to produce the right kind of development opportunities. Be careful about this. In my work as a recruiter, I meet too many ambitious candidates who have come to regret hasty decisions to change jobs. They have little or nothing to tell me about their achievements: they didn't give themselves time to make any.

Conversely, those who have passively waited years for promotion have often let golden opportunities pass them by and got stuck in roles without interest or challenge. They appear at interview as bored, frustrated, negative and narrow, and seldom get short-listed. So even if you are perfectly content, it makes sense to keep a routine eye on the outside world. Read the business press to keep in touch with major developments in the economy and the market; read technical or professional journals to keep up with advances in your field; read the industry press to learn about developments in pharmaceuticals. Monitor the job advertisements—not so much to find a new job—more so that you understand trends in the employment market and the kinds of things on offer.

Bear in mind that a lot of vacancies are filled by networking—shrewd recruiters often start by asking around their industry and professional contacts for advice about potential candidates. This is another reason why you should be active in professional societies and clubs, at symposia and at meetings. Just as your contacts may seek your advice, so they may also alert you to opportunities that are maybe only at the planning stage. Include the reputable recruitment consultancies in your network, but avoid the cowboys. If you don't keep the serious recruiters up-to-date with changes in your career situation and plans (or your new address and 'phone number!) they'll be less likely to contact you when they're briefed to fill a vacant job. And if you are actively seeking a new job, have a mobile 'phone and leave an answering machine or voicemail on at home.

And of course, if you've done your 'Book of My Life' properly, you'll find it easy to prepare convincing CVs—in the plural because you'll certainly need more than one. First, you'll need a general one that can be produced at a moment's notice in response to unexpected requests. This one should be short—just a single page will do. Head it with your name, main professional qualifications and your contact details—postal and e-mail address, home and mobile 'phone and fax numbers. Show your current or last employer and job first, with two or three lines to describe the main features. Then show previous jobs in reverse chronology, with diminishing amounts of description. Finish with a brief statement of other personal information that might be relevant to any job application—for example, details of your family, relevant academic qualifications and your activities outside work.

Second, you'll need to prepare special editions of your CV to back up your applications for specific jobs. In these, give no more information and no less than is asked for in the job advertisement or headhunter's brief. Show the information clearly and concisely. Make sure it's professionally presented and pleasing to look at, with good layout and simple typography. If you don't have access to a skilled typist, it's worth paying a bureau to ensure a quality production. Avoid jargon and fancy language. Keep sentences short. Stick to the relevant facts. Remember you can always fill in gaps if you've said too little, but you can't recall information that the reader sees as superfluous, irrelevant, inaccurate or counterproductive. Avoid rhetoric and hype: they may be reassuring to you, but they just might make the reader giggle or snort. Check and double-check it before sending it in: get your best friend to check it a third time. Remember that many organisations now scan CVs into their databases—so avoid shading, boxes, tables, photographs and fancy graphics that might get in the way of this. If e-mailing, send as a Word attachment—most systems can cope with this. If snail-mailing, send it flat and unbound—that way it's easy to copy, distribute and file. Make sure the CV is attached to a covering letter addressed to the right person with his/her correct job title (if you don't know—'phone and check), and referring to the vacancy you're applying for. Above all, remember that though the only purpose of a CV at this stage is to get you an interview, a future employer is entitled to treat it as a legally-significant document. So don't tell any lies.

But before you start job hunting, and certainly before you apply for any job, you should have a shopping list based on a clear vision of the key features you need to see in any new role if it's to justify a decision to move. When a new job mirrors or closely approximates to this vision, you can justify the investment of some serious time to explore the prospects. If the initial exploration generates too many doubts, back off. If not, continue to explore it. Go carefully: remember you are approaching a multi-million pound decision which could have a profound transforming influence not only on your own life and fortunes, but also on those people—colleagues and friends as well as family—who depend on you. But don't hold back if everything is going the right way for you. If a new position matches most or all the key criteria in your plan—go for it!

Bibliography

Francis, D. (1985) *Managing Your Own Career*, Fontana-ATM, London.

Golzen, G. and Garner, A. (1992) *Smart Moves*, Penguin, London.

Maslow, A. (1970) *Motivation and Personality*, Harper & Row, New York.

Nelson Bolles, R. (1985) *What Colour is Your Parachute?*, Umbrella Publishing, London.

Nicholson, N. and West, M. (1988) *Managerial Job Change: Men and Women in Transition*, Cambridge University Press, Cambridge.

Sheehey, G. (1977) *Passages: Predictable Crises of Adult Life*, Bantam, New York.

Yeager, N. (1991) *The Career Doctor*, John Wiley, New York.

The market for your product

de Bono, E. (1980) *Opportunities*, Pelican, Harmondsworth.

McCormack, M.H. (1984) *What They Don't Teach You at Harvard Business School*, Collins, London.

Mintzberg, H. (1993) *The Nature of Managerial Work*, Prentice-Hall, Englewood Cliffs, NJ.

Townsend, R. (1971) *Up the Organisation*, Coronet, London.

Whyte, W.H. (1980) *The Organisation Man*, Penguin, Harmondsworth.

27

Opportunities for Education and Training in the Pharmaceutical Industry

Peter D. Stonier[1] and Gareth Hayes[2]

[1]AXESS Ltd, Richmond, Surrey, UK
[2]nrg pathway, Cumbria, UK

Introduction

Training and education in the pharmaceutical industry can be considered from two viewpoints: from the position of the trainer or from the position of the trainee. Whilst the role of the trainer (supervisor, coach, facilitator, mentor, manager) has increased in scope and value over recent years, the skills required to perform such a function are largely transferable across industries and not necessarily specific to pharmaceutical work. The importance of training and development to support individual career needs and pharmaceutical company quality standards cannot be underestimated.

This chapter focuses on meeting the needs of the trainee. The term 'trainee' may seem pejorative to those who embark on industry careers with high levels of educational qualifications, experience and expertise, and who have gained their positions through competitive selection and expectations of effective contribution. It is used firstly because there is no ready alternative and secondly because in the context of the rapidly changing technological, managerial and organisational industrial setting, continuing education and training are an inherent career-long learning process, regardless of seniority, longevity or trajectory: 'we are all trainees now!'

This chapter is inevitably different in format to others featured in this book, focusing as it does on training opportunities currently available and recommended to those selected pharmaceutical disciplines discussed, which in the space available cannot possibly be exhaustive. The best source of discipline-specific training

Careers with the Pharmaceutical Industry, Second edition. Edited by P. D. Stonier.
© 2003 John Wiley & Sons Ltd. ISBN 0 470 84328 4

originates from the professional bodies that support that role. These organisations provide much source material. However, many commercial training companies run competitive alternatives and the trainee is advised to consider all options appropriate to their individual training needs, company policies and experiences of others.

The desire to learn through continuous improvement is matched by the desire to improve through continuous learning. Adequate training can fulfil this need, but it is important to apply rules of measurement and evaluation. Only by assessment of training through competency measurement can the trainee be nurtured into a position of excellence.

The curriculum vitae offers a simple way to keep track of training received but a more detailed record should be kept by trainees themselves to illustrate specific examples of how the skills and knowledge gained from training have been implemented. With this information the individual can identify outstanding training needs and, more significantly, highlight achieved goals thus increasing their career opportunities.

All trainees should become aware of the expected training cycle and their learning needs with the scope of the career options. A proactive trainee should insist on an induction programme when starting a new company, whatever their status and experience.

The Training Cycle

A simple cycle of events can be assessed continually as part of an active career plan. Continuing professional development demands that, at whatever level, training is reviewed and acted upon. There will never be a situation when there are no training needs, and this is a worthwhile exercise to apply to all activities when considering training opportunities.

Relating the essential components of learning, knowledge, skills, attitude and understanding to the learning cycle of experience, reflection and deliberate testing can help clarify training needs within career objectives:

- Identify training needs;
- Analyse training needs;
- Set training objectives;
- Design and implement training;
- Evaluate training.

The evaluation of training, set against the original objectives, should allow a competency level to be assigned. This may be set by the manager or employer, if not, it is worthwhile to include a grade in a personal development plan (e.g. aware, basic, competent, distinguished, expert). Personal development plans should feature a combination of performance assessment, career plan and business need.

Induction

Following a training needs analysis, built around experience, curriculum vitae and job description, an induction programme for a new post can be developed. As trainee, trainer or manager it is worthwhile applying a simple template to ensure that key information is understood and all new staff are benchmarked to accepted quality standards. A review of training needs will highlight unfamiliar tasks that must be taken on board quickly and efficiently. This will benefit all parties.

A knowledge and skills profile offers the best headlines for an induction template. It is important that the extension of knowledge and skills goes beyond the simple 'doing of the job'. If not, there is a training need. There are five main characteristics to cover.

1. General knowledge at the corporate level, for example:

   - Pharmaceutical business (local and global);
   - Organisation of company (national and international);
   - Product portfolio.

2. Job-specific roles and responsibilities, for example:

   - Sales techniques;
   - Clinical research practices;
   - Regulatory requirements.

3. Therapeutic and product knowledge, for example:

   - Indications and related disorders;
   - Physiology and pharmacology;
   - Formulations and competitors.

4. Other technical requirements, for example:

   - Marketing plans;
   - Medical responsibilities;
   - Statistics, pharmacokinetics.

5. Transferable skills, for example:

   - Presentation skills;
   - Time management;
   - Team building, leadership.

Such an induction programme cannot be immediate, unless the company organises a full two to four-week induction programme prior to starting the job. It is essential that the many topics to be covered are prioritised by setting key objectives. Other aspects to consider are resources, including budget, and specialised needs. Self-development may well be essential, when resources are limited, but care must be taken to be efficient with training opportunities and not cause conflict with active roles and responsibilities. Development of competency comes with time and experience.

There is a subtle difference between competence and competency worthy of clarification. Competence is a standard obtained with a particular skill while competency reflects a manner of behaviour in performing said skill. As such competences refer to ranges of skills whereas competencies refer to the behaviours adopted in competent performance. As the individual measures his or her competences and competencies they, and their trainer, must be aware of the difference.

Appraisal and Personal Development

Following induction, the individual and sponsor company have joint responsibility for ensuring personal development. The benefits to both parties may be obvious yet progress must be monitored continually to guarantee that both parties are satisfied with agreed goals and targets. In the event of dissatisfaction, continual review allows prompt action and reassessment of goals. Measurement of training needs is usually performed at appraisal and the individual should expect appraisals to be stretching and challenging, if performed properly. Appraisals should decide a career plan based on knowledge, skills and performance to date, i.e. recorded competencies.

The sponsor company will consider training an investment. It does not wish to train the individual to take a career step out of the company but must take the risk that this may occur. Appraisal will measure the adequacy of training for the role or for the future role of the appraisee. The sponsor company will want to be sure that the training has a clear link to corporate business needs, that training is the most effective solution to a learning need and, through continued appraisal, realise that benefits of training are evaluated beyond 'course satisfaction'.

The usual appraiser will be the line manager of the appraisee although it is important that a relationship exists between these two and the sponsor company departments of human resources and training. Often the latter belong to the same department. A company template for appraisal and subsequent training plans—in other words, a career plan—is likely to be in place to enable consistency and efficient measurement across individuals, teams and departments. If working individually without a career plan it may be worth using such an example as a guide. Whether an appraiser or an appraisee, the first training to be undertaken may indeed be a short course ensuring everyone uses the appraisal process in the same manner.

The appraisal will cover many more areas than training and development needs, e.g. performance output, relationships, yet ultimately outcomes from appraisal will focus around the career plan and what has to be done to achieve agreed goals. The training cycle remains the same and the five categories listed under 'Induction' may also be used to cover more focused training needs. At appraisal it is important to recognise that it is not only the appraisee who is being measured. It is an opportunity to record and discuss support and performance of the appraiser, other staff and the training personnel; this is often referred to as a 'three hundred and sixty degree' appraisal.

Continuing professional development

A personal syllabus will develop through frequent appraisals leading to a continual personal development programme. When this begins to include further qualifications or formally evaluated course work it may be called a Continuing Professional Development (CPD) plan. Many supporting professional bodies, listed later in this chapter, provide extensive literature on personal CPD plans, some of which are mandatory.

CPD is a useful tool for identifying and measuring 'lifelong learning', in other words it can be described as the data that supports the snapshot curriculum vitae and gives direction to the career plan. Lyness (2002) describes CPD as:

- Allowing time to focus on development needs and career ambitions;
- Increasing awareness of potential career options;
- Analysing strengths and weaknesses;
- Planning short-term learning needs;
- Recognising previously unseen learning opportunities;
- Involving the employer to marry personal needs with business needs;
- Collating a portfolio of evidence to demonstrate commitment;
- Keeping up-to-date within chosen profession;
- Collating a portable record of progress and achievements;
- Promoting self-awareness and self-motivation.

Principles of learning

Many objective corporate needs will be resolved through knowledge and skills training. A change of therapeutic area will impact on knowledge training and the inevitable introduction of new IT systems will impact on computer skills training. The hardest development area to assess, by both appraiser and appraisee, will be in the area of transferable skills: those affecting attitude and behaviour. The individual's capabilities can be summarised as follows:

- Knowledge: What I know
- Skills: What I can do
- Attitude: What I believe
- Experience: What I have done
- Network: Who I can call on to help me

The latter category may be one of the most important as it determines how far the individual will go in terms of self-development. Whether through reading, videos, self-sponsored courses, computer-based training or open learning activities, there is a finite resource for self-development. People can be the best resource and a good manager can also be the best coach. Observing someone doing the job, as well as reading the books, can often provide the best results. The appraisee must not look solely to the appraiser for development direction, even though they may hold wisdom in many areas.

Training styles

The ideal trainer may be found in a number of contacts and it is up to the individual to draw on the best sources. Trainer managers may be described as one or more of the following.

- Instructor (building competence): Good instructors plan meticulously, conveying instructions slowly and precisely ensuring comprehension; they use repeating methods to confirm that trainees have learnt to a pre-agreed level.
- Coach (building performance): The coach gets much closer to the trainee taking a shared, but not necessarily equal, responsibility for the 'issue'. Good coaches give encouragement with the right mix of observed direction and delegation.
- Mentor (building lives): Mentors focus more on feelings and emotions, especially those that result in drive and motivation; providing an example to the trainee, good mentors develop attitude and behaviour in the trainee, and whereas the coach may prompt 'How?' the mentor will ask 'Why?'.

Learning styles

It is commonly accepted that adults learn when they are actively involved in the learning process and interested in the subject. Whilst this may be thought to be inherently the case when being trained on a subject directly affecting the career, different learning styles and types have a significant impact on what is learnt.

- Resistance: As a trainee it is important not to attend training programmes with resistance, although for whatever reason—tutor, location, topic—this situation may arise. Others may also feel that training goals and objectives run counter to their needs. It may also be a simple case of insecurity through ignorance or lack of self-belief. A good trainer will create the right atmosphere for training yet it is vital that the trainee comes prepared to be trained. Again it is in the trainee's hands to have the right attitude.
- Active/passive: Learning is not the passive reception of impressions through the direct *tabula rosa* method commonly associated with school memories. Active

or Socratic learning has much more impact as it involves the trainee and makes them open to learning.

- Association: New learning should best be tied in with what the trainee already knows. Blending what is to be learnt with what is already familiar provides a two-way interaction and a positive environment for learning.

Learning types

The trainee should know what sort of learner they are. This will not only help them select the most appropriate training programmes but be aware of their potential contribution and expectations when attending compulsory development courses. There are four key types of learners and it is possible to be a combination of types.

- Action learner: Action learners are enthusiastic and comfortable with judging by immediate experience. They will like visual and practical learning methods such as exercises and case studies.
- Thinking learner: Thinking learners collect data and may be cautious about putting things into practice in haste. They prefer lectures and visual materials like books and videos.
- Modelling learner: Modelling learners attempt to fit their observations into logical theories and models. They think in a step-by-step way needing rules to be obeyed. They like plans, flowcharts and diagrams to support the learning material.
- Practical learner: Practical learners like to consolidate learning by practising what has been learnt. They are problem solvers who act in a more structured way than action learners. They too like case studies, exercises and simulations.

The learning environment

The learning environment, subject and trainer are governed by the resources available and without preparation the trainee may find themselves in an unsuitable environment for their learning needs. When choosing a training programme it is worthwhile to investigate the environment and learning style to be approached. In addition it is useful to find out who else, and how many others, will be attending. Different companies employ different methods to train and this may be based on 'numbers through the door' rather than an effective training method. The most effective training programmes will use a variety of training methods.

- Lecture: While this can be a one-way communication, suited to some thinking learners, it can be useful for large numbers and also to provide introductory knowledge information.

- Discussion: This is very effective in smaller groups of two to 10 trainees satisfying action, modelling and practical learners in discussion regarding skills, knowledge and experience.
- Demonstration: Although a one-way communication it involves the trainee through observation of skill and experience.
- Exercise: One of the most effective training methods, if evaluated properly, this can involve all trainees at an individual and group level. It is useful for all types of learners.
- Simulation: Involving all the learning types this is a favourite of modellers. With two-way communication, in groups or individually, simulations use knowledge, skills and experience.
- Case study: The most direct and relevant method of training, and often the hardest to do, this involves all aspects of the principles of effective learning.

Regulations and Training Records

Aside from personal development needs and the business requirements of corporate progress, the pharmaceutical industry is one of the most highly regulated in the world. The strict regulation extends to matters concerning training and development and the majority of disciplines will find themselves governed by formal guidelines and legal requirements for the quality and quantity of training before and during the specific function. In the scientific areas these are usually described as GxPs such as Good Laboratory Practice—GLP—and Good Clinical (Research) Practice—GCP; whilst sales and marketing personnel have to strictly adhere to Codes of Practice; and regulatory staff must clearly be completely aware of, and work within, all aspects across the legal framework. The medical profession is incorporating Continuing Medical Education (CME) and Continuing Professional Development (CPD) into plans for a demonstration of continuing competence to practise, based on annual appraisals and a five-yearly assessment for revalidation in order for a practitioner to remain on the general medical register. Everyone should undertake a professional and ethical obligation to remain up-to-date with best practice standards in the role that they perform.

Apart from direct observation, which must also be undertaken, the sponsor company management, sponsor company auditors, and external inspection units can only be sure of correct adherence to formal training requirements by correct and meticulous record keeping. All training and development in the pharmaceutical industry must be recorded and maintained.

The responsibility for keeping the training logs of staff vary from company to company, being held either by the human resources or training departments, or by the manager of the department to which the individual belongs. However, it is recommended that each individual keeps a copy of their own records where they can; this can form part of their personal CPD plan and is inherently part of the information supporting their curriculum vitae. It is important to be able to verify the effectiveness of the training undertaken. The simplest form of record, which details title, date and attendees, does not inform an inspector, of any kind, whether the training was of value. The most usual method of tracking value is by comparing the training data against actual performance changes at appraisal. Again this may be viewed as purely a 'top level' assessment and they can raise more questions than they answer. It is recommended to introduce a direct competency measurement to the evaluation of training. Here a manager, coach or trainer will identify the training need, prior to training, and through witnessing the trainee 'put into practice' what they have learnt, be able to verify through dated signature the success or failure of the training. It is important, however, that the training records are not made too complex leading to a maze of information, which serves to confuse rather than clarify.

Training Sources

Whether self-supporting or with the aid of a 'training aware' sponsor company, the ambitious trainee has a number of options available in order to satisfy the identified training needs. Most of the larger sponsor companies will run consolidated in-house courses covering a vast array of topics from specific skills training, e.g. GxPs, therapeutic areas, IT, to challenging transferable skills, e.g. problem solving, time management, cultural communication. In addition, their training programmes will be indexed to competency measurement and appraisal. In the smaller companies and as individuals such in-house programmes may not be available. This need not be a disadvantage. A greater spectrum of training experience may give greater value to a personal portfolio and offer a wider outlook of the 'bigger picture'. The marketplace offering commercial courses to support any of the training needs for all of the pharmaceutical disciplines is huge.

Commercial courses are not usually inexpensive and application to become a delegate must be a considered decision made from previous experience or advice from another source. As has been highlighted under 'Principles of learning' above, networking in the industry is essential. Training may be competitive between the commercial companies themselves but information on 'good' and 'bad' courses is usually freely shared across sponsor companies. Human resources or the heads of specific departments are good sources of relevant information. The most effective commercial training companies are often those who can tailor their training material to the needs of the trainees and when a group or team is involved this material can be customised to highly specific sponsor company requirements. Clearly the best source of specific training comes from the professional bodies supporting each discipline. In the majority of cases their primary objective is education-based in order to maintain the highest possible standards for their profession.

Education and Training Offered by Professional Bodies

Institute of Clinical Research (ICR)

Website: www.instituteofclinicalresearch.org
(See also: Association of Clinical Research Professionals (ACRP) www.acrpnet.org)

The ICR education programme aims to provide practice-based education and training that is relevant to the profession, up-to-date and flexible enough to facilitate the professional development and career advancement of its members whether they be study site coordinators, CRAs or other groups. The academic recognition that many of the ICR courses now offers is allowing it to offer recognised professional qualifications that provide a nationwide and Europe-wide standard for the clinical research profession.

The Institute also runs one-off study days, discussion meetings and networking opportunities which are publicised on an individual basis. All education days and courses within the framework of the professional development and postgraduate programmes are available to be taken as education opportunities in their own right. There is no obligation to register with the university or to take the assessments, but many participants do so, in order to make the most of the education opportunity.

Clinical Research Certificate of Professional Development (CCR)

A one-year part-time course designed specifically by and for study site coordinators and related professionals. It is also suitable for clinical trial pharmacists. The course comprises six mini-modules that run in pairs and in all modules include coursework and assessments. The intake usually runs from September with modules running in September, February and June. The CCR is integrated into the rest of the Institute postgraduate programme and successful participants in the CCR who wish to continue on to the Postgraduate Certificate can enter directly, so avoiding the need to complete the first two compulsory modules 'Introduction to Clinical Trials and Clinical Trial Practice' or 'Clinical Trial Management and Organisation'.

Postgraduate Certificate

The Postgraduate Certificate is available for the successful completion of four compulsory modules normally undertaken within the first year of study. These are:

1. Introduction to Clinical Trials and Clinical Trials Practice;
2. Clinical Trial Management and Organisation;
3. Research Methods;
4. Structured Project: a thesis on a clinical research project.

Postgraduate Diploma

The Diploma qualification follows on from the Postgraduate Certificate and the award is granted for the achievement of passes in a further four modules chosen from six options:

1. Research Methods;
2. Applied Pharmacology and Therapeutics;
3. Ethics and Regulation;
4. An Introduction to Health Economics and Quality of Life;
5. Clinical Laboratory Investigations;
6. Toxicology and Adverse Events.

Successful completion of the Postgraduate Diploma provides immediate entry to the MSc.

Master's Degree in Clinical Research

This highest level of the Institute's programme is normally for successful participants in the Postgraduate Diploma who by completing the MSc project, full-length dissertation, oral presentation and *viva voce* examination can gain the MSc award. Exceptionally, applicants with a minimum of five years' certified experience of clinical trial management and organisation at a sufficiently high level will be admitted directly. In order to enrol for the Diploma Programme, applicants must complete the application form and attend for interview. They must also provide evidence that employers will allow 12 to 15 days of study leave per year in order to attend the course and associated examinations and that they will allow a suitable member of their staff to act as tutor/mentor. Applicants should be working in a clinical research environment and satisfy one of the following criteria:

- Hold an honours degree in science or exceptionally, an honours degree (or equivalent) in any subject;
- Have obtained the Clinical Research Certificate in Professional Development;
- Have at least two years' experience of clinical trial organisation in the pharmaceutical industry or a recognised academic or NHS clinical research centre backed by certification.

Other selected courses, seminars and workshops

Introduction to Clinical Trials and Clinical Trial Practice
So You're Thinking of Going Freelance?
First Steps to Management

Research Methods
Clinical Research Project Management
Effective Accompanied Field Visits
Introduction to GCP Audits
An Introduction to Clinical Trial Administration

The British Association of Pharmaceutical Physicians (BrAPP)

Website: www.brapp.org
(See also: Faculty of Pharmaceutical Medicine www.fpm.org.uk; International
Federation of Associations of Pharmaceutical Physicians (IFAPP) www.ifapp.org)

The British Association of Pharmaceutical Physicians (BrAPP) is the professional
association for doctors in the industry. It was founded in 1957 to encourage professional development and organise training for doctors in the industry, and has had a
long involvement in training and development of pharmaceutical physicians.

The association was instrumental in establishing the Diploma in Pharmaceutical
Medicine of the Royal Colleges of Physicians in 1976, and in a Joint Advisory
Committee with the ABPI established a postgraduate training course in pharmaceutical medicine which was transferred to the University of Wales, Cardiff. BrAPP
is the co-organiser of this two-year course, which has five residential sessions each
year, aiming to cover the core elements of the faculty's syllabus in pharmaceutical
medicine for the Diploma.

The University of Surrey's MSc courses in pharmaceutical medicine and clinical
pharmacology additionally cover the syllabus for doctors wishing to take the
Diploma in Pharmaceutical Medicine.

BrAPP also runs its own training workshops and has periodic meetings which are
recognised for Continuing Medical Education (CME) accreditation.

Before joining the industry

Doctors considering a career move to the pharmaceutical industry in the UK should
be fully registered with the General Medical Council (GMC) or its equivalent,
which must be recognised by the GMC. This is essential. It is also essential that
they should have completed a period of post-registration clinical work, namely
General Professional Training (GPT), through senior house officer posts in hospital
practice.

In the UK this is at present a minimum of two years. In other countries, the
equivalent of GPT may be shorter or longer than two years and its relationship
with the time of entry to the medical register may differ. Doctors from outside the
UK should check with the Faculty of Pharmaceutical Medicine that they have
completed the appropriate period of GPT, before joining the industry.

Scientific degrees, e.g. BSc, MSc, PhD are desirable, but not essential, additional qualifications. Postgraduate clinical diplomas and degrees, e.g. MRCP, MRCGOP, MD are also desirable but not essential, unless specifically sought by an employer.

Pharmaceutical medicine has come of age over the last 40 years, and is now a medical specialty in its own right, having, since 1989, established its own Faculty of Pharmaceutical Medicine in the UK's Royal Colleges of Physicians.

Background to education and training for pharmaceutical physicians

Doctors joining the pharmaceutical industry are encouraged to undertake training in pharmaceutical medicine with a view to obtaining the Faculty's Diploma in Pharmaceutical Medicine.

Education and training in pharmaceutical medicine is likely to take on an even higher profile now that pharmaceutical medicine has been recognised by the Department of Health as a listed medical specialty, since 17 April 2002.

A programme of Higher Medical Training (HMT) will be available under the auspices of the Royal Colleges of Physicians Joint Committee on Higher Medical Training (JCHMT) and the Faculty of Pharmaceutical Medicine. This will lead to a Certificate of Completion of Specialist Training (CCST-UK) in pharmaceutical medicine.

This will be a four-year programme undertaken by doctors employed as pharmaceutical physicians and will include the Diploma in Pharmaceutical Medicine, which covers the syllabus in pharmaceutical medicine (knowledge base).

It will also include seven modules of training in practical aspects of the specialty, in order to demonstrate competency to practise as a specialist. Six of the modules, at least two of which must be undertaken on-the-job in the workplace, cover Medicines Regulation, Clinical Pharmacology, Clinical Development, Drug Safety Surveillance, Statistics and Data Management, and the Healthcare Marketplace. The seventh module, which derives from the other six, will cover aspects of management and interpersonal skills relevant to the practice of pharmaceutical medicine, and must also be undertaken in the workplace.

Other courses

Any postgraduate course is not all-inclusive and participants are encouraged to extend their knowledge by personal study and the attendance at other relevant courses.

Courses are organised and run by a number of bodies, including BrAPP, the ABPI, university departments of clinical pharmacology, and a considerable number of specialist training organisations for the pharmaceutical and related industries. In addition industry encourages its doctors to attend and participate in therapeutic area symposia and congresses, which enable them to be at the forefront of the advancing knowledge in their particular area.

Another most important aspect of training is that which occurs on the job. Instruction from senior medical and technical staff within an organisation is the basis of this, each covering their area of expertise by personal instruction or small group activities. The development of management and communication skills may also be covered in this or more formally by in-house or external courses.

At a time when HMT and Specialist Certification for Pharmaceutical Medicine are scheduled for introduction in 2002/3, BrAPP has a major role in ensuring that its members' interests are represented in the development and implementation of these programmes.

British Institute of Regulatory Affairs (BIRA)

Website: www.bira.org.uk
(See also: European Society of Regulatory Affairs www.esra.org; Regulatory Affairs Professional Society www.raps.org)

The Institute covers the whole field of regulatory affairs and offers an integrated training and personal development programme for regulatory affairs professionals, devised and run by experienced professionals working in the same areas. The aim is to provide 'cradle to grave' training, and this commences with our acclaimed intro- ductory course and continues with training days and one-day training courses. The pinnacle of the education programme is the Diploma course, which leads to the Master of Science degree in Regulatory Affairs, validated by the University of Wales. Much of the training is held in an interactive setting, enabling learning and discussion to take place.

The Institute also provides management briefings to update all concerned with new and ongoing developments in regulatory affairs.

Basics of regulatory affairs

A one-day introductory course for PAs, secretaries, newcomers to regulatory affairs and allied disciplines such as marketing, project managers, etc. who require a basic knowledge of the subject.

The introductory course

This course—the original of its kind—has developed a very high reputation and has been run on over 20 occasions. It is an annual six-day intensive residential course, providing a thorough background to the major areas of knowledge required by a person entering regulatory affairs. The course exposes the participants to an unparalleled gathering of regulatory affairs knowledge. It combines over 30 formal lectures with a number of relevant case studies and participants receive a substantial handout as a reference. Objectives can be summarised as follows:

- To introduce participants to regulatory affairs, the working party and to explain the course structure.
- To achieve familiarity with basic European legislation and requirements for submission of dossiers.
- To gain knowledge of product development and of the European dossier covering aspects such as:
  o The active ingredient;
  o Pharmaceutical development;
  o Validation and stability testing;
  o Pre-clinical safety evaluation studies;
  o Clinical trial applications;
  o Detailed content and tips concerning parts II, III and IV of the dossier;
  o The post-marketing support functions of a registration department including variations, renewals, post-marketing surveillance, summary of product characteristics, labelling, advertising and patient information leaflets.
- To gain in-depth knowledge of potential routes (centralised, decentralised, national) and strategic considerations for achieving an approval covering the pros and cons of each option.
- To provide an insight into the registration of specialised products covering biotech/hi-tech products, devices and providing an insight into future changes for the requirements of a European dossier.

Originally aimed at new entrants to the profession, the course is of equal interest to persons wishing to retrain in regulatory affairs following an in-company redeployment or a change of career. It is recommended that entrants should have been working in a regulatory affairs function for at least three to six months, to gain maximum benefit.

Training days

This programme comprises a series of one-day workshops intended to provide a comprehensive grounding in theory and practice of regulatory affairs, leading on from the introductory course. However, they are also of value to experienced persons who require a refresher in particular areas. Although designed as an ongoing course to cover all aspects of regulatory affairs, it is possible to attend a single training day as each subject matter will be complete in itself. The training days make the greatest possible use of 'hands-on' experience of BIRA members and practical case studies feature prominently during the day. This series of meetings is particularly suitable for more junior regulatory affairs professionals.

Management training

New developments—legislative, technical and political—occur all the time and may well impact on the company's regulatory function. This series of meetings is designed to be organised quickly to provide delegates with information 'as it happens' along with opportunities for networking. There is usually a review meeting held towards the end of the year to assess the events of the previous year and their impact on the forthcoming one.

Biotech workshops

The BIRA Biotech Group has been formed to inform members of the regulatory issues involved in the biotechnology industry. The workshops and conferences are designed to address the scientific issues associated with the regulatory requirements and submissions for biological and biotechnologically derived pharmaceuticals throughout their development. With advances in analytical technology and the rapidly changing biotech regulatory environments, these workshops are intended to extend the ability of regulatory affairs staff both to appreciate the data they handle and to use the information appropriately in submissions.

Diploma and MSc in Regulatory Affairs

These part-time courses are designed to meet the postgraduate educational and vocational needs of personnel employed in the field of regulatory affairs in the pharmaceutical and allied industries. Four or five modules are held per academic year. Thirteen modules have been established and examples are as follows:

Module 1 Management of Regulatory Affairs and Strategic Planning
Module 2 Regulatory Strategy for a New Active Substance
Module 3 Regulatory Requirements for a New Active Substance
Module 4 Core Clinical Studies—The Regulatory Input
Module 9 Registration of Biological and Biotechnology Products
Module 11 USA—The Regulatory Environment
Module 12 Medical Device Regulatory Affairs

The Diploma and MSc are organised and operated by the British Institute of Regulatory Affairs; both are validated by the University of Wales and the qualifications are awarded by the University of Wales. To obtain the Diploma a student, who may enrol at any module, must take eight modules over a maximum period of five years and satisfy the other requirements stated in the schedule of assessment. Students wishing to study further to obtain the MSc must first successfully complete the Diploma course and then add a research-based dissertation to qualify for the MSc.

The Diploma in Regulatory Affairs was established in 1989 and has continued very successfully. The MSc in Regulatory Affairs was introduced during 1995. BIRA takes full responsibility for the operation and management of both courses. The course is fully validated and approved by the University of Wales and the Diploma and MSc qualifications are awarded by the University of Wales. The course of study and the content of each module are continually reviewed to ensure that the subjects covered are up-to-date and relevant to the needs of regulatory affairs professionals. Candidates would normally have worked in regulatory affairs for a minimum of two years and be Members or Fellows of BIRA or another equivalent professional regulatory body. They must also satisfy the requirements laid down in the University Matriculation Regulations. These state that a candidate shall have qualified for a degree of an 'approved' university or of the Council for National Academic Awards. A person who does not satisfy this requirement but is considered sufficiently well qualified and experienced to pursue the course may be admitted to candidature subject to the Regulations.

Both the Diploma and MSc courses consist of the same series of free-standing modules. Four or five modules are offered per year. The aim is to provide flexibility and choice for candidates but candidates cannot attend more than four modules per year. Students are required to attend eight modules within a minimum of two years and a maximum of five academic years. Students are also required to complete course journals, written assessments and to submit a project (of between 5000 and 10 000 words) to obtain the Diploma. To obtain the MSc, students must successfully complete the Diploma and then submit an MSc-level dissertation of 12 000–20 000 words. The MSc qualification subsumes the Diploma qualification.

Statisticians in the Pharmaceutical Industry (PSI)

Website: www.psiweb.org
(See also: European Federation of Statisticians in the Pharmaceutical Industry www.efspi.org)

PSI's many activities are generally planned, organised and implemented by its various subcommittees, which operate under the direction of the PSI Main Committee. Supported by the Executive Office, the Main Committee comprises 11 members with at least one representative from each PSI subcommittee. Main Committee meetings are held six to eight times each year. PSI aims to maintain a balance within the membership of Main Committee, in terms of areas of work activity, job role and type of company worked for, reflecting the diversity of the overall membership of PSI as far as possible.

The training subcommittee organises about three training courses each year designed specifically to bring statisticians working within the pharmaceutical industry up-to-date in a particular subject area. PSI training courses are generally of one or two days' duration, with presenters often chosen from academia. Each course provides a broad state-of-the-art overview of the topic with the main focus on application, but also with sufficient theory to clarify the concepts behind the techniques. Courses are designed to be informal, and delegate numbers are generally limited to 30 to encourage questions and discussion. In addition the training subcommittee works in collaboration with other professional groups, and runs an annual training course for statisticians new to the industry.

The training course for statisticians new to the industry, widely known as the 'Introduction to Industry Training Course', has been running since 1986. It aims to broaden the participants' knowledge and appreciation of the drug development process from discovery through to marketing. It enables participants to learn about the role and interaction of statistics with other disciplines within the industry and also allows them to meet and exchange ideas with statisticians of a similar level of experience. There are six sessions (Research, Toxicology, DM/ CROs, Clinical Trials, Pharmacy and Production, Marketing) hosted by six companies, each lasting one or two days. Each session includes talks by relevant specialists, workshops to encourage active involvement from the participants and guided tours of relevant work areas.

The scientific and conference subcommittee organises a number of one-day scientific meetings as well as joint meetings with other professional bodies each year. The topics of these meetings include statistical techniques, applications in pre-clinical and clinical trials, therapeutic areas, as well as regulatory and management issues.

British Association of Research Quality Assurance (BARQA)

Website: www.barqa.com
(See also: German QA Group www.dggf.de; US QA Association www.sqa.org)

The primary purpose of BARQA is to assist members in the understanding, interpretation and implementation of national and international regulations covering Good Laboratory Practice (GLP), Good Clinical Practice (GCP) and Good Manufacturing Practice (GMP). Since its inception the Association has grown and developed to reflect the changes taking place in regulatory requirements and government inspections, and has recognised the needs of industry by promoting an extensive training syllabus.

Professional development courses

Quality assurance training to specific, in-depth courses as listed under BARQA Professional Development Courses (www.barqa.com). There are courses to suit all levels, abilities and disciplines. Most of the courses are residential over two or three days and run twice a year. They are well established and recognised. Therefore, they are all extremely well attended by delegates from the UK and abroad.

The Good Practices Programme is a range of courses covering various aspects of regulatory good practice. There are courses relevant to those just starting out as well as those at more senior levels. Prior to every course all material is updated to reflect current regulatory changes. Each course combines lectures with workshops arming delegates with practical skills whilst extending their knowledge base.

The Auditing Skills Programme is made up of four courses that together provide full training on the role of an auditor. The tutors have a mix of personal skills experience and technical QA experience. The courses can be attended on an individual basis or in sequence.

The Personal Skills Programme is a relatively new addition that seeks to provide training in this area whilst grounding the experience in regulated research and development.

The auditing course

This course is specifically designed to develop auditing skills and to give an insight into the role of the audit programme in achieving regulatory compliance and quality improvement. The course has been designed to complement BARQA's research quality assurance courses: Research Quality Assurance for Good Laboratory Practice, Good Clinical Practice Auditing—A Practical Approach and Good Manufacturing Practice for Investigational Medicinal Products.

The course is applicable to any area of regulated research and development. It is particularly valuable where there is a quality system (e.g. GCP, GLP, GMP, ISO 9000) requirement for audit. In order to benefit from the course, personal experience of audit is essential. Benefits include improved organisation of the audit programme to maximise its contribution to quality audit planning and conduct and effectiveness in communicating audit outcomes. The course is structured to encourage delegates to discuss and develop ideas, to solve problems and to exchange information. A major feature of the course is a series of practical workshops. Working in small syndicate groups, delegates will be able to put into practice the skills learned during the lectures. Between them, the course tutors have vast experience of quality audit in the pharmaceutical, agrochemical and chemical industries under Good Laboratory, Clinical and Manufacturing Practice codes and against ISO and related quality management standards.

Regulatory compliance and computer systems

This course provides guidance on the introduction and operation of high-quality computer systems in Good Clinical, Laboratory and Manufacturing Practice regulated environments. The course is designed for quality assurance personnel, computer scientists, and those involved in the introduction and use of computer systems. Benefits include improved understanding of the interpretation and application of Good Practice regulations to computer systems, practical experience of developing documentation and procedures for the control of systems and improved audit capability. Access to an experienced panel of speakers with experience of both European and US regulatory environments is available. A major feature of the course is a practical project to reinforce the lecture material. Working in small syndicate groups the project will provide the opportunity to develop a better understanding of the requirements for regulatory compliance in relation to computer system use.

Audit analysis and report writing

Having completed the observation and recording phase of the audit and gathered all the evidence, how are findings and conclusions communicated? This course will explore principles and best practice in the analysis and reporting of audit findings through informative presentations and practical exercises. The course will develop auditor confidence and job satisfaction, give auditors the tools necessary to improve their efficiency and improve the effectiveness, focus and credibility of the audit programme.

Diploma of Credit in Research Quality Assurance

The Diploma is primarily intended for the auditor community, providing candidates who have about two years' relevant experience with a broad knowledge and understanding across non-clinical research, clinical research and the manufacture of clinical trials supplies, governed by GLP, GCP, GMP and GCP (Veterinary) in the international environment. The course is a work-based programme of self-managed study at distance. There are two three-day residential teaching sessions in Cambridge during the course. The one-year programme is fully assessed. Successful completion leads to a nationally recognised graduate qualification. The candidate gains a broader understanding of quality and quality assurance in the research and development domain. Other benefits include personal development in such areas as critical analysis, problem solving, communication, interpersonal skills, research, writing and organisation skills. The employer gains directly by the accelerated development of the professional, their enhanced skill set and breadth of learning, and vital flexibility in the dynamic work environment. They also gain through the work-based project, which each candidate has to complete.

The Master's Programme

The Master's Programme takes this professional development to a higher level and to a wider audience, including all those with responsibility for managing the quality processes which contribute to successful R&D. A flexible, work-based programme of self-managed study at distance, which can be completed within three years. It comprises compulsory core modules, options to suit particular interests and modules reflecting students' prior experience and qualifications. The focus is on industry specifics; international quality standards in scientific research and development, best practice in regulated scientific research and development, and safety and efficacy assessment. The syllabus also encompasses research techniques, quality management, international operations and general management. The programme offers candidates a unique recognition at Master's level in this rapidly developing and challenging field. For the employer, participation demonstrates an organisation's commitment to quality improvement.

PhD in Research Quality Assurance

Quality professionals wishing to undertake independent research at doctoral level. A research programme usually work-based and completed in four to five years on a part-time basis under the supervision of the Applied Sciences Research Committee of the University. Recognition at doctoral level based on the presentation of a thesis and a *viva voce* examination.

Association for Clinical Data Management (ACDM)

Website: www.acdm.org.uk
(See also: Society for Clinical Data Management, Inc. www.scdm.org)

The Association for Clinical Data Management aims to lead the development and appreciation of the essential activities of the clinical data management (CDM) profession. ACDM provides explicit settings for the membership to develop standards within the profession. We also seek to enhance the individual skills, knowledge and professional development of our members. The intent is to equip them to participate more effectively in the mainstream of drug development.

Introduction to Clinical Data Management

The longest running of all the ACDM's courses, the Introduction to Clinical Data Management was set up in 1990. There are usually three presenters, one pharmaceutical industry consultant and two experienced data managers.

Intermediate Clinical Data Management

For those with one to three years' experience in clinical data processing, these three-day courses are held two or three times per year to fill the gap between Introductory and Advanced courses. Lectures and workshops provide an appreciation of the role of statistics in clinical trial design, and an understanding of the results of statistical analyses. They provide increased understanding of the design of case report forms, and an appreciation of the different aspects of laboratory data handling with respect to clinical data management.

Advanced Clinical Data Management

An annual three-day course for ACDM members or other associated organisations, for data management professionals with at least two years' experience in clinical data processing, who are either in, or intending to pursue, a supervisory or management position. Interactive presentations, discussion groups and exercises aim to increase understanding of issues relating to a total quality concept within clinical data management, to provide an overview of the issues that should be considered in relation to clinical data management systems, and to demonstrate tools available to maximise efficiency of project co-ordination within clinical data management. Course topics include Project Management, Computerised Clinical Data Processing Systems, Data Quality Systems, Training Strategies and Interaction between the Pharmaceutical Company and the CRO.

Staying Ahead of the Game

Set up in 1995, this one-day workshop offers a participate review of current guidelines which affect the discipline of clinical data management. Three widely respected lecturers currently present it from both the pharmaceutical company and CRO sectors of the industry. Delegates are offered the opportunity to develop their own interpretation of guidelines, whilst basing such interpretations on the experience and knowledge of not only the lecturers but also the other delegates attending the workshop. The workshop focuses on potentially contentious topics taken from ICH and European GCP guidelines. These cover areas such as the use of computerised systems, the maintenance of an audit trail of database changes and corrections to CRFs. Predefined scenarios are provided to discuss such requirements in the context of our everyday jobs, set against current data management working practices within the pharmaceutical industry. The workshop also incorporates a section on the EU Data Privacy Directive and an overview of European regulatory options, including regulatory requirements to be in place before data collection activity can begin. Finally the workshop takes a look at quality management systems and techniques that can be used to improve quality.

Part-time Postgraduate Studies in Clinical Data Management

The aim of the programme is to provide a formal education leading to an academic and professional qualification for CDM personnel. Alternatively, modules for the scheme can be taken singly as short courses for training purposes. The programme provides those attending a stimulating and enjoyable opportunity to develop both as individuals and as professionals, increasing their efficiency, effectiveness, capacity and competence, and building on the skills and knowledge gained from valuable work experience. It also represents a great chance to meet others from different parts of the industry to share experiences and build up a network of friends and contacts.

The qualifications are intended to:

- Provide a known standard of professional qualification;
- Facilitate the recruitment of experienced staff;
- Enhance career opportunities within CDM.

Initial development and subsequent changes to the courses involve extensive consultation with the industry as this is a joint venture between the Association for Clinical Data Management (ACDM) and Kingston University (KU), where the courses operate within the university-wide Postgraduate Credit Framework.

Awards:

- Postgraduate Certificate in Clinical Data Management;
- Postgraduate Diploma in Clinical Data Management;
- MSc in Clinical Data Management.

Awards are gained on the successful completion of a set number of modules. The Certificate requires four core modules and the Diploma four optional modules. The MSc additionally requires a substantial research project or dissertation.

Modules are either core or optional. Most modules are three-day courses with additional individual study and assessment work, although variations in format appropriate to the topic area exist. Modules are run throughout the year. Individual modules may be taken as short courses by those interested in increasing their knowledge of a particular topic without registering for a formal qualification. Students who have successfully completed the assignments associated with the modules subsequently may apply to register for the qualification. Example modules are:

- GCP and the Regulatory Process;
- Statistical Thinking for Data Managers;
- Application of IT in CDM;
- CRF Design and Electronic Data Capture;
- Data Handling (Coding, Entry, Data Validation, Reporting);
- Quality Management and Control.

The research project or dissertation will require students to use a variety of skills including report writing, interview techniques and presentations to produce a project/dissertation of approximately 10 000 words in length. It is expected to require approximately 600 hours total effort and is equivalent to four taught modules. The subject selected by the student must be relevant to CDM and may be based on the student's current field of employment. Supervision will be undertaken by university staff and CDM experts. Applicants for the MSc should normally have a degree in a life science, mathematics or computing discipline from a British university or its equivalent. Applications will also be considered from candidates who have a degree in another area, a healthcare-related qualification or who have appropriate work experience. Candidates without previous qualifications may be required to submit written work to demonstrate an ability to attain the required standards of the course and will register for the Certificate in the first instance.

National Vocational Qualification (NVQ) in Clinical Data Management

National Vocational Qualifications are a government run scheme. The qualifications are designed to be vocational in nature. They demonstrate the candidate's ability to perform the job they are in. They therefore provide assurances in the ability of an employee to perform well. This can be of benefit in employment of new staff and audits where a company is required to provide evidence that an employee is fully qualified and trained to do the job they are doing.

NVQs are already in place for a number of different industries. There are often common elements in NVQs across different job functions. All of this ensures that an NVQ, once obtained, is recognised both within and outside the industry. If an employee moves to another industry and wishes to qualify for an NVQ in this industry, in completing an NVQ in CDM, they may find they have already completed some of the units required. The NVQ is being set up by the ACDM Clinical Data Management Qualification Working Party, with the help of the National Training Organisation for the pharmaceutical industry: the ABPI. Once set up, it will be run through an awarding body. In order to maintain the currency of the NVQ, the content will be reviewed at regular intervals and may have to be revised. There are five different NVQ levels available in the scheme. The ACDM propose to use three of these levels for the NVQ in CDM: levels 2, 3 and 4. Although the qualifications are vocational rather than academic in nature, and cannot truly be equated with academic qualifications, the following, broad equivalents will give a basic idea of the level of each qualification:

- Level 2: Data entry level personnel ($\sim$ 5 GCSEs equivalent);
- Level 3: Data manager, technical area/supervisor ($\sim$ HNC equivalent);
- Level 4: Data manager, management level (degree equivalent).

Each level will be made up of a number of units of competence. Some of these units will be compulsory, others a choice from a variety of options. Within data management, there are varied practices. In some companies, data managers may work on a variety of data management tasks. In others, they may work in specialised areas of data management. The structure of the qualification is intended to ensure that it is relevant to as many people as possible, so the core modules are general requirements, such as health and safety, using SOPs, etc., rather than specific data management-related tasks, to allow as much flexibility as possible. Anyone can start an NVQ at whichever level they feel is suitable. It may be suitable to immediately apply for level 4, for example. Alternatively, a candidate may wish to first qualify at level 2, and then add to their knowledge, moving up to further levels at a later stage.

Senior Clinical Data Managers' Forum

The ACDM Senior Clinical Data Managers' Forum is sponsored by the ACDM Training Sub-Committee. Under the guidance of this Sub-Committee, meetings are set up on a quarterly basis to share the experiences and discuss specific items of interest. Each meeting is held in London from midday and continuing into the evening. Past topics have included:

- Motivating a Composite Workforce;
- Cultural Awareness in International Teams;
- Developing and Assessing Personal Skills in Data Managers;
- Cost Effective Data Management Strategies for the Future.

Members of the forum group are required to have been working in clinical data management for a minimum of five years and have either line or project management experience.

The Association of Information Officers in the Pharmaceutical Industry (AIOPI)

Website: www.aiopi.org.uk
(See also: Drug Information Association (DIA) www.diahome.org)

The Association of Information Officers in the Pharmaceutical Industry exists to support and assist its members in the development of their professional skills and responsibilities. AIOPI is the professional organisation for individuals in the pharmaceutical industry who are involved in the provision and management of information.

MSc in Pharmaceutical Information Management

Run jointly by AIOPI and City University, this modular course covers all aspects of information management within the pharmaceutical industry and is applicable to both medical information and research information workers. This course provides postgraduate level education in pharmaceutical information management to students wanting a specialist qualification in the subject. The course is primarily, though not exclusively, designed for those engaged in pharmaceutical information work in industry or the health services. Certificate or Diploma qualifications are achieved by completing four or eight modules respectively, and a Master's degree by subsequent completion of a research project and dissertation.

The aim of the course is to enable a student to gain a good understanding of the basic principles of information science and information management, and of their relevance to pharmaceutical information systems and services, and to obtain detailed insight into some particular areas. The course should complement the practical experience gained by students in the workplace.

Information services of various kinds are fundamental to the discovery, development and use of medicines. Within the pharmaceutical industry, often regarded as the epitome of the 'information intensive' industry, research information units provide both external and internal information provision and management to discovery and development programmes, while medical information units provide in-depth information on the company's products to external doctors, pharmacists, etc., and commercial information units handle information on competitors, marketing data, etc. Additionally, information personnel are involved in activities such as records management and archiving, regulatory affairs, data administration, IT support, and many more. Within the NHS, drug information pharmacists provide information services on effective use of medicines to all healthcare professions, and are also involved in database compilation, records management, current awareness, etc. The move towards evidence-based medicine, with consequent need for evaluation and presentation of information, is of obvious importance to this group. Other sectors with a heavy reliance on the handling of pharmaceutical information and knowledge include publishing, database production, software services, and consultancy of varied kinds. The course is actively supported by three relevant professional bodies:

- Association of the British Pharmaceutical Industry (ABPI) (www.abpi.co.uk);
- UK NHS Drug Information Pharmacists Group (DIPG) (www.ukdipg.org.uk);
- Association of Information Officers in the Pharmaceutical Industry (AIOPI) (www.aiopi.org.uk).

Attaining a recognised academic qualification is becoming increasingly important for career progression in all aspects of pharmaceutical information work. This course also offers immediate practical benefits, in terms of applicable knowledge and skills, and of networking contacts with fellow students and practitioner lecturers, as well as insight into a wide range of possibilities for career development. There are already several examples of students of this course gaining promotion, or wider responsibilities, partly attributable to their training at City.

Entry qualification is generally an honours degree in any subject from a British university, or equivalent. Candidates with other qualifications—e.g. pass degree, HND, HNC, BTEC, relevant Diploma—are also admitted, providing they are engaged in pharmaceutical information work at a level appropriate for a graduate, and have additional substantial professional work experience. Although no degree subject is specified in the admission requirements, some background scientific knowledge is necessary, as would be gained from working in any pharmaceutical environment. Students should also have a good knowledge of spoken and written English. Current employment in a position involving pharmaceutical information handling is required. Exceptionally, students are admitted who are not in such employment, e.g. during a career break, providing they have had at least two years' relevant experience, with less than a two-year gap. Given the part-time nature of the course, most students are from the UK. However, the block release format permits attendance by students based elsewhere in Europe, and we particularly welcome such students.

The basic qualification is the Diploma. Successful completion of the Diploma course requires the student to successfully complete eight modules, within three years from initial registration. Students who successfully complete four modules within two years, and who do not intend to proceed to a Diploma, are eligible for the award of a Certificate. Conversion of a Diploma to a Master's degree by submission of a research-based dissertation may follow completion of the taught component.

Thirteen modules are currently offered. Pharmaceutical Information Foundation is taken initially by all students, except in exceptional circumstances, and followed by its Basic Skills distance learning component. This module runs in September each year. Modules are offered with a frequency depending on demand, subject to students always being able to complete the required number of modules within the time period required by the regulations.

Methods of teaching and learning vary according to the nature of the material being covered, and will therefore differ from module to module. In general terms there is a mix of formal lecture presentation with discussion/seminar and individual student work, allowing for exchange of experience and building on the experience and knowledge of each student. Several of the modules are led by expert practitioners, and visiting practitioner lecturers contribute to all modules, ensuring that latest developments from the world of practice are covered. Assessment is on a module-by-module basis, each module being assessed separately; there are no 'final exams'. Modules are assessed according to the nature of the material being covered, but assessment generally includes both short examinations/practical exercises/presentations during the module, and also coursework, of varied form, but generally essay-style.

Reference

Lyness, V. (2002) *Clin. Res. focus*, **13**(4), June.

Useful Information

Recruitment/Employment

Association of the British Pharmaceutical Industry, Health Industry Information Officer, ABPI, 12 Whitehall, London SW1A 2DY, UK
Tel: +44 (0)20 7930 3477; Fax: +44 (0)20 7747 1411; Web: www.abpi.org.uk

AXESS Limited, Parkshot House, 5 Kew Road, Richmond, Surrey TW9 2PR, UK
Tel: +44 (0)20 8560 2300; Fax: +44 (0)20 8560 2033
Email: info@axess.co.uk; Web: www.axess.co.uk

Eames Jones Judge Hawkings, 29 High Street, Welwyn, Hertfordshire AL6 0EE, UK
Tel: +44 (0)1438 840 984; Fax: +44 (0)1438 840 429
Email: partners@ejjh.co.uk

Euromedica plc, Enterprise House, Vision Park, Histon, Cambridge CB4 9ZR, UK
Tel: +44 (0) 1223 235333; Fax: +44 (0) 1223 235305; Web: www.euromedica.com

Recruitment and Employment Confederation (REC), 36–38 Mortimer Street, London W1W 7RG, UK
Tel: +44 (0)20 7462 3260; Fax: +44 (0)20 7255 2878; Web: www.rec.uk.com

RSA Search and Selection, The Melon Ground, Hatfield Park, Hatfield, Hertfordshire AL9 5NB, UK
Tel: +44 (0)1707 259 333; Fax: +44 (0)1707 271366
Email: service@pharmarecruit.com; Web: www.pharmarecruit.com

Talentmark Search and Selection, King House,
5–11 Westbourne Grove, London W2 4UA, UK
Tel: +44 (0)20 7229 2266; Fax: +44 (0)20 7229 3549
Web: www.talentmark.net

Professional & Educational

Association for Clinical Data Management (ACDM), PO Box 129, Macclesfield, Cheshire SK11 8FG, UK
Tel: +44 (0)1625 511 818; Fax: +44 (0)1625 511 750
Email: admin@acdm.org.uk; Web: www.acdm.org.uk

Association of Clinical Research Professionals (ACRP),
Global Headquarters, 500 Montgomery Street, Suite 800, Alexandria, VA 23314, USA
Tel: +1 703 254 8100; Fax: +1 703 254 8101
Email: office@acrpnet.org; Web: www.acrpnet.org

Careers with the Pharmaceutical Industry, Second edition. Edited by P. D. Stonier.
© 2003 John Wiley & Sons Ltd. ISBN 0 470 84328 4

European Office, Fountain Court, 2 Victoria Square, St Albans, Hertfordshire AL1 3TF, UK
Tel: +44 (0) 1727 884 884; Fax: +44 (0) 1727 884 800
Email: EURoffice@acrpnet.org

Association of Independent Clinical Research Contractors (AICRC), PO Box 1055, Oadby, Leicester LE2 4X2, UK
Tel: +44 116 271 9727; Fax: +44 116 271 3155
Web: www.aicrc.org.uk

British Association for Research Quality Assurance (BARQA), 3 Wherry Lane, Ipswich IP4 1LG, UK
Tel: +44 (0)1473 221 411; Fax: +44 (0)1473 221 412
Email: info@barqa.com; Web: www.barqa.com

British Association of Pharmaceutical Physicians (BrAPP), Royal Station Court, Station Road, Twyford, Reading RG10 9NF, UK
Tel: +44 (0)118 934 1943; Fax: +44 (0)118 932 0981
Web: www.brapp.org

British Institute of Regulatory Affairs (BIRA), 7 Heron Quays, Marsh Wall, London E14 4JB, UK
Tel: +44 (0)207 538 9502; Fax: +44 (0)207 515 7836
Web: www.bira.org.uk

Clinical Research Nurses Association (CRNA), Department of Neurology, 6th Floor Queen Mary Wing, National Hospital for Neurology and Neurosurgery, Queen Square, London WC1N 3BG, UK
Tel: +44 (0)207 837 3611; Fax: +44 (0)207 676 2044
Web: www.man.ac.uk/rcn/ukwide/crna

European Medical Writers Association (EMWA), Association Head Office, 40–44 High Street, Northwood, Middlesex HA6 143, UK
Web: www.emwa.org

European Society of Regulatory Affairs (ESRA), 7 Heron Quays, Marsh Wall, London E14 4JB, UK
Tel: +44 (0)207 515 7673; Fax: +44 (0)207 515 7836
Web: www.esra.org

Faculty of Pharmaceutical Medicine, 1 St Andrews Place, Regents Place, London NW1 4LB, UK
Tel: +44 (0)207 224 0343; Fax: +44 (0)207 224 5381
Email: fpm@f-pharm-med.org.uk; Web: www.fpm.org.uk

Institute of Clinical Research (ICR), PO Box 1208, Maidenhead, Berkshire SL6 3GD, UK
Tel: +44 (0)1628 829900; Fax: +44 (0)1628 829922
E-mail: info@instituteofclinicalresearch.org; Web: http://www.instituteofclinicalresearch.org

International Federation of Associations of Pharmaceutical Physicians (IFAPP), Rendementsweg 24 E-1, 3641 SL Mijdrecht, The Netherlands
Tel: +31 297 285 144; Fax: +31 297 256 046
Email: ifapp@plante.nl; Web: www.ifapp.org

Royal College of Nursing (RCN), 20 Cavendish Square, London W1G 0RN, UK
Tel: +44 (0)845 772 6100
Web: www.rcn.org.uk

Royal Society of Medicine (RSM); 1 Wimpole Street, London W1G 0AE, UK
Tel: +44 (0)207 290 2900
Email: sections@rsm.ac.uk
    memberships@rsm.ac.uk
Web: www.roysocmed.ac.uk

Royal Statistical Society (RSS), 12 Errol Street, London EC1Y 8LX, UK
Tel: +44 (0)20 7638 8998; Fax: +44 (0)20 7256 7598
Email: rss@rss.org.uk; Web: www.rss.org.uk

Statisticians in the Pharmaceutical Industry (PSI), PSI Executive Office, Resources for Business, South Park Road, Macclesfield SK11 6SH, UK
Tel: +44 (0)1625 511 750; Fax: +44 (0)1625 267 879
Email: admin@psiweb.org; Web: www.psiweb.org

The Association for Information Officers in the Pharmaceutical Industry (AIOPI), PO Box 297, Slough PDO, SL1 7XT, UK
Email: aiopi@aiopi.org.uk; Web: www.aiopi.org.uk

Regulatory

European Agency for the Evaluation of Medicinal Products (EMEA), Eudranet Helpdesk, 7 Westferry Circus, Canary Wharf, London E14 4HB, UK
Tel: +44 (20)27 18 84 00; Fax: +44 (20)74 18 84 16
Email: mail@emea.eu.int; Web: www.eudra.org

Medicines Control Agency (MCA), Market Towers, 1 Nine Elms Lane, Vauxhall, London SW8 5NQ, UK
Tel: +44 (0)207 273 0000; Fax: +44 (0)207 273 0353
Email: info@mca.gsi.gov.uk; Web: www.mca.gov.uk

Miscellaneous/General Industry

Drug Information Association (DIA), Europe DIA, Postfach 4012, Basel, Switzerland
Tel: +41 61 386 9393; Fax: +41 61 386 9390
Email: diaeurope@diaeurope.org; Web: www.diahome.org

European Federation of Pharmaceutical Industry Associations (EFPIA), Rue du Trône 108, B-1050 Brussels, Belgium
Tel: +32 (0)2 626 2555; Fax: +32 (0)2 626 2566
Email: info@efpia.org; Web: www.efpia.org

InPharm, First House, Park Road, Guildford, Surrey GU1 4XB, UK
Tel: +44 (0)1483 515 311
Email: info@inpharm.com; Web: www.inpharm.com

Pharmafile, First House, Park Road, Guildford, Surrey GU1 4XB, UK
Tel: +44 (0)1483 515 300; Fax: +44 (0)1483 515 301
Email: publishing@pharmafile.co.uk; Web: www.pharmafile.com

PharmiWeb, Abbey House, Grenville Place, Bracknell, Berkshire RG12 1BP, UK
Tel: +44 (0)1344 667 433; Fax: +44 (0)1344 667 434
Email: frontdesk@pharmiweb.com; Web: www.pharmiweb.com

Index

Note: Page numbers in *italics* refer to figures; page numbers in **bold** refer to tables; 'n' after a page number signifies a footnote.

ABPI, *see* Association for the British Pharmaceutical Industry
absorption, distribution, metabolism, elimination (ADME) 179, 184
academic clinical pharmacology, contribution to medicines research 17–25
Academic Specialty in Pharmaceutical Medicine, Complutense University of Madrid, Spain 13
ACDM, *see* Association for Clinical Data Management
acebutolol, acetyl metabolite of 21
N-acetyl-transferase, activity of 22
Aconitum sp. 178
ACRP, *see* Association of Clinical Research Professionals
ACRPI, *see* Association for Clinical Research in the Pharmaceutical Industry
Adair, J. 146
ADME, *see* absorption, distribution, metabolism, elimination
adrenalin, introduction of 4
8-adrenoceptor antagonists 22
ADRs, *see* adverse drug reactions
Advanced Monitoring Skills, ICR course 73
adverse drug reactions (ADRs) 180–181, 213, 215, 228, 256, 259
pharmacists as monitors of 160
adverse events (AEs) 91, 104, 165, 195
advertising 89, 140, 211
law, and the 257
Advertising Directive, EC 257
AEs, *see* adverse events
Africa 205
agrochemicals 161, 185
AIDS 30

AIOPI, *see* Association of Information Officers in the Pharmaceutical Industry
albumin, diminished synthetic ability for 22
American Medical Writers Association (AMWA) 12, 243
training by 243
amiloride 21
AMWA, *see* American Medical Writers Association
anaesthetics 48, 63, 181
analgesics 21
analyst 72, 85
analytical chemistry 40
analytical chemists 157
Anderson, S. 159
angina pectoris 18–19
animal metabolism 158
animal models, knockout mouse 37
animal technicians, veterinary supervision of 180
animal welfare and husbandry 180–181
anti-asthma drugs 33
antianginal effects 18
antibiotics 5, 14, 70
antihistamines, non-sedative 24
antihypertensives 19
APIL, *see* Association of Personal Injury Lawyers
applicable regulatory requirement(s) 188
Applied Pharmacology and Therapeutics, CCR module 321
appraisal
annual 145
personal development, and 314–318
archiving 86, 91, 169
arthritis 21
ASA Committee on Training of Statisticians for Industry 107
Asia 272

assessment 248
centre 131
assessors, MCA 248
assistant brand manager 131
assistant medical director 62
associate medical director 62
Association for Clinical Data Management (ACDM) 116, 331–335
Advanced Clinical Data Management Course 330
topics for 330
CDM Qualification Working Party 332
Intermediate Clinical Data Management Course 330
Introduction to Clinical Data Management Course 330
National Vocational Qualification (NVQ) in CDM 332–333
level of qualification 333
Part-time Postgraduate Studies in CDM 331–332
modules for 332
MSc in CDM 331
Postgraduate Certificate in CDM 331
Postgraduate Diploma in CDM 331
requirements for 332
Senior Clinical Data Managers' Forum 333
topics for 333
Staying Ahead of the Game Workshop 330–331
Training Subcommittee 333
website 12, 337
Association for Clinical Research in the Pharmaceutical Industry (ACRPI), UK 68, 87
journal 75
website 12
Association for Victims of Medical Accidents (AVMA) 26

Careers with the Pharmaceutical Industry, Second edition. Edited by P. D. Stonier.
© 2003 John Wiley & Sons Ltd. ISBN 0 470 84328 4

Association of Clinical Data
   Management (ACDM) 301
   website 12
Association of Clinical Research
   Professionals (ACRP),
   USA 68, 77, 97, 318
   website 318
Association of Clinical Research,
   USA 12
   website 12
Association of Information Officers
   in the Pharmaceutical Industry
   (AIOPI) 12, 224, 231, 334–335
   Certificate 335
   Diploma 335
      modules for 335–336
   MSc in Pharmaceutical
      Information Management
      334–336
   Postgraduate Diploma/MSc in
      Pharmaceutical
      Information Management
      231
   Postgraduate Diploma/MSc in
      Pharmacovigilance 231
   Specialist Interest Group for
      Adverse Reactions 231
   website 12, 334–335
Association of Personal Injury
   Lawyers (APIL) 264
Association of the British
   Pharmaceutical Industry
   (ABPI) 75, 160–161, 224, 278,
   321, 335, 337
   Joint Advisory Committee 320
   Medical Representative's
      Examination 139
   website 76, 335
astemizole 24
atenolol 18, 22
audit/auditing 8, 86, 112, 188
   certificate 188
   conduction of 195–196
   focus on 199–200
   growth area of 211
   report 188
   systems 195, 198
      examples of 195
   trail 188
   trial specific 195
auditors 12, 71, 91, 94, 194
   career pathways 200–201
   education and qualifications
      of 196
   continuing 198–199
   interactions of 197
   knowledge base, skills and
      competences of 196
   linguistic abilities of 196
   personal attributes of 197
   training 198, 200–201
      continuing 198–199
      focus on 200
Australia 204, 241, 248, 262,
   270

Australian Pharmaceutical Benefits
   Scheme 270
automated mass spectrometry 39
Autonomous University of
   Barcelona, Spain, Postgraduate
   Diploma in Pharmaceutical
   Medicine 13
autoradiography 41
AVMA, see Association for Victims
   of Medical Accidents

B-TECH 113
BARQA, see British Association of
   Research Quality Assurance
Bayesian methods 109
Belgium 13
bendrofluazide 17
benoxaprofen 19
   hazards of 21
benoxyprofen 6
   hepatic side-effects 6
benzodiazepines 19, 23
   elderly and 21
   hangover effects of 21
   legal claim involving 261, 263
   physicians as defendants,
      and 261
benzothiadiazine (thiazide)
   diuretics 17–18
beta-blockers 33
biochemistry 61, 94, 151, 207
biochemists 37–38, 40–41, 43
bioinformatics 34
biologists 38, 40–41, 50
   discovery 102
   pre-clinical 48
biology 37–38, 155
biomarkers 104
biostatisticians 99
biotechnology 253
   companies 42, 62, 236, 285
   emergence of 29
   products 207
BIRA, see British Institute of
   Regulatory Affairs
blood 207
   products, legal claim
      involving 261
   tests 24
BMedSci, pharmacology 47
Bohaychuk, W. 201
Bolvidon 258
Bradford Hill, Sir A. 4
bradycardia 22
brand
   management, career in 129–136
   manager 129–130
      assistant 131
   career of 131–132
      progression 135–136
   'fit' in organisation 135
   key personal attributes 130
   role of 132–135
   strategy, market aligned 132
   team 132, 135

leader 135, 136
   'virtual' 134
   value 130, 133
branding 130
   introduction of 5
BrAPP, see British Association of
   Pharmaceutical Physicians
British Association of
   Pharmaceutical Physicians
   (BrAPP) 11, 278, 321, 338
   courses with other bodies 321–
      322
   essential registration 320–321
   Joint Advisory Committee 320
   meetings 320
   Postgraduate Training Course in
      Pharmaceutical
      Medicine 320
   website 320
   workshops 320
British Association of Research
   Quality Assurance
   (BARQA) 12
   Audit Analysis and Report
      Writing Course 328
   Auditing Course 327
   Diploma of Credit in Research
      Quality Assurance 328–330
   Master's Programme 330
   PhD in Research Quality
      Assurance 330
   Professional Development
      courses 327
      Auditing Skills
         Programme 327
      Good Practices
         Programme 327
      Personal Skills
         Programme 327
   Regulatory Compliance and
      Computer Systems
      Course 328
   Research Quality Assurance
      courses 327
      Good Clinical Practice
         Auditing A Practical
         Approach 327
      Good Manufacturing
         Practice for Investi-
         gational Medicinal
         Products 327
      Research Quality Assurance
         for Good Laboratory
         Practice 327
   website 12, 326–327
British Institute of Regulatory
   Affairs (BIRA) 11, 12, 205,
   322–325
   Basics of Regulatory Affairs
      course 322
   Biotech Group workshops 324
   Diploma course 322, 324–325
      modules for 324
      requirements for 325
   Regulatory Affairs, in 208

fellowship of 325
introductory course 208, 322–323
objectives of 323
management training 324
Master of Science (Regulatory Affairs) 322, 324–325
modules for 324
requirements for 325
membership of 325
training days 323–324
website 12, 322
British Pharmacopoeia 4–5
Brown, C. 6
BSc 70, 73, 321
BTEC 335
bufuralol, nausea and vomiting due to 22
burden of disease studies 271–272
Burley, D. 6
business
development 43
information 133
management 86
philosophy 130
buying signal 140

caffeine 23
Calcis Consultants, training by 73
calcium channel blocking drugs 19, 23
Cambridge, UK 330
Canada 204
cancer 30
treatment 272
Cancer Act (1930) 5
candidate compounds 179
captopril 18
carbamazepine 23
carcinogenic potential 179
carcinogenic testing 181–182
carcinogenicity studies 183
cardiac arrhythmias, dosage titration in control of 19
Cardiff University, UK, continuing education courses at 74
cardiovascular medicine, drugs in 19
career development 11–14, 41–43
aims and objectives, definition of 303–304
'Book of My Life' 302–303, 305
CRAs, for 74–75
data management, in 115–116
defining self as product 302–303
field-based opportunities for 74
leading on from discovery 42–43
outside the organisation 305–306
pharmaceuticals, in 301–306
within research 41–42
within the organisation 304–305
working process for 302
career planning 289–300
career progression 287–336

carers
bodies supporting 130
groups 134
Case Record Form (CRF) 69–70, 331
design 113, 112
electronic data capture, and ACDM course module in 332
Case Report Form (CRF) 81, 85, 90–91, 99, 195
transmission 90
CCR, *see* Clinical Research Development
Certificate of Professional Development
CCST-UK, *see* Faculty of Pharmaceutical Medicine, Certificate of Completion of Specialist Training
CCST-UK, *see* Royal Colleges of Physicians, Certificate of Completion of Specialist Training
CD-ROMS 240
CDM, *see* Clinical Data Management
cell biologists 37–38, 40
central nervous system (CNS), drugs in 19
cephalosporins 33
Certificate in Clinical Research 94
Certificate of Completion of Specialist Training (CCST-UK) 54, 321
modules for 323
Certificate of Professional Development 86
John Moore's University, Liverpool, UK 13
certificates of credit 199
Chartered Institute of Marketing 129
Diploma in Marketing 131
Chemical Industries Association (CIA) 161
chemical weapons 178
chemistry 151, 155, 204
computational 34
high throughput 31
chemists 38, 40–43, 48
analytical 43
computational 41
discovery 102
high-throughput 41
organic 36, 41
physical 41, 43
chemophobia 183
chief pharmacists 142, 153
chlorthalidone 17
chlorzoxazone 23
CIA, *see* Chemical Industries Association
ciclosporin 23–24
cimetidine 23
citrus juices, interaction with 23

City University, London, UK 334–335
Diploma in Information Management 13
MSc in Pharmaceutical Information Management 334–336
requirements for 335
Postgraduate Diploma/MSc in Pharmaceutical Information Management 231
civil servants 248
clinic nurse 87
clinical audit facilitator 171
clinical audits, nurses 163, 168, 171–173
clinical data coordinator/manager 113
Clinical Data Management (CDM) 329, 331–332
clinical development 133
clinical document scientist 241
clinical endpoints 104, 109
clinical experience, importance of 63
clinical governance 152, 174
committees 152
community pharmacy, and 152
defined 152
Clinical Laboratory Investigations, CCR module 319
clinical liaison 140
teams 131
clinical pharmacologists 21, 99, 157
career development 53
personal attributes and roles of 48–53
coordination role in Phase I 51
management responsibilities 52–53
multi-tasking and time management 52
regulatory activities 51
research and discovery 48
qualifications of 47–48
role of 8, 17
training and continuing education 54
transferable skills 50–51
clinical pharmacology 9, 31, 75
career in 47–54
certificate module, as 321
commercial support 50
defined 47
exploratory 48–49
infrastructure 52
management responsibilities 52–53
personal attributes and roles in 48–53
exploratory 48–49
research and discovery 48

clinical pharmacology (*cont.*)
    Phase I studies 49
    discontinuation of 49
    regulatory 50
    training 63
Clinical Project Assistant
    (CPA) 80, 86
    CRA trainee role 80
Clinical Quality Assurance (CQA)
    auditors, qualification and skill
        of 196
    career in 187–200
        pathways 200–201
    education of auditors 196
        continuing 198–199
    interactions 197
    knowledge base of auditors 196
    management 200–201
    personal attributes
        required 197
    personnel, responsibilities
        of 194–196
        conducting audits 195
        managing SOPs 194
        training and consulting 196
    role and responsibility of 193–
        194
        expanding 199–200
    skills and competences of
        auditors 196
    training 198, 200–201
        continuing 198–199
        focus on 200
clinical research 40, 103–105, 112,
    116, 220–221, 225, 244
    careers in 45–126
    ethical issues, and 259–260
    head of 117
    key roles in 79–95
    postgraduate courses in 13
    quality requirements in 190–192
    scientists 238
Clinical Research Associate
    (CRA) 67–76, 79–80, 86, 90–
    91, 94, 163, 168–171, 196, 200,
    295, 318
    background to post 67–68
    career path, development and
        opportunities 74–75, 169–
        170
    challenges 75
    education and
        qualifications 69–70
        background reading 71
        continuing 73–74
    freelance 75
    head 85
    in CROs 123
    interactions 71–72
    interpersonal skills 71
    job description 68–69
    knowledge base, skills,
        competencies 67, 70–71
    personality attributes 72–73, 170
    pharmacists as 160

    role and responsibilities 168–169
        skills required 170
    team 85
    training and qualifications 73,
        170–171
Clinical Research Certificate of
    Professional Development
    (CCR) 320
    modules for 320
clinical research coordinator 68, 88
Clinical Research Executive
    (CRE) 68
Clinical Research Focus 74
    (*CRfocus*) 74
Clinical Research for All 68
Clinical Research Manager (CRM)
    68, 74, 72–73
clinical research monitor 68
Clinical Research Nurse (CRN) 87,
    163–168, 174
    career path 165–167
    conflict of interest 165
    employment brief 164
    network for 167
    personality attributes of 167
    portfolio 168
    role and responsibilities 164–
        165
        skills required 166
    training and qualifications 167–
        168
    unit nurse 165
clinical research physicians 157
Clinical Research Scientist (CRS)
    68
clinical research skills 93
clinical research staff 12
clinical research standards, global
    79
clinical research unit nurse 165
clinical resource nurse 171
clinical studies
    marketing oriented 58
    physicians, and 57
Clinical Therapeutic Trials (CTTs)
    163–164, 167–169
    skills required 164
clinical toxicology 185
Clinical Trial Certificate
    Exemptions (CTXs) 278
clinical trial coordinator 88
Clinical Trial Management and
    Organisation, CCR
    module 320
Clinical Trial Management, ICR
    event 93
clinical trial officer 88
Clinical Trial Practice the Industry
    Benchmark, ICR event 93
clinical trial practices 86
clinical trial supplies 158–159
    pharmacist 72, 85
Clinical Trials Administrator
    (CTA) 79–87, 70, 72, 90, 94
    background reading 84

career development and
    opportunities 86–87
    centrality within project 83–85
    education and
        qualifications 83–84
        continuing 85
    interactions 84–85
    job description 81–83
    knowledge base, skills,
        competencies 84
    personality attributes 85
    role and responsibility 79, 81
    training 84, 85–86
Clinical Trials Administrator
    Forum 86
Clinical Trials Directive 79–80
clinical trials, execution of 94
clinical trials, multi centre,
    multinational 169
Clinical Trials, PSI course on 326
clinicians 113
    difficult 71
clinics 153
close-out visit 91
closing 140
    on brand or product 137
CME, *see* Continuing Medical
    Education
coaching 115, 139, 314
Code of Practice Authority 278
collagen vascular disease 18
commercial directors, pharmacists
    as 160
commercial liaison, physicians
    and 61
commercial trainee scheme, fast-
    track 131
Commission for Health
    Improvement 130
Committee for Proprietary
    Medicinal Products
    (CPMP) 249–250, 257–258
    Good Clinical Practice
        Guidelines 260
    Notice to Applicants and
        Guidelines 257
    working parties of 250
Committee on Safety of Medicines
    (CSM) 25, 248–249
Common Technical Document
    (CTD) 8, 206, 212
communication 83, 166
    skills 235
    regulatory affairs, and 207
    nurses 167
    verbal and non-verbal 167
    written and oral 94
communications agencies
    medical writers, and 235, 239–
        241, 243–244
    specialist 134
communications manager 244
community pharmacist 151
    prescribers, and 152
    professional colleagues, and 152

stock control 152
training 152
wholesale purchasing 152
community pharmacy 151–153
clinical governance, and 152
compassionate-use studies 102
compensation for injury 260
Compensation Guidelines, ABPI 260
competitor analysis 132
competitor awareness 134
compliance 24, 188
estimation of 24
forms of 24
Complutense University of Madrid, Spain, Academic Specialty in Pharmaceutical Medicine 13
computer literacy, need for 113
computerisation and data management, advances in 117
Computerised Clinical Data Processing Systems, ACDM course topic, as 330
computers, physicians and 61
confidentiality, issues of 93, 119, 180
Conium maculatum 178
consent
documents 89
procedures 180
consultancy 25, 154
business plan 279
characteristics and qualities for success 280–281
areas of expertise 280–281
networks 280
resourcefulness 281
work ethic 281
default option, as a 277
mission statement 279
pitfalls and minefields 283–285
buffers 284
conflict of interest 285
operation size 283–284
speaking 284–285
planning for 277–280
product characteristics 277–278
resources 278–280
reasons for going into 275–277
benefits of 276–277
risks of 276
statistical 107–108
types of work 281–283
bridging a gap 283
experience, gaps in 282
expertise, gaps in 282–283
head count, gaps in 282
consultants 120, 144
pharmaceutical medicine, in 275–285
Consumer Protection Act, UK (1987) 264
contingency fees 265
continuing education 73–74

Continuing Medical Education (CME) 219, 252, 316, 320
registration, and 219
Continuing Professional Development (CPD) 219, 252, 309–310, 313, 316
contract laboratory services 82
Contract Research Organisations (CROs) 9, 51, 53, 67, 88, 119–124, 163, 187, 197, 251, 275, 291
ambiguity in 122
career pathways in 123–124
current guideline review 330
education and qualifications required by 121–123
skills and personal attributes 122–123
medical writers, and 235–236, 241, 243
project costing and 120
regulatory affairs, and 205, 210
roles and responsibilities in 120
staffing levels of 120
training in 123
transfer fees levied by 124
working in 119–124
Contract Sales Organisations (CSOs) 138–139
contrast media, legal claim involving 261
Control of Substances Hazardous to Health (COSHH) 211
core technologies 34
Coronary Heart Disease (CHD) 268
corporate affairs 221
corporate appraisal process 131
corporate planning 211
COSHH, *see* Control of Substances Hazardous to Health
cosmetics 185
cost-effectiveness 80, 270
counselling 115
CPA, *see* Clinical Project Assistant
CPD, *see* Continuing Professional Development
CPMP, *see* Committee for Proprietary Medicinal Products
CQA, *see* Clinical Quality Assurance
CRA, *see* Clinical Research Associate
CRE, *see* Clinical Research Executive
CRF, *see* Case Record Form; Case Report Form
CRfocus 290
criminal sanctions 256
CRM, *see* Clinical Research Manager
CRN, *see* Clinical Research Nurse
CROs, *see* Contract Research Organisations
CRS, *see* Clinical Research Scientist

CSM, *see* Committee on Safety of Medicines
CSOs, *see* Contract Sales Organisations
CTA, *see* Clinical Trials Administrator
CTD, *see* Common Technical Document
CTTs, *see* Clinical Therapeutic Trials
CTXs, *see* Clinical Trial Certificate Exemptions
curriculum vitae 292–296, 302, 310–311
content 293–294
covering letter 295–296
presentation 295
structure 293
training, and 310
cyclopenthiazide 17
cytochrome isoenzymes
CYP1A2 23
CYP2B6 23
CYP2C 23
CYP2D6 22–23
CYP2E1 23
CYP3A 23
CYP3A4 23
P450 (CYP2D6) 22–24, 49
inhibitors of 23
substrates for 23
cytotoxic drugs 165

Daily Telegraph 139
Dangerous Drugs Act (1930) 5
Danol 152
Daonil 152
data analysis, practical issues 104
data analyst 115
data cleaning 122
data coordinator 115
data entry clerk 113
Data Handling, ACDM course module in 334
data inspection 7–8
data management 39, 291
careers in 111–117
development 115–116
range of 112–115
certificate module, as 323
director/head of 113–115 (*114*)
functions of 111–112
data processing and analysis 112
design 112
project management 112
review 111–112
future of 116–117
postgraduate courses in 13
reporting structure in *114*
team 72, 85
training 115
data managers 12, 50, 69, 108, 196, 200, 295
data monitor 115

data processing and analysis 112
Data Protection Act, UK 290
Data Quality Systems, as ACDM
   course topic 330
data streams, management of 117
databases 90, 116
   clinical study 113
   design of 112
   systems 84
debrisoquine 23
   4-hydroxylation of 22
   orthostatic hypotension, and
      22
degrees 337
   biochemistry 228
   biological 184
   biomedical 241
   honours science 319
   life science 113, 228
   medical 92
   pharmacology 228
   pharmacy 207
   physiology 228
   science 91
delegation 92–93, 115
Denmark 270
dentists 152
Department of Health, UK 152,
      177n, 248, 258
   Ethics Committee Guidelines
      260
   notices 257
   pharmaceutical medicine as
      listed specialty 321
Department of Regulatory
   Affairs 205
desk-top publishing 113
Developing New Brands 129
development 120–121
   medicines 1–44
development director 62
diabetes 268
diagnostic companies 62
DIBT, see Diploma of the Institute
   of Biology
Dictionary of Drug Development
   68
diethylene glycol 5
digoxin 155
dihydropyridine 19
Dip Pharm Med 54
DIPG, see NHS Drug Information
   Pharmacists Group
diplomacy 71
Diplomas 335
   East Anglia Polytechnic
      University, UK 13
   Information Management,
      City University, London,
      UK 13
   Institute of Biology (DIBT), UK
      184
   Marketing 131–132
   Pharmaceutical Information
      Management 229, 231

Pharmaceutical Medicine 11,
      63, 252–253
   University of Wales Institute
      of Science and
      Technology, UK 13
   Pharmacoepidemiology 252
   Regulatory Affairs 208
   University of Wales, UK 13
directors 132
   assistant/associate 62
   medical 62
discovery research, entry
   requirements for 40–41
Distillers 6
District Pharmaceutical Managers
   153
diuretics 17–18
DM/CROs, PSI course on 328
DNA
   cloning 34, 38
   damage 182–183
   sequencing 34
doctors 70, 91, 130, 138, 140, 179,
      320
   hospital 152–153
   qualified in pathology 179
documentation 89
   management 200
dogs 179
L-dopa 21
dosages 153
   form 157
dose–response relationships
   studies on 17–19
dose level 157
dose range 159
Drug Information Association
   (DIA) 14, 334, 339
   website 336
Drug Safety Executive 215
Drug Safety Physician 215–216, 220
drug(s)
   absorption 39, 159
   accountability and laboratory
      90–91
   action, assessment 103
   administration 165
   alternative 30
   availability 157
   bioavailability 157
   committees 226
   delivery 153
   design 30
   development 32–33
      contracting out of 34
      cost and complexity of 8–9
      dangers of isolation from
         discovery 34
      key ingredients 33
      management of 33–35
      statisticians in 102–105
   discovery 31–32, 102
      career in 29–43
      dangers of isolation from
         development 34

innovative working climate,
      and 31
   management of 33–35
   process of 35–40
   target identification 36–37
distribution 39, 159
driving, and 250
effects, duration of 154
elimination 39, 159
inactivity 64
information services 60
   Association 14, 334, 339
   director 62
   physicians, and 60
pharmacist 142
interactions 50
   studies of 23–24
licensing 9
metabolism 39, 41, 43
   pre-systemic 19
new 144
   analytical development of 153
pharmacokinetics/dynamics
      157
reconstitution 165
registration 203
regulation 58
regulatory affairs 60
   physicians, and 60
regulatory authority 53
safety 74, 225, 232
   assessment 52
   careers in 213–222
   certificate module, as 321
   executive 215
   officer 94
   physician 215–216, 220
safety monitors 174
   nurses as 163, 168
shelf life 157
stability 155
supply 165
targeting 154
therapy 270
toxicity 64
trials, early 5
withdrawals 213

e-mail 289
East Anglia Polytechnic University,
      UK
   Diploma 13
   MSc 13
eClinical processes, future
   adoption of 111, 117
economics 268
ecotoxicologists 180
ecotoxicology 185
EDC, see Electronic Data Capture
editorial executive/assistant 241
education and training 11–14, 61
   pharmaceutical industry, in the
      309–336
   pharmaceutical physicians, for
      321

physicians, and 61
professional bodies, by 319–336
programmes 135
efficacy 270
EFSPI, see European Federation of
Statisticians in the
Pharmaceutical Industry
elderly
adrenoceptor sensitivity, change
in 20
baroreceptor function, decline
in 20
care of 142
non-steroid anti-inflammatory
drugs and 21
sleep disturbances in 21
Electronic Data Capture
(EDC) 111
electronic data submission, growth
area of 211
Electronic Systems for Transmission
of Regulatory Information
(ESTRI) 8
gateways 8
Electronic Territory Management
Systems (ETMS) 141
electrophysiologists 40
electrostatic potential 38
EMEA, see European Medicines
Evaluation Agency
EMWA, see European Medical
Writers Association
End of Marketing as We Know It,
The 130
England 260–262, 270
courts 258
Law Society 264
enzyme inhibitors, angiotensin-
converting 18
enzymologists 41
epidemiology 60, 261, 266
physicians, and 60
epileptics 23
Eraldin 260
erythromycin 23–24
Escherichia coli 38
ESRA, see European Society of
Regulatory Affairs
ESTRI, see Electronic Systems for
Transmission of Regulatory
Information
ethics 25, 51, 93, 171, 180
committees 69, 158, 260
guidelines for 192, 260
issues of, clinical research and
259–260
problems of 255
regulations and 140
standards of 166
Ethics and Regulation, CCR
module 319
Ethics and Regulations, ICR
event 93
ETMS, see Electronic Territory
Management Systems

Europe 4–6, 8–9, 11, 43, 68, 75, 94,
116, 120, 124, 130, 204–206,
211–212, 225, 243, 248–249,
252, 255–256, 266, 271–272,
278, 319, 329, 335
controls in 256
European Clinical Trials
Directive 69, 159, 171
European Community 253, 258
Commission 281
directives 171, 256–258
legislation 255, 257–258
licensing 256
European Course in Pharmaceutical
Medicine, University of Basel,
Switzerland 13
European Diploma in
Pharmaceutical Medicine
(EUDIPHARM), University of
Lyon, France 13
European Federation for Good
Clinical Practice 12
European Federation of Statisti-
cians in the Pharmaceutical
Industry (EFSPI) 100
website 327
European GCP guidelines 332
European law 259
provisions of 258
European legislation 228, 325
European licensing system 253
European Medical Writers
Association (EMWA) 12, 243
training by 243
European Medicines Evaluation
Agency (EMEA) 212, 248–250
European regulatory options 333
European Society of Regulatory
Affairs (ESRA) 12, 205, 322
introductory courses 208
website 324
European Union (EU) 79–80, 99–
100, 155, 192
GCP guideline 192
Data Privacy Directive 331
Excel 241

Faculty of Pharmaceutical
Medicine 11, 63, 252, 278,
300, 320–321, 338
Certificate of Completion of
Specialist Training (CCST-
UK) 321
modules for 321
Diploma 321
Higher Medical Training
Programme 321
Specialist Certification for
Pharmaceutical
Medicine 322
website 320
failure to research 265
failure to warn 265
learned intermediaries, and
265–266

Far East 205
FDA, see Food and Drug
Administration
felodipine 23
field visits, sales 134
field-based nurses 169, 171
finance 61
department 72
fine chemicals 161
Finland 270
First Steps to Management, ICR
course 73
fixed-dose procedure 182
FOIL, see Forum of Insurance
Lawyers
Food and Drug Administration
(FDA), USA 5, 7, 248, 270–
271, 278
Code of Federal Regulations
(CFR) 192, 198
New Drug Application
(NDA) 192, 199
Food and Drugs Acts, USA (1906;
1912) 203
forensic toxicology 185
formularies, care and 271
Formulary Committee 142
formulation
design 156–157
new drugs, of 153
clinical trials, and 154
optimum 103
stability of 157–158
formulator 160
Forum of Insurance Lawyers
(FOIL) 264
France 9, 13, 260
pharmacy training in 155
Francis, D. 301
FRCS 251
Free University of Brussels, Belgium
(ULB), Postgraduate
Programme in Pharmacology
and Pharmaceutical
Medicine 13
freelance writers 241, 244–245
Future Systems, EC 258

GCP, see Good Clinical Practice
GCRP 115
GCSEs 113
gene chip technology 34
gene therapy products 14
gene therapy treatments 171
General Medical Council (GMC)
4, 253
registration 251, 322
general practice 63, 251
General Practitioners (GPs) 142,
144, 152
representative 141–143
General Professional Training
(GPT) 322
genes
abnormal 37

genes (cont.)
  under/over expressed 37
genetic polymorphism 22–23
  drug oxidation reactions, and 22
  metabolic ability, and 22
  substrates, and 22
genetic toxicity 182
genetic-orientated companies 62
geneticists 41
genetics 102
  research 75
genomics 30–31, 34, 37, 42, 75, 117,
  119, 253
Germany 6, 9, 13
  pharmacy training in 155
  QA Group
  website 328
  thalidomide marketed 6
Glaxo plc 160
GLP, see Good Laboratory
  Practice
glucose intolerance, long-term 18
GMC, see General Medical Council
GMP, see Good Manufacturing
  Practice
Good Clinical Practice (GCP) 14,
  68, 70, 73, 80, 84, 86, 92, 169,
  188, 189–190, 193–194, 196–
  197, 199, 219, 237, 283, 316,
  326–328
  guidelines 260
  quality management
    requirements in 192–193
  regulatory process, and the
    ACDM course module in
    332
  veterinary 328
Good Laboratory Practice
  (GLP) 158, 181–182, 189–190,
  199, 316, 326–328
  inspectors 181
Good Manufacturing Practice
  (GMP) 158, 189–190, 199,
  326–328
government 130
  agencies 220
  schemes, voluntary 256
GPs, see General Practitioners
GPT, see General Professional
  Training
graduates 179
  life science 131, 138
  qualified in pathology 179
granulocytosis 18
Great Britain, thalidomide
  marketed 6
growing market share 135
Guideline on GCP 79–80, 86, 91,
  99–100
Guidelines for Standards in Medical
  Information 224
Guidelines on Research, RCP 260
Guildford University, UK,
  continuing education courses
  at 74

GxPs 189, 316–317
gynaecology 252

Hansch analysis 36
Harmonised Tripartite Guideline of
  Good Clinical Practice 69
health and safety at work, growth
  area of 211
Health Care Education, training
  by 73
health centres
  chiropodist 153
  dentist 153
  GP surgery 153
  pharmacy 153
health economics 75, 268
Health Economics and Quality of
  Life, Introduction to, CCR
  module 319
health economists 268, 273
  educational background 268
  work of 268–272
    clinical trials 269
    commercial 271
    cost-effectiveness 270–271
    international 272
    marketing 271–272
    supply 272
Health Maintenance Organisations
  (HMOs) 267, 271
health promotion 152
healthcare
  benefit providers 140
  companies 29–30
  Marketplace, as certificate
    module 323
  paradigm 267
  professionals 137–138, 224–225
    bodies supporting 130
    role of the pharmacist in 151–161
Helsinki Declaration 192, 198
hepatocyte metabolism 41
high-street chemist 151
  communication with
    professional colleagues 152
    prescribers, and 152
  stock control 152
  training 152
  wholesale purchasing 152
high-throughput chemistry 39
  enabling developments 39
high-throughput screening 119
Higher Medical Training
  (HMT) 11, 63
  Programme 323–324
historical documents, retention
  of 90
HMOs, see Health Maintenance
  Organisations
HNC 337
HND 70, 73, 337
hormone pregnancy test 261
hospital(s) 141, 153
  doctors 152–153
  pharmacists 144

pharmacy 153
  representative 142, 144
HPLC 41
human genome 14
human insulin, legal claim
  involving 261
human resources 72–73, 85, 146–
  147, 289, 293, 301
  officers, pharmacists as 160
  training, and 314, 318–319
human testing, requirements for
  204
hybridisation, in situ 34
Hydra 182
hydralazine 22
hyperkalaemia 21
hypertension 22
  treatment of 17–18
hypokalaemia 18
hypotension, orthostatic 22

ICI 260
ICR, see Institute of Clinical
  Research
IEC, see Independent Ethics
  Committee
IFAPP, see International Federation
  of Associations of
  Pharmaceutical Physicians
immune-inflammatory diseases 30
immunohistochemistry 34
immunological products 207
immunologists 40
incentives 145
indemnity 180
Independent Ethics Committee
  (IEC) 81–82, 90, 190
  submission 89
industrial chemicals 185
Industrial Pharmacists Group 161
industry interfaces 7–8
infectious diseases 252
information 74
  leaflets 69
  management 230
    postgraduate courses in 13
  Information Managers in the
    Pharmaceutical Industry 12
  information pharmacist 94, 224
  information technology (IT) 79,
    112, 200, 211, 217, 221, 224,
    245, 294, 313, 317
    CDM, application in
      ACDM course module in 332
    group 113
    management 233
    skills 84–85, 94, 166
    specialists 41
    support 334
  informed consent 190, 260
    process 165
  inspection, independent 90
  inspectors 71
  Institute of Chartered
    Accountants 11

Institute of Chartered Surveyors 11
Institute of Clinical Research (ICR),
    UK 11, 12, 68–69, 73–74, 77,
    84, 86–87, 92–94, 96, 167, 338
    accreditation schemes 74
    Clinical Research Certificate of
        Professional Development
        (CCR) 318–319
        modules for 318
    courses 93
    education and training 318–320
    courses, seminars and work-
        shops 319–320
    journal of 74
    Master's Degree in Clinical
        Research 319
    Postgraduate Certificate 318
        modules for 318
    Postgraduate Diploma 319
        modules for 319
    SSC subcommittee 94
    training courses 73
    website 76, 318
Institutional Review Board
    (IRB) 190
intellectual property law 255
interaction 23, 50, 58–60, 71–72,
    84–85, 92–93, 152, 159, 197,
    217–218, 242, 249
Interaction Between
    Pharmaceutical Companies
    and CROs, ACDM course
    topic 330
International Conference on
    Harmonisation (ICH) 8–9,
    68, 79–80, 86, 91, 99, 101, 188,
    189, 192–193, 198, 237
    Expert Groups 158
    good clinical practice 14, 170,
        188, 189, 192–193, 195–196,
        198
    guidelines 330
    E6 guideline 99
    E9 guideline 99–100
International Federation of
    Associations of
    Pharmaceutical Physicians
    (IFAPP) 12, 338
    website 320
international medical affairs 244
International Society of
    Pharmacoeconomic and
    Outcomes Research 12
International Standards
    Organisation (ISO) 188, 196,
    199
    ISO 9000 327
international symposia 134
Internet 281, 289–290
interpersonal skills 85, 130
    CRAs 71
interviews 115, 296–300
    arrival at 298
    behaviour after 299–300
    behaviour during 298

personal presentation in 297–298
    questions, interviewee 299
    questions, interviewer 298–299
    types of 297
intrauterine devices, legal claim
    involving 261
intravenous administration 165
Introduction to Clinical Trials and
    Clinical Trial Practice, CCR
    module 318
Introduction to Clinical Trials, ICR
    event 93
Introduction to ICH GCP for Study
    Site Personnel 93
Introduction to Industry Training
    Course, PSI 326
    sessions of 326
investigational product 82
investigator(s) 67, 72, 82–83, 90
    Site File (ISF) 90–91
IRB, see Institutional Review Board
Ireland 260, 262
ISF, see Investigator Site File
ISO, see International Standards
    Organisation
isoniazid 22
isoxicam, pharmacokinetics of 21
isozymes, see cytochrome
    isoenzymes
ISPE 12
IT, see Information Technology

Jack, D., Director Glaxo plc 160
Japan 8–9, 43, 51, 99–100, 120,
    204–205, 212, 248, 278
jaundice 22
JCHMT, see Royal Colleges of
    Physicians, Joint Committee
    on Higher Medical Training
job hunting 289–300, 337–339
job interview 139
John Moore's University, Liverpool,
    UK 84, 86, 94
    Certificate of Professional
        Development 13
    Postgraduate Certificate 13
    Postgraduate Diploma 13
    MSc 13, 84, 86, 94
Jones, T., Director ABPI 160

Karolinska Institut, Sweden,
    Pharmaceutical Medicine
    Course 13
ketoconazole 23
key accounts 136, 141
    management 143
    managers 144
King, S. 129
Kingston University, Surrey, UK
    Postgraduate Certificate 13
    Postgraduate Credit Framework
        331
    Postgraduate Diploma 13
    MSc 13
knowledge and skills profiles 311

Labelling Directive, EC 257
labelling, changes to 216
laboratory 83
    technician/assistant 92
laboratory animals 179
Lasix 152
Latin America 272
Law Society Gazette 261
LD50 method 182
leadership model 146
learning, principles of 315–316
Legal Aid Board 261, 264, 266
    franchise proposals by 264
legal and ethical issues 43, 94, 221,
    255
    see also ethics
Letter of Indemnity 89
library storage 39
licensing 43, 61, 120–121
    applications 237
    physicians, and 61
ligand affinity and structure 38
Lilly 5
lipophilicity 38
litigation 283
    international dimensions of 262
    multiple claims 263–266
liver
    disease, effects of 22
    failure
        ascites, and 22
        encephalopathy, and 22
Liverpool University, UK,
    continuing education courses
    at 74
    see also John Moore's University,
        Liverpool
London Pharmacopoeia 4
London School of Hygiene and
    Tropical Medicine, UK 252
    Diploma in Pharmaco-
        epidemiology 252
Losec 152
Lundbeck 272

MA, see Marketing Authorisation
MAA, see Marketing Approval
    Application
macrolides 24
macromolecular science 34
MAHs, see Marketing
    Authorisation Holders
MAIL, see Medicines Act
    Information Letters
management and interpersonal
    skills, certificate module,
    as 323
management and organisation 86
manager(s)
    account 144
    brand 129–130
        assistant 131
    CRM 68, 71–74
    data 12, 50, 69, 108, 113, 196,
        200, 295

managers(s) (*cont.*)
　departmental 231
　information 12
　marketing 72, 135
　　development 135
　MCA 248, 251
　NHS 140, 143–144
　pharma product 129, 153
　pharma sales 73, 138
　pharmacovigilance 220
　product, *see* brand
　project 8, 121, 169, 196, 200
　RBM 136, 141–142
　sales 137, 140–141, 144–145
　　directorial 143–144
　　district 144
　　first-line 136, 141, 143, 147
　　national 143–144, 147
　　regional 143–144, 147
　　role of 143–146
　　second-line 143, 147
Managing Your Own Career 303
market analysis/segmentation 132
market awareness 134
market development manager 135
market research 132
market trends, tracking of 132
marketing 57–58, 60, 62, 87, 94,
　221
　assistant 131
　campaign 133
　defined 129–131
　economists, and 269
　executives 131, 157
　management, second-line 146
　manager 135
　PSI course on 326
　research 75, 94
　sales, and 43
　support 102
　team 142
　the site 88
　trainee 131
Marketing Approval Application
　(MAA), Europe 50–51
Marketing Authorisation
　(MA) 204
　application for, main parts of
　　204
　updates to 205
Marketing Authorisation Holders
　(MAHs) 248, 250
mass spectrometry 41
Master's degree 268
　University of York, UK 268–
　　269
Master of Business Administration
　(MBA) 132
mathematical modelling 101, 103
mathematicians 41
mathematics 155
matrix management 121
　roles 58
MBA, *see* Master of Business
　Administration

MCA, *see* Medicines Control
　Agency
MD 63, 323
MDA, *see* Medicines Devices
　Agency
media interest, litigation and 263
media publicity 216
media scheduling companies 133
Medicaid, USA 271
medical affairs scientist 241
Medical Assessor 215, 247–254
medical communications 237
medical defence organisations,
　rising fees for 262
medical degree 92
medical department 68, 73, 133,
　142
medical device companies 62
medical devices 75
medical director 62, 72, 117
Medical division director 62
medical editor 241
medical education 140
medical graduate 215
medical information 12
　careers in 223–233
　department of 133, 140
　executive 224
　role content in 227–228
　　answering enquiries 227
　　current awareness 227–228
　　product safety 228
　　promotional material
　　　approval 228
　　provision of information to
　　　staff 227
medical information officer
　career course 231–232
　external 232
　lateral moves 232
　job content 225–227
　　current awareness
　　services 226
　　information requests from
　　　company staff 226, 232
　　internal expert advisory
　　　service 226, 232
　　knowledge-base mainte-
　　　nance 226
　　library and archives 227, 232
　　medical information
　　　service 225–226
　　review of promotional mate-
　　　rial 226
　　training 227
　　writing 227
　numbers and distribution 225
　pharmacists as 160
　qualifications and personal
　　attributes 228–230
　　information management
　　　230
　role of 224
　　expansion of 233
　　training and education 230–231

medical marketing 220
medical negligence 255
Medical Reform Act (1858) 4
Medical Representative's
　Examination 139
medical representatives 137–139
　career 138–143
　　development 141–143
　commercial responsibility 141
　nurses as 163
　position in the organisation 141
　reason for 137–138
　role of 139–140
　trial shadowing of 139
medical sales management
　career in 137–147
　development 147
　role of 143–147
medical sales reps 144
medical sales, career in 137–147
medical services 61
　physicians, and 61
medical writers 12, 69, 72, 85, 241
　career pathways, development
　　and opportunities 243
　challenges, opportunities and
　　changing course 245
　education and qualifications
　　241–242
　interactions 242
　introduction of 6
　job description 240–241
　knowledge base, skills and
　　competencies 241–242
　materials prepared by
　　marketing 236
　　conference communica-
　　　tions 239
　　papers for publication
　　　238–239
　　product monographs
　　　239–240
　　specialist areas 240
　　support materials 240
　　regulatory 236
　　end-of-study reports 237
　　expert reports 237
　　investigator's
　　　brochure 238
　　protocols 238
　nurse as 168, 171
　personal attributes 242–243
　role and responsibilities 236–
　　240
　training 243
medical writing 74, 116
　career, as a 235–245
　regulatory affairs, and 116, 207
Medicare, USA 271
medicinal chemistry 38–39
medicinal chemists 38, 40–43
medicine(s) 216
　children and 250
　disposal of 152
　Faculties of 11

interactions with 152
internal 63
pharmaceutical
  specialist discipline 3–14
regulation
  career opportunities in 247–254
certificate module, as 321
research and development 1–44
academic clinical pharma-
  cology, contribution
  of 17–25
regulatory roles and responsibilities in 208–209
role and responsibilities
  in 156–159
side-effects of 152
variables influencing effects of
  24
Medicines Act, UK (1968) 131,
  228, 256, 259
Information Letters (MAIL)
  256–258
legislation 258
Medicines Commission 25
Medicines Control Agency (MCA),
  UK 155, 247n, 249, 253, 258,
  281
career development and
  opportunities 250–251
Clinical Trials Unit 248
education 251–252
continuing 252–253
interactions 249
management opportunities 251
hierarchy of 251
mission statement 247
operational divisions
  Inspection and Enforcement
  248
Licensing 248, 250–251
Post-Licensing 248, 250–252
personal qualities 252
qualifications 251–252
revalidation 252–253
staff roles and
  responsibilities 248–250
assessors 248, 251
Chief Executive 251
directors 251
inspectors 248
managers 248, 251
training 252–253
Medicines Devices Agency (MDA)
  253
meetings 60, 82
'mega' brands 135
Members of Parliament, UK 249
mentor 316
meta-analyses 104
metabolism 103
drug 151, 159
metabolites, comparative toxicity
  of 179

metoprolol 22–23
mianserin 258
mice 179
microbiologists 40
microbiology 70, 207
microphysics 157
Microsoft Access® 84
Middle East 205
molecular biologists 36
molecular biology 37
molecular modellers 36, 40
molecular modelling 38
monitors 68–69, 72
international team of 72
morbidity 271
MRCGOP 321
MRCP 48, 251, 321
MRCPath, see Royal College of
  Pathologists, Member of
MRPhS, see Royal Pharmaceutical
  Society, Member of
MSc 70, 73, 199, 319, 321
East Anglia Polytechnic
  University, UK 13
Information Science, in 229
John Moore's University,
  Liverpool, UK 13
Pharmaceutical Information
  Management, AIOPI 229,
  334–336, 339
Pharmaceutical Medicine,
  University of Surrey, UK 13
Kingston University, Surrey,
  UK 13
toxicology, in 184
University of Hertfordshire, UK
  13
University of Wales, UK 13
multi-tasking 85
musculoskeletal system, drugs for
  19

National Health Service (NHS),
  UK 7, 75, 124, 130, 144, 152,
  223–224, 231, 251, 270, 319,
  334
Drug Information Pharmacists
  Group (DIPG), UK 335
website 335
hospitals 140
liaison 131, 135–136
manager 143–144
specialists 142
managers 143
primary care trusts 140
representatives 142
teams 143
trusts 172, 174
national health strategy 152
National Institute for Clinical
  Excellence (NICE) 7, 130,
  144–145, 223, 226, 270
Appraisal Committee 270
National Prescribing Centre 144
national sales director 141

National Service Frameworks
  (NSFs) 142, 267
clinical guidelines 163, 171, 174
National Training Organisation for
  the Pharmaceutical Industry,
  see under Association of The
  British Pharmaceutical
  Industry
National Vocational Qualification
  (NVQ) in CDM 332–333
Nature 244
nausea and vomiting 22
NDA, see New Drug Application
negotiation 71, 93, 115
nephrologists 21
Netherlands 270
networking 94, 167, 292, 307
neurodegenerative disease 30
neurology 63
new chemical entities 30
New Drug Application (NDA),
  USA 50–51, 204, 206
New Drugs Panel 142
New Scientist 75, 244, 290, 292
New University of Lisbon, Portugal,
  Pharmaceutical Medicine
  Course 13
New Zealand 204, 262
NICE, see National Institute for
  Clinical Excellence
nifedipine 19, 23
pharmacology in elderly 19–20
plasma concentration of 18–19
NMC, see Nursing and Midwifery
  Council
non-steroidal anti-inflammatory
  drugs
elderly and 21
legal claim involving 261
North America 5, 8, 11, 120, 124,
  243, 262, 265, 272
Northern Ireland 261–262
Notice to Applicants and
  Guidelines, CPMP 257
NRG (training) Consultants,
  training by 73
NSFs, see National Service
  Frameworks
nuclear magnetic resonance 41
analysis 39
nuclear medicine 63
nurse(s) 67, 130, 138, 140, 228
advisor 163, 168, 171–174
career pathway 172–173
personality attributes 173
role and responsibilities 172
training and qualifications
  173–174
careers with the pharmaceutical
  industry 163–174
clinic 87, 165, 171
auditing 163, 168, 171–173
courses for 167
field-based 169, 171
managerial skills 167

nurse(s) (cont.)
  patient care 174
  post-registration education 166
    higher degrees 167–169
  practice 144
  publications by 166
  registered 91, 165, 167
    RGN/RMN 173
  research 87, 94, 165
  specialist 144
  see also clinical research nurse
nursing 216
  graduates 215
  homes 153
  qualifications 113
  skills 93
  staff 72
Nursing and Midwifery Council
  (NMC) 92, 97, 172
nutritionists 228
NVQ, see National Vocational
  Qualification

obstetrics 252
occupational toxicology 185
off-patent products 134
oncology 51, 141, 145
ophthalmic products 207
ophthalmology 63
opinion leader advisory boards 135
opium 178
oral contraceptives, legal claim
  involving 261
Organon 258
osteoarthritis 21
osteoporosis 30
outcomes analysis 268
outcomes research 102
outsourcing
  core competency, as a 124
  professionals 121
over-the-counter products 29

paediatrics 63
Pan-European Federation of
  Regulatory Affairs Societies
  (PEFRAS) 205
Papaver somniferum 178
Paracelsus 177
paramedics 138
Parke Davis 4
Parkinson's disease 19, 21
patent agents 43
patent, law 255
patents 5, 29, 61, 211
pathologist, in toxicology 179
pathology 266
patient information, growth area
  of 211
patient records 172
  auditing 172, 174
  software for 152
patients
  bodies supporting 130
  groups 134

recruitment 122
PCTs, see Primary Care Trusts
PEFRAS, see Pan-European
  Federation of Regulatory
  Affairs Societies
penicillin 5, 33
people management 115
Periodic Safety Update Reports 249
Periodic Safety Update Reviews
  (PSURs) 215–217
personal development 131, 310,
  312–316
personal injury litigation 255
personnel management 52
pertussis vaccine 261
pesticides 185
pharma marketing 129, 135
pharma product manager 129
pharmaceutical analysis 151, 157–
  158
Pharmaceutical Analysis Group 161
Pharmaceutical and Medicines
  Information Management.
  Principles and Practice 231
Pharmaceutical Chemist (PhC) 154
pharmaceutical chemistry 155
pharmaceutical companies 119–121,
  220, 247
  current guideline review 330
  economics of 7
  emergence of 4
  employment 275
  organisation of 10
  proposed nationalisation of 6–7
  structure of 10
  sub-specialisation 9–10
  types of 62
  USA, in 62
  'virtual' 120
pharmaceutical development
  scientist 160
pharmaceutical factors and
  medicine effectiveness 24
pharmaceutical industry 153–154,
  251
  adoption of new techniques by
    29
  careers for nurses in 163–174
  careers for physicians in 55–64
    areas of work 60–61
    challenges 61–62
    characteristics required in
      63–64
    interactions 58–60
    opportunities for advance-
      ment 61–62
    dual ladders 61
    reasons for joining 55–57
    reasons for not joining 64
    roles 57–58, 59
  directorial positions in 62
  economics of 7
  education, opportunities
    for 311–338
  European 257

general careers with 149–285
  globalisation 253
  importance of interactive,
    flexible groups in 31, 33
  innovativeness categorised 30
  knowledge of 71
  medical departments 57
  medical writers, and 235, 243
  regulation in 255–259
  statisticians in 99–109
  training, opportunities for 311–
    338
Pharmaceutical Industry Code of
  Practice 131, 134, 140, 228
pharmaceutical innovations 157
pharmaceutical law, a growing legal
  speciality 255–266
pharmaceutical medicine
  consultant in 275–285
  postgraduate courses in 13
  specialist discipline 3–14
  toxicologists in 177–185
Pharmaceutical Medicine Course,
  Karolinska Institut, Sweden
  13
Pharmaceutical Medicine Course,
  New University of Lisbon,
  Portugal 13
pharmaceutical physicians 12, 238,
  320
  education and training,
    background to 321
pharmaceutical R&D strategy, key
  elements in 30–33
pharmaceutical
  representatives 140, 160
pharmaceutical sales managers
  138
pharmaceutical scientists 157
Pharmaceutical Society of Great
  Britain 154
pharmaceutical trade
  magazines 139
pharmaceuticals, career
  development in 301–306
pharmaceutics 155
Pharmacia 272
pharmacists 67, 71, 72, 130, 138,
  140, 225, 228
  career pathways 159–161
  chief 142, 153
  job description 151–154
    academic 154
    community pharmacy 151–
      153
    hospital pharmacy 144, 153
    pharmaceutical
      industry 153–154
  prescribing 156
  role in healthcare 151–161
  role in R&D 156–159
  section heads 160
pharmacodynamic factors and
  medicine effectiveness 24
pharmacodynamics 8, 49

pharmacoeconomics 12, 206, 267, 269, 272–273
pharmacoeconomists 268, 273
  educational background 268
  industry careers for 267–273
  work of 268–272
    clinical trials 269
    commercial 271
    cost-effectiveness 270–271
    international 272
    marketing 271–272
    supply 272
pharmacoepidemiology 6, 216–217, 219–222, 252
pharmacognosy 155
pharmacokineticists 50, 157
pharmacokinetics 8, 24, 31, 41, 43, 49–50, 52, 103, 159, 238, 251
pharmacologists 37–38, 40–41, 43, 48
  see also clinical pharmacologists
pharmacology 49, 61, 94, 155, 204, 207, 221, 238, 266
  see also clinical pharmacology
pharmacovigilance 12, 200, 248–249, 252, 258–259
  careers in 213–222
  defined 213
  education and qualifications 216–217, 219
  interactions 217–218
  job description 214–215
  knowledge base, skills and competences 217
  personal attributes 218
  postgraduate courses in 13
  practice of 6
  professional development 219
  role and responsibility 214–216
    expanding the scope of 220–221
  training 219
pharmacovigilance associate 215, 219–220
pharmacovigilance manager 220
pharmacovigilance physician 215
pharmacy 40, 82–83, 204, 216
  background to profession 154–156
  continuing professional development 155
  cross-sector experience in 155
  degree 151
  graduate 215
  laboratories 89
  origins of 4
  postgraduate practical training 155
  practice issues 154
  technician/assistant 92
  the law, and 155
pharmacy and production 102
  PSI course on 328
PharmiWeb 292, 302
Phase I 159, 165, 278

research, lack of legislation 260
  studies 31, 33, 49, 51, 75, 102–103
Phase II
  studies 49, 58, 102–103, 159, 278
Phase III 158–159, 278
  studies 50, 102–103, 108
PhC, see Pharmaceutical Chemist
PhD 63, 70, 121, 153, 170, 199, 228, 251, 321
phenytoin 23
Phlexglobal Ltd 97
phocomelia 6
physicians 50, 68, 99, 101, 121, 250
  career opportunities for 55–64
  challenges 61–62
  interactions 58–60
  opportunities for advancement 61–62
  reasons for 55–57
  roles 57–58, 59
  desirable characteristics of 63–64
  law qualifications, and 266
physics 155
physiology 94
plan presentation 132
planning 244
  tracking, and 86
Poison Laws, UK 203
polymers 161
poor performance 145–146
portfolio management 102
Portugal 13
Post Registration Education Professional Practice (PREPP) 173
post-marketing studies 102–103
post-registration training 63, 166
postdoctoral training 63
Postgraduate Certificate
  Clinical Trial Administration, in 84, 86
  John Moore's University, Liverpool, UK 13
  Kingston University, Surrey, UK 13
Postgraduate Diploma
  John Moore's University, Liverpool, UK 13
  Kingston University, Surrey, UK 13
  Pharmaceutical Medicine, Autonomous University of Barcelona, Spain 13
Postgraduate Programme in Pharmacology and Pharmaceutical Medicine, Free University of Brussels, Belgium (ULB) 13
postgraduate qualifications 199
Postgraduate Study Course in Pharmaceutical Medicine, University of Witten/Herdecke, Germany 13

PowerPoint 239, 241
practice nurses 144
practolol 6, 260
pre-clinical research, careers in 45–126
pre-clinical sciences, physicians and 61
PREPP, see Post Registration Education Professional Practice
prescriptions, computer generated 152
presentation skills 71, 115, 130
primary care 130, 141–142, 144, 163, 167, 171
Primary Care Trusts (PCTs) 130, 142–143, 145, 152
Primodos litigation 261
Principles of Medical Statistics [4]
proactivity, importance of 73
problem solving 71, 93, 115
procainamide 22
process improvement 102
process research 40
process-oriented pharmacy 154
product adviser 224
product development, certificate module, as 321
product liability 260–266
product management 143
  career in 129–136
  first line 147
product manager, see brand manager
product marketing 138
product registration
  career in 203–212
  job description 204–205
product specialist 224, 231, 233
product types and medical information 225
production scheduling 133
production, large-scale 103
products 205
products experts 224, 231, 233
professional bodies, education and training by 320–338
Professional Portfolio for Study Site Personnel 94
professional support 10–11
programme team 40
programmers 72, 85, 113
project and time management 115
project coordination 60–61
  director 62
project coordinator/planner 60
project leaders 58
project management 52, 72, 87, 211
  ACDM course topic, as 330
  data management and 112–113
  skills 166
project managers 8, 58, 60–62, 196, 200
  marketing 72

project managers (cont.)
nurses 169
profile in CRO 121
project team, work of 40
promotion, requirements for 42
promotional budget 133
propafenone 23
propranolol 18, 22
protein biochemistry 37
proteomics 14, 34, 253
protocols 164–166, 169–170, 180–
181, 192, 194, 204, 282
care, and 271
design 99–100
feasibility 88
review 111–112
PSI, see Statisticians in the
Pharmaceutical Industry
PSURs, see Periodic Safety Update
Reviews/Reports
psychiatry 63, 266
psychology 268
public relations 232
publications 102, 166, 278

QA, see Quality Assurance
QC, see Quality Control
QM, see Quality Management
QSARs, see quantitative structure–
activity relationships
QT interval 49
quality 188, 270
Quality Assurance (QA) 8, 74, 86,
112, 116, 187–200 (188, 191),
244, 283
growth area of 211
postgraduate courses in 13
Quality Assurance Journal 201
Quality Control (QC) 103, 153,
188, 189, 191, 192–194
Quality Management (QM) 188,
189–190, 191, 192–194
requirements in GCP 192–193
Quality Management and Control,
ACDM course module in 334
quality of life 58, 269
quality requirements in clinical
research 190–192
quantitative structure–activity
relationships (QSARs) 102
quinidine 23

R&D, see Research and
Development
radiochemistry 151
radiology 63
radiopharmaceuticals 153
RAPS, see Regulatory Affairs
Professional Society
rashes 18
rats 179
RBM, see Regional Business
Manager

RCN, see Royal College of Nursing
REC, see Recruitment &
Employment Confederation
receptor theory 14
H2-receptor antagonists 33
reconciliation 91
recruitment 289–292
agencies 244
campaign planning 290–292
advertisement sites 291–292
aims 291
networking 292
relocation 291
Internet age, in the 289–290
law, and the 290
offers and beyond 300
subject 89–90
Recruitment & Employment
Confederation (REC) 337
referral services 88, 90
Regional Business Manager
(RBM) 136, 141–142
regional director, sales 141
regional pharmaceutical
managers 153
regional sales manager 73
regional sales trainer 142
regional therapy area specialists 131,
142, 144
registration 54
fast track to 119
registration executives, pharmacists
as 160
registration officer 160
regulation 255–259
regulatory affairs 74, 112, 133, 200,
220, 225, 232, 244, 259
career in 203–212
course of 208
development 209–211
specialisation 210
director 62
education and training 207–208
job content 205–206
divisions of 205–206
expansion of 211
job description 204–205
personnel 205
postgraduate courses in 13
qualifications and personal
attributes 206–207
roles and responsibilities
medicines research and
development, in 208–
209
Regulatory Affairs Journal 208
Regulatory Affairs Professional
Society (RAPS), USA 205,
324
courses 208
website 324
Regulatory affairs societies,
European 205
regulatory agencies 180–181, 218,
221

regulatory authorities 69, 104,
215–216, 237, 257
economists and 269
regulatory bodies 25
careers with 210
presentation to 204
regulatory control 256
regulatory documents 89
medical writers, and 235
regulatory executives 12
introduction of 6
regulatory guidelines 106
effect on statistical
methodology 101
regulatory medicine 249, 252
regulatory personnel, numbers and
distribution 205
regulatory requirements 79, 119
regulatory submission 157
regulatory support 102
remote data capture 124
renal artery stenosis 18
renal dysfunction 21
renal failure 21–22
report review 112
reports 69, 99, 241
research 112
medicines 1–44
PSI course on 328
research and development 5–7,
9–10, 14
academic societies, and 11
director 62
Research and Development 61,
156, 158–159, 291
companies 62
core technologies in 34
costs 30
development phase 31, 40
contracting out of 34
dangers of isolation from
discovery 34
key ingredients 33
management of 33–35
director 161
discovery phase 30
dangers of isolation from
development 34
innovative working climate,
and 31
management of 33–35
discovery process 35–40
research organisation and
management 35–36
career development in
41–43
entry requirements for
40–41
genetics research in 35
team structures in 35
local hospital 89
medical writers, and 237, 241
product licensing in 35
regulatory affairs, and 208–209,
211

research alliances in 35
research projects
 birth of 36–40
 career development in 41–42
 target identification and
  research 36–40
 biology 37–38
 high-throughput chem-
  istry 39
 medicinal chemistry 38–
  39
 statisticians in 99
 strategy, key elements in 30–33
 teamwork, importance of 31,
  33, 40
 necessary elements in 32
research associates,
 pharmacovigilance 221
research coordinator 88
Research Methods, CCR
 module 318–319
research nurse 87
 junior 165
 role 94
research site 88
respiratory medicine 252
response surface methodology 103
results 80
resuscitation training 165
retail chemists 141, 144
riboflavin, urine screening, and
 24
Right Medicine, The, Scottish
 initiative for pharmaceutical
 care 156
risk-sharing agreements, CROs
 and 124
Robson, A.S. 231
Rostrum Training, training by 73
Royal College of Nursing (RCN)
 92, 94–95, 97, 164, 301
Royal College of Pathologists
 (MRCPath), membership of
 185
Royal College of Physicians of
 London, Guidelines on
 Research 260
Royal Colleges of Physicians,
 UK 321
 Certificate of Completion of
  Specialist Training (CCST-
  UK) 321
 modules for 321
 Diploma in Pharmaceutical
  Medicine 320
 Faculty of Pharmaceutical
  Medicine 6, 12, 53
 Higher Medical Training
  programme 321
 Joint Committee on Higher
  Medical Training
  (JCHMT) 321
Royal Pharmaceutical Society 152,
 161
 Member of (MRPhS) 154–155

Royal Society of Medicine (RSM)
 339
Royal Statistical Society (RSS) 339
RSM, see Royal Society of Medicine
RSS, see Royal Statistical Society

S+ software 106
safety 270
 data sheets (COSHH), growth
  area of 211
 profile 103
salaries and perks in CROs 122
sales 87, 94
 careers in 127–147
 director 147
 force 131, 133, 134
 management 131, 143
 line levels of 138
 manager 137, 140–141, 144–145
 directorial 143–144
 district 144
 first-line 136, 141, 143, 147
 national 143–144, 147
 regional 143–144, 147
 role of 143–146
 second-line 143, 147
 marketing, and 75, 120
 medical writers in 235, 240
 recruitment agencies 139
 representative 137
 medical 144
 targets 135, 140
 teams 140
 territory 141
 track record 138
 training 143
sampling inspection 103
Sanofi-Synthelabo 272
SAS software 106
satellite symposium 134
Scandinavia 272
Schering AG 272
Schering Plough 269
Schools of Pharmacy, UK 155
 degrees from 155
 entry requirements for 155
science graduate 215
scientific adviser 224
scientist(s) 101
 clinical document 241
 discovery 102
 research 105
Scotland 156, 261–262
screening, high throughput 30–31,
 37–40, 42
Scrip 296
secondary care 130, 163, 167, 171
section head, pharmacists as 160
Selective Serotonin Reuptake
 Inhibitors (SSRIs) 24
senior brand manager 135
senior clinical associate 170
senior managers 132
Senior Pharmacovigilance
 Associate 220

senior product manager 135
senior sales role 131
shareholder expectations 143
sheep dip, legal claim involving 261
SIGAR, see Specialist Interest
 Group for Adverse Reactions
site coordination 89
site investigator 87
site monitor 68–69
Site Monitoring Organisation
 (SMO) 163
site physicians 87
site preparation 89
site visits 89
slide kits 240
smart cards, patient 221
Smart Moves 301
SmithKline, French litigation 258
SMO, see Site Monitoring
 Organisation
Society for Clinical Data
 Management, Inc. 329
 website 329
Society of Pharmaceutical
 Medicine 14, 278
Socrates 178
software packages 106, 115
SOPs, see Standard Operating
 Procedures
source documentation
 verification 90
South Africa 204
South America 205
Spain 13
special groups, studies in 19–23
 elderly patients 8, 19–21, 50
 children 8
 liver disease 22, 50
 renal disease 21–22, 50
specialist agencies 134
Specialist Certification for
 Pharmaceutical Medicine 324
Specialist Interest Group for Adverse
 Reactions (SIGAR) 231
Specialist Registrar 48
specialists 231
spectinomycin 5
sponsor company 79–81, 83–84, 87,
 88–89, 91, 93
SSC, see Study Site Coordinator
SSRIs, see Selective Serotonin
 Reuptake Inhibitors
stability tests 153
staff supervision 83
Standard Operating Procedures
 (SOPs) 8, 68, 71, 73, 81, 83–84,
 86, 89, 106, 169, 187, 188, 192–
 194, 196, 198, 219, 237, 283,
 333
 purposes of 193
standards 11–14
statin, use of 268
statistical data 94
statistical methodology, clinical
 trials, and 99–100, 106

statistical personnel 69
statistical thinking for data
    managers, ACDM course
    module in 332
statistical/modelling
    approaches 23
statisticians 12, 41, 48, 50, 58, 72,
    85, 113
    activity, areas of 102
    consultancy 107–108
    drug development, in 102–105
    clinical research 103–105
    methodological challenges,
        variety of 100–102
    pharmaceutical industry, in
        the 99–109
    skills required by 105–109
    communication skills 107,
        109
    knowledge of the context
        106
    project management skills
        108–109
    technical foundation 105–
        106
Statisticians in the Pharmaceutical
    Industry (PSI) 12, 100, 339
    committee structure of 325
    Introduction to Industry
        Training Course 326
    sessions of 326
    training courses 326
    website 325
statistics 52, 251
    certificate module, as 321
    data processing, and 60, 62
    physicians, and 60
statutory requirements 237
steering committee 69
steroids, legal claim involving 261
strategic health authorities 130,
    142, 145
strategic planning 132, 211
strict liability 264
structure–activity
    relationships 40
Structured Project: Thesis, CCR
    module 318
study budget 82, 89
study documents 81
study drug 82
study site 82
    team 85
Study Site Coordinator (SSC) 72,
    79–80, 82, 87–94, 163–168
    career development and
        opportunities 94
    path 165–167
    centrality within project 92–93
    conflict of interest 165
    continuing education 94
    evolution of role 80
    interactions 92–93
        with subject or patients 80,
            92

job description 88–91
    knowledge base, skills,
        competencies 91–92
    nursing background 80
    personality attributes 93, 167
    portfolio 168
    role and responsibility 87–88,
        164–165
    skills required 166
    temporary contracts and
        unsecured funding 95
    training and qualifications 93–
        94, 167–168
study team leader 85
subjects 90, 94
    consent form 69
    medical notes 91
sulphanilamide 5
sulphonamides 22
summary of product
    characteristics 249
Supplementary Protection
    Certificate Scheme,
    Europe 211
supply and demand 133
support materials, sales force 133
support staff, managing 74
Sweden 9, 13, 48
Switzerland 9, 13
syncope 22

tachycardia 20
tactical promotion plan 133
Tagamet, generic copies of 258
target audience 137
target organs 179
target validation 30–31
teachers 138
teaching 154
team(s)
    leaders 231
    management, aspects of 145
    members 90
    on-site 72
    player abilities 63, 72
    skills 94
    worker 130
        pharmacovigilance, and
            217
teratogenicity 261
teratology 266
terfanadine 24
testosterone 23
tests 178
    psychometric, verbal,
        numerical 139
    short-term 179
thalidomide 6, 178, 203, 256, 260
The CTA Qualification 86
The Monitor 75
theophylline 23
therapeutic audits, field based 163
therapeutic clinical trials 94
therapeutic committees 226
therapeutic index 204

therapeutic ratio 49
Therapeutic Substances Act, UK
    (1925) 5, 203
therapeutics 14
therapies 30
    gene-based 54
Therapy Review Specialist 171
time management, writers and 242
timing 80
TMF, see Trial Master File
To Be A CRA 69
tolbutamide 23
tolerance 159
Total Quality Management (TQM)
    188, 190, 191
toxic side effects, monitoring of 172
toxicokinetics 184
toxicologists 48, 50
    in pharmaceutical
        medicine 177–185
    qualities and abilities
        required 182–184
    study director, as 180–181
    work of 178–182
toxicology 40, 61, 102–103, 158,
    177, 204, 207, 221, 266
    clinical 185
    defined and explained 177–178
    forensic 185
    ecotoxicology 185
    occupational 185
    pharmaceutical 178
    PSI course on 328
    technicians 180–181
    training and careers in 184–185
Toxicology and Adverse Events,
    CCR module 321
TQM, see Total Quality
    Management
tracking systems 82–85
trademarks 43
    law, and 255
trainees, meeting the needs of 311–
    338
training and education 73, 74, 84,
    85–86, 93–94, 160, 282–283
    competence and
        competencies 312
    continuing professional
        development 309–310,
        313, 316
    CROs, in 123
    events 54
    knowledge and skills
        profiles 311
    learning environment 315–316
    case-study 316
    demonstration 316
    discussion 316
    exercise 316
    lecture 315
    simulation 316
    learning styles 314–315
    active/passive 314
    association 315

resistance 314
learning types 315
  action learners 315
  modelling learners 315
  practical learners 315
  thinking learners 315
on the job 73
personal development
  appraisal, and 312–316
  plans for 310
pharmaceutical industry, in
  the 309–336
pharmaceutical physicians,
  for 321
principles of learning 313–314
professional bodies, education
  and training by 319–336
regulations and training
  records 316–317
training cycle, the 310
training needs analysis 311
training sources 317
  commercial courses 317
  in-house courses 317
  professional bodies 318–336
training styles 314
  coach 314
  instructor 314
  mentor 314
training cycle, the 310
training needs analysis 311
training programme, sales 139
Training Strategies as ACDM
  course topic 330
training, data management 115
  management skills 115–116
training, pharmacovigilance 219
training, regulation 252–253
training, writers 243
Trial Master File (TMF) 81, 90
trial training 89
triazolam 23
tricyclic antidepressants, CNS
  toxicity and 22–23
trizolam, plasma concentration of
  21
tumorigenesis 183

UKCAPS 161
United Kingdom 4–5, 7, 9, 13, 33,
  48, 54, 63, 68, 81, 87, 94, 100,
  130, 138–140, 152–154, 156,
  159, 183, 224–225, 241, 244,
  247–249, 253, 256–258, 260–
  262, 265, 267, 269, 272, 275,
  289, 320, 327, 335
United Kingdom Central Council
  for Nursing, Midwifery and
  Health Visiting (UKCC) 92
United States of America 5–6, 9,
  29, 33, 43, 60, 62, 68, 88, 99–
  100, 183, 204–206, 212, 225,
  241, 256, 262, 265–267, 269,
  270–272, 278, 328
Federal Government 271
Senate Committees of 6
University of Basel, Switzerland,
  European Course in
  Pharmaceutical Medicine 13
University of Hertfordshire,
  UK 231
  MSc 13
  postgraduate diploma/MSc in
    pharmacovigilance 231
University of Lyon, France,
  European Diploma in
  Pharmaceutical Medicine
  (EUDIPHARM) 13
University of Surrey, UK, MSc
  courses in pharmaceutical
  medicine 13, 320
University of Wales at Cardiff,
  UK 322, 324–325
  Diploma in Regulatory
    Affairs 13, 208
  MSc 13
  Postgraduate Training Course in
    Pharmaceutical Medicine
    320
University of Wales Institute of
  Science and Technology, UK,
  Diploma in Pharmaceutical
  Medicine 13
University of Witten/Herdecke,
  Germany, Postgraduate Study

Course in Pharmaceutical
  Medicine 13
University of York, UK 268–269
  Master's degree 268
urine tests 24
US QA Association
  website 326

vaccines 207
ventricular tachycardia, torsade de
  pointes form of 24
vets 179
videos 240
visual aids 239
vomiting and nausea 22

Wales 13, 270
ward pharmacy 153
web design staff 8
websites, useful 12, 76, 96, 125,
  152, 175–176, 202, 222, 234,
  246, 318, 320, 322, 325–327,
  329, 334–335, 337–339
Wellcome Foundation 261
wholesalers 141
wholesaling 154
Winslade, J. 68
Word 241
World Wide Web 8
writers, medical
  agency 236
  completer–finishers as 242
  freelance 236–237, 241, 244–
    245
writing 282

X-ray 72

yeast cells 38
Yellow Card reporting system 249

Zyman, S. 130

Index compiled by Lewis N. Derrick